D0743034

Statistics for Biology and Health

Springer

New York
Berlin
Heidelberg
Barcelona
Hong Kong
London
Milan
Paris
Singapore
Tokyo

Statistics for Biology and Health

Brian Everitt   Sophia Rabe-Hesketh

Analyzing Medical Data Using S-PLUS

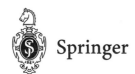 Springer

Brian Everitt
Sophia Rabe-Hesketh
Institute of Psychiatry
Biostatistics and Computing Department
De Crespigny Park
Denmark Hill
London SE5 8AF
United Kingdom

Series Editors

K. Dietz
Institut für Medizinische Biometrie
Universität Tübingen
Westbahnhofstrasse 55
D-72070 Tübingen
Germany

M. Gail
National Cancer Institute
Rockville, MD 20892
USA

K. Krickeberg
Le Chatelet
F-63270 Manglieu
France

J. Samet
School of Public Health
Department of Epidemiology
Johns Hopkins University
615 Wolfe Street
Baltimore, MD 21205-2103
USA

A. Tsiatis
Department of Statistics
North Carolina State University
Raleigh, NC 27695
USA

Library of Congress Cataloging-in-Publication Data
Everitt, Brian.
    Analyzing medical data using S-PLUS / Brian Everitt, Sophia Rabe-Hesketh.
        p. cm. — (Statistics for biology and health)
    Includes bibliographical references and index.
    ISBN 0-387-98862-9 (alk. paper)
        1. Medical statistics—Computer programs.   2. S-Plus.   I. Rabe-Hesketh, S.   II. Title.
    III. Series.
    RA409.5 E94 2001
    610'.285—dc21   2001020445

Printed on acid-free paper.

Production managed by A. Orrantia; manufacturing supervised by Jerome Basma.
Photocomposed copy prepared by Macrotex, Savoy, IL.
Printed and bound by Maple-Vail Book Manufacturing Group, York, PA.
Printed in the United States of America.

9 8 7 6 5 4 3 2 1

ISBN 0-387-98862-9   SPIN 10728668

Springer-Verlag   New York Berlin Heidelberg
A member of BertelsmannSpringer Science+Business Media GmbH

Preface

Medicine's progress from dogmatic, even mystical, certainty to scientific uncertainty, which began in the 17th century, continues almost unabated to the present day. The key to this progress has been the collection and valid interpretation of evidence, particularly quantitative evidence, provided by the application of statistical methods to medical investigations. In the last two decades, the field of medical statistics has grown rapidly and complex statistical procedures are now a routine part of medical research. This is possible because of the wide and increasing availability of an extensive variety of statistical software packages. Which package medical statisticians or medical researchers use is probably, initially at least, largely serendipity—what is readily available in their place of work, for example. But over time, experience with a number of packages usually leads to a favorite. We make no bones about it, S-PLUS is one of our favorites for reasons of flexibility, convenience, power and, yes, fun; working with S-PLUS on a project is usually most enjoyable and entertaining. And to convince readers that we are not alone in our regard for the package, the following are quotations from other users of S-PLUS for medical research:

> I can implement algorithms much faster than I can write them in C and get the final output graphed much better than SPSS. I would say it transfomed my professional life (Dr Gary Gunkemeier, Starr-Wood Cardiac Group)

> I've added routines to SAS and it is difficult. How difficult? Almost two orders of magnitude harder than S-PLUS. Something that will take me 2-4 hours in S-PLUS, will take me 2-4 days in

SAS. The last time I wrote a procedure in SAS was just before I learned to write functions in S-PLUS. It is unmatched as an environment for coding functions. (Dr Terry Therneau, Mayo Clinic).

In this book, we will try to illustrate why we feel that such claims are merited, by using S-PLUS to apply a wide variety of statistical methods, from simple to sophisticated, to a range of data sets. The necessary mathematical background for all but the most basic techniques is also included. Each chapter ends with a set of exercises that will hopefully develop the reader's expertise with S-PLUS so that they can use the package to undertake 'tailor-made' analysis of their data sets.

We hope that this book will be useful to many categories of medical statisticians from graduate students in MSc and doctoral programs to those working in reseach institutes and the pharmaceutical industry. In addition, we like to think that the book will appeal to medical researchers who, although not primarily statisticians, undertake statistical analysis using a particular package. If we convert some of these, at least, by convincing them that S-PLUS provides an ideal and exciting environment in which to attack their data analysis problems, then we shall deem our efforts in writing this book a success.

Brian Everitt and Sophia Rabe-Hesketh, London

Contents

Prologue: Medical Statistics

Introduction

As we enter the first few months of the New Millenium, the majority of papers published in medical journals continue to contain a substantial amount of statistical material. And this has been true for at least the last 20 or 30 years. The majority of clinicians now accept that the key to progress in medicine is the collection and valid interpretation of evidence, particularly quantitative evidence in the form of numerical observations and measurements. The proper use of statistical methods is central in this process.

But acceptance of the role of statistics in medical research has not always been so widespread. Bradford Hill in his *Principles of Medical Statistics* quotes the following question posed by the writer of an article on statistics in medical journals in 1921:

> Is the application of the numerical method to the subject-matter of medicine a trivial and time-wasting ingenuity as some hold, or is it an important stage in the development of our art, as others proclaim?

Such a question could hardly be asked today. And not so long ago an eminent psychiatrist wrote the following in a letter to that august journal the *Lancet* in respect of a clinical trial of a treatment for depression:

> One must go on repeating the fact that if, in the past thirty years, one had ever paid very much attention to statistics, es-

pecially when they were not supported by clinical bedside findings, treatment progress in this country would not have got very far.

Such questions and doubts about the usefulness of statistics in medicine now look increasingly foolish when, fortunately, a 'facts speak louder than statistics' attitude is increasingly rare among clinicians; most are well aware of the contribution that statistics and statisticians have made to medical research, although some controversy remains. Not everyone, for example, is convinced by the claims of modern evidence-based medicine (see Sackett *et al.*, 1991), although to us they seem entirely reasonable and desirable. Nor is every clinician yet convinced by the need for experimental approaches (including randomization) in the evaluation of all forms of intervention, whether they be surgical procedures, psychotherapies or healthcare reforms. But thankfully there remain only a tiny minority of clinicians who fail to appreciate what developments in statistical methodology can offer to medical research.

Statistics in Medicine

Statistics are ubiquitous in medical research. Journals and magazines for clinicians are increasingly filled with statistical topics, because statistics are increasingly a part of medical practice. No doctor can escape the demands of audit, resource allocation, hospital utility, vaccination uptake and the like. Neither can they avoid the statistical results from research papers often quoted in promotional materials for drugs and other medical therapies. And as research in medical statistics continues apace, the sophistication and complexity of the statistical techniques applied to medical data has increased accordingly. Logistic regression is now commonplace in the medical literature as are Cox's model for survival data, generalized linear models, the bootstrap, factor analysis, random effects models for longitudinal data and Bayesian methods. Such widespread use of methods requiring, in many cases, heavy computation, would clearly not be possible without the use of computers or statistical packages. With a moderately priced PC and a relatively moderately priced package, a researcher can now apply most of the techniques of modern (and not so modern) statistics almost routinely. And with a package such as S-PLUS, even the most recently developed methods can often be implemented without a great deal of difficulty.

S-PLUS

S-PLUS is a language and an interactive programming environment for data analysis and graphics. Its origins lie in AT&T's Bell Laboratories in the

1980s from where it has developed into an extensive and coherent collection of tools for graphical displays and statistics. It also offers an effective object-orientated programming language that provides very flexible and powerful possibilities for implementing newly created statistical methods. One of its great strengths is that functions written to allow recently described techniques to be used can employ as building blocks any of the procedures already available in the language.

S-PLUS can be used in a variety of ways. In this book, we shall concentrate on using the command language in the form of script files, but 'dialogues' are also available that make the application of many methods extremely straightforward, and examples of using these will be given in Appendix A.

But it is the command-line style of the script files that we feel is of most importance for readers who wish to become serious users of S-PLUS. And in support of this view, we give the following quotation from a statistician who has been involved with computers for over 40 years, John Nelder:

> I am very much aware that for the modern student the menu mode is the one preferred, and indeed the only one known. I am, however, not convinced that the menu mode is optimum for all users or for all usages. The freedom of being able to say what you want, instead of responding to given lists, is to me worth having. Imagine how restrictive conversation would be, if instead of making your own points for yourself, you were restricted to pointing at sets of alternatives defined by the person you were talking to. The frustrations would soon become apparent.

We make no claim that our script files are as elegant as they could be, and it may be a useful exercise for readers to improve them as they see fit. Nevertheless, they get the job done, and for the statistician, it is this that is of most importance. Unlike most other texts dealing with statistics and S-PLUS, all code for the analysis described in a chapter is listed at the end of the chapter, rather than scattered throughout the text. We chose this structure because it enables readers to learn about the statistical techniques and their application and to assess the potential of S-PLUS, without being distracted by 'chunks' of software with which they may be unfamiliar.

At the end of the chapter, the code used in each section is explained and detailed comments are included in the script. Together with the introductory chapter, this should allow readers who are not yet users of S-PLUS to understand the code and to carry out the exercises. The commands that complete the figures or tables of the chapter are clearly highlighted, enabling readers who are familiar with S-PLUS to quickly find out how a particular graph or analysis has been produced.

For those wishing to work through the chapters' code in detail, we recommend that they download the script files from our website and recreate graphs and analyses on their PC as they read through the chapters simply by running the relevant part of the script file.

All script files can be downloaded from the following website

http://www.iop.kcl.ac.uk/IoP/Departments/BioComp/splusBook.stm

1
An Introduction to S-PLUS

1.1   Introduction

S-PLUS is a language designed for data analysis and graphics developed
originally at AT&T's Bell Laboratories. It is described in detail in Becker, *et
al.* (1988), Chambers and Hastie (1993), Venables and Ripley (1997) and
Krause and Olson (2000). In addition to providing a powerful language,
the most recent versions of the software, S-PLUS 2000 and S-PLUS 6, also
include an extensive graphical user interface (GUI) on Windows platforms
(this is not available in UNIX). The GUI allows routine analyses to be
carried out simply by completing various dialogue boxes and allows graphs
to be produced and edited by a 'point-and-click' procedure.

In this chapter, we will describe how to use the S-PLUS command line
language and say a little about the GUI. In subsequent chapters, we shall
concentrate on the S-PLUS language and return, in a little more detail, to
the GUI in Appendix A.

1.2   Running S-PLUS

In this section, we describe how S-PLUS is run on Windows platforms.
All subsequent sections except the last apply equally to S-PLUS on UNIX
platforms. S-PLUS is opened by double-clicking into the file (or shortcut
for) SPLUS.exe. The result is an S-PLUS window containing a **Commands**
window or an **Object Explorer** window. During a session, **Graphics**

windows may be opened and often output will be sent to a **Report** window, by changing the default for text output routing in the Options list. The windows seen in a typical S-PLUS session are as in Figure 1.1.

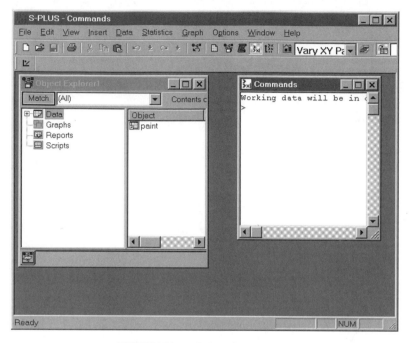

FIGURE 1.1. S-PLUS windows.

Commands can be typed into the **Commands** window, next to the > prompt, and any resulting output appears below.

S-PLUS is a language for the manipulation of objects. Data sets (called *data frames* in S-Plus), vectors, matrices and lists are passed to functions and returned by functions. The content of these objects may be viewed by simply typing the name of the object. (This is equivalent to passing the object to the **print()** function.) The **Object Explorer** window displays objects of the current session by object category. This window can be opened by clicking into ![icon]. At the end of a session, the user can select which objects created within the session should be saved within the 'current directory' or database. By default, this is the _data subdirectory of the directory where the S-PLUS files are located, e.g., in c:\Program Files\sp2000_data. The command **search()** lists the current directory under [1].

Because it is usually preferable to keep the data for different projects in different directories, it is a good idea to start the S-PLUS session by setting the directory in which any objects are to be saved and which may contain relevant objects from a previous session. This is done by 'attaching' the directory at the first position of the *search path* using the command

```
> attach("c:/project/_data", pos = 1)
```

Note that forward slashes / were used in the directory path instead of the usual backward slashes \. Two backward slashes \\ may also be used.

Another way of ensuring that any S-PLUS work relating to a particular project is stored in the relevant directory is to produce a separate shortcut to S-PLUS for that project that will cause S-PLUS to start in the correct directory. This may be done by editing the target box of the shortcut tab of the properties dialogue shown below

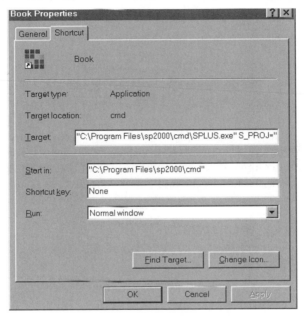

to contain

```
"C:\Program Files\sp2000\cmd\SPLUS.EXE"  S_PROJ="c:\project"
```

where the path of SPLUS.EXE may be different depending on where it has been installed.

1.3 Elementary commands

Elementary commands consist of either expressions or assignments. For example, typing the expression

```
> 42 + 8
```

in the **Commands** window and pressing Return will produce the following output:

```
[1] 50
```

In the remainder of this chapter, we will show the command (preceded by the prompt >) and the output as they would appear in the **Commands** window together like this:

```
> 42 + 8
[1] 50
```

Instead of just evaluating an expression, we can assign the value to a scalar using the syntax `scalar` $< -$ `expression`.

```
> x <- 42 + 8
```

An alternative symbol to the '$< -$' characters for an assignment is an 'underscore' (not used in this book):

```
> x _ 42 + 8
```

Longer commands can be split over serveral lines by pressing Return before the command is complete. To indicate that S-PLUS is waiting for completion of a command, a '+' occurs instead of the > prompt. For illustration, we break the line in the assignment above:

```
> x<-
+ 42+8
```

In practice, it is however more convenient to type the commands into a *Script file* shown in Figure 1.2.

A Script file (*.ssc) is an ASCII text file that may be opened within S-PLUS to build and keep a sequence of commands required for a particular analysis. This way, the entire analysis can be repeated at the press of a button if necessary, for example, if a data entry error is detected. The whole Script file may be executed by selecting Script and Run from the menu bar or by pressing F10. Alternatively, one or more commands may be selected and run by highlighting the relevant text within the Script file and pressing the triangle ▸. A new command must begin on a new line or after a semicolon. Line breaks in the middle of a command are allowed. S-PLUS ignores lines whose first character is a hash symbol #. Comments can therefore easily be included anywhere in the script file. If S-PLUS is busy executing a command, it can be interrupted by pressing the [Esc] button.

Each chapter of this book contains an annotated Script file for the examples used in that chapter. (These script files are also available at the website mentioned in the Preface.)

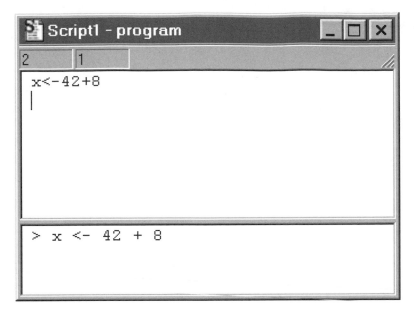

FIGURE 1.2. Script file.

1.4 Vectors

A commonly used type of S-PLUS object is a vector. Vectors may be created in several ways, of which the most common is via the concatenate function, c(), which combines all values given as arguments to the function into a vector.

```
> x <- c(1, 2, 3, 4)
> x
[1] 1 2 3 4
```

Here, the first command created a vector and the second command, x, a short-form for print(x), causes the contents of the vector to be printed. (Note that S-PLUS is case sensitive, and x and X are different objects.)

The number of elements of a vector can be determined using the length() function:

```
> length(x)
[1] 4
```

The c() function can also be used to combine strings denoted by enclosing them in " ". For example,

```
> names <- c("Brian", "Sophia", "Harriett")
> names
[1] "Brian"     "Sophia"     "Harriett"
```

The c() function also works with a mixture of numeric and string values, but in this case, all elements in the resulting vector will be converted to strings.

```
> mix <- c(names, 55, 33)
> mix
[1] "Brian"    "Sophia"   "Harriett" "55"       "33"
```

Vectors consisting of regular sequences of numbers can be created using the seq() function. The general syntax of this function is seq(lower,upper, increment). Some examples are given below:

```
> seq(1, 5, 1)
[1] 1 2 3 4 5
> seq(2, 20, 2)
 [1]  2  4  6  8 10 12 14 16 18 20
> x <- c(seq(1, 5, 1), seq(4, 20, 4))
> x
 [1]  1  2  3  4  5  4  8 12 16 20
```

When the increment argument is one, it can be left out of the command. The same applies to the lower value. More information about the seq() function and all other S-PLUS functions can be found using the help facilities; for example,

```
>help(seq)
```

shows a help page. Help can also be obtained by selecting Help from the top menu bar and selecting Search S-PLUS Help. This opens a window listing all items on which help is available in alphabetical order (see Figure 1.3).

Sequences with increments of one can also be obtained using the syntax first:last, for example,

```
> 1:5
[1] 1 2 3 4 5
```

A further useful function for creating vectors with regular patterns is the rep() function, with general form rep(pattern, number of times). For example,

```
> rep(10, 5)
[1] 10 10 10 10 10
> rep(1:3, 3)
[1] 1 2 3 1 2 3 1 2 3
> x <- rep(seq(5), 2)
> x
 [1] 1 2 3 4 5 1 2 3 4 5
```

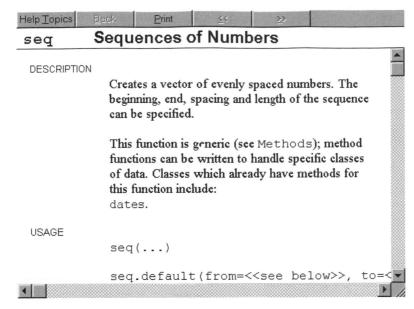

FIGURE 1.3. Part of help file for `seq()`.

The second argument can also be a vector of the same length as the first argument to indicate how often each element of the first argument is to be repeated:

```
> x <- rep(seq(3), c(1, 2, 3))
> x
[1] 1 2 2 3 3 3
```

Increasingly complex vectors can be built by repeated use of the `rep()` function.

```
> x <- rep(seq(3), rep(3, 3))
> x
[1] 1 1 1 2 2 2 3 3 3
```

We can access a particular element of a vector by giving the required position in square brackets.

```
> x <- 1:5
> x[3]
[1] 3
```

A vector containing several elements of another vector can be obtained by giving a vector of required positions in square brackets:

```
> x[c(1, 3)]
```

TABLE 1.1. Arithmetic operators

Operator	Meaning	Expression	Result
$+$	plus	$2 + 3$	5
$-$	minus	$5 - 2$	3
$*$	times	$5 * 2$	10
$/$	divided by	$10/2$	5
^	power	2^3	8

TABLE 1.2. Common functions

S-PLUS function	Meaning
sqrt()	square root
log()	natural logarithm
log10()	logarithm base 10
exp()	exponential
abs()	absolute value
round()	round to nearest integer
ceiling()	round up
floor()	round down
sin(),cos(),tan()	sine, cosine, tangent
asin(),acos(),atan()	arc sine, arc cosine, arc tangent

```
[1] 1 3
> x[1:3]
[1] 1 2 3
```

We can carry out any of the arithmetic operations described in Table 1.1 between two scalars, a vector and a scalar or two vectors as follows:

```
> 1 + 2
[1] 3
> x <- 1:3
> x + 2
[1] 3 4 5
> x + x
[1] 2 4 6
> x * x
[1] 1 4 9
```

An arithmetic operation between two vectors returns a vector whose elements are the results of applying the operation to the corresponding elements of the original vectors. We can also apply mathematical functions to vectors, such as the square root or logarithm, and the others listed in Table 1.2. The functions are simply applied to each element of the vector. For example,

```
> x <- 1:3
> sqrt(x * x)
[1] 1 2 3
```

1.5   Matrices

Matrix objects are frequently needed in S-PLUS and can be created by the
use of the **matrix()** function. The general syntax is

```
matrix(data,nrow,ncol,byrow = F)
```

The last argument specifies whether the matrix is to be filled row by row
(the alternative being column by column) and takes on a logical value. The
expression **byrow = F** indicates that **F** (false) is the default value.

```
> x <- c(1, 2, 3)
> y <- c(4, 5, 6)
> xy <- matrix(c(x, y), nrow = 2)
> xy
     [,1] [,2] [,3]
[1,]   1    3    5
[2,]   2    4    6
```

Here, the number of columns is not specified and so is determined by
simple division.

```
> xy <- matrix(c(x, y), nrow = 2, byrow = T)
> xy
     [,1] [,2] [,3]
[1,]   1    2    3
[2,]   4    5    6
```

Here, the matrix is filled row-wise instead of by columns by setting the
byrow argument to T for True.

A square bracket with two numbers separated by a comma is used to
refer to an element of a matrix. The first number specifies the row, and the
second specifies the column.

```
> xy[1, 1]
[1] 1
```

The [i,] and [,j] nomenclature is used in S-PLUS to refer to complete
rows or columns of a matrix and can be used to extract particular rows or
columns.

```
> xy[1, ]
[1] 1 2 3
```

```
> xy[, 2]
[1] 2 5
> xy[, c(1, 3)]
     [,1] [,2]
[1,]    1    3
[2,]    4    6
```

As with vectors, arithmetic operations operate element by element when applied to matrices.

```
> xy * xy
     [,1] [,2] [,3]
[1,]    1    4    9
[2,]   16   25   36
```

Matrix multiplication is performed using the %*% operator.

```
> xy %*% t(xy)
     [,1] [,2]
[1,]   14   32
[2,]   32   77
```

Here, the matrix xy is multipled by its transpose (obtained using the t() function). Matrix multiplication of xy by xy would, of course, result in an error message.

(It is usually extremely helpful to attach names to the rows and columns to a matrix. This can be done using the dimension() function. We shall illustrate this in Section 1.7 after we have covered list objects.)

As with vectors, matrices can be formed from numeric and string objects, but in the resulting matrix, all elements will be strings.

```
> Mix <- matrix(c(names, 55, 32, 30), nrow = 2,
+ byrow = T)
> Mix
        [,1]      [,2]        [,3]
[1,] "Brian"  "Sophia"  "Harriett"
[2,] "55"     "32"      "30"
```

Higher dimensional matrices with up to eight dimensions can be defined using the array() function.

1.6 Logical expressions and subsetting matrices and vectors

So far, we have mentioned values of type numeric or character (string). When a numeric value is missing, it is of type NA. (Complex numbers are

TABLE 1.3. Logical operators

Operator	Meaning
<	less than
>	greater than
<=	less than or equal to
>=	greater than or equal to
==	equal to
!=	not equal to
&	and
|	or
!	not

also available.) Another type in S-PLUS is logical. S-PLUS has two logical values, T (true) and F (false), and a number of logical operations that are extremely useful when making comparisons and choosing particular elements from vectors and matrices.

The symbols used for the logical operations are listed in Table 1.3. We can use a logical expression to assign a logical value (T or F) to x:

```
> x <- 3 == 4
> x
[1] F
> x <- 3 < 4
> x
[1] T
> x <- 3 == 4 & 3 < 4
> x
[1] F
> x <- 3 == 4 | 3 < 4
> x
[1] T
```

In addition to logical operators, there are also logical functions. Some examples are given below:

```
> is.numeric(3)
[1] T
> is.character(3)
[1] F
> is.character("3")
[1] T
> 1/0
[1] Inf
> is.numeric(1/0)
[1] T
```

```
> is.infinite(1/0)
[1] T
```

Logical operators or functions operate on elements of vectors and matrices in the same say as arithmetic operators:

```
> is.na(c(1, 0, NA, 1))
[1] F F T F
> !is.na(c(1, 0, NA, 1))
[1] T T F T
> x <- seq(20)
> x < 10
 [1] T T T T T T T T T F F F F F F F F F F F
```

A logical vector can be used to extract a subset of elements from another vector as follows:

```
> x[x < 10]
[1] 1 2 3 4 5 6 7 8 9
```

Here, the elements of the vector less than 10 are selected as the values corresponding to T in the vector x < 10. We can also select elements in x depending on the values in another vector y:

```
> x <- seq(50)
> y <- c(rep(0, 10), rep(1, 40))
> x[y == 0]
 [1]  1  2  3  4  5  6  7  8  9 10
```

1.7 List objects

List objects allow any other S-PLUS objects to be linked together. For example,

```
> x <- seq(10)
> y <- matrix(seq(10), nrow = 5)
> xylist <- list(x, y)
> xylist
[[1]]:
 [1]  1  2  3  4  5  6  7  8  9 10

[[2]]:
     [,1] [,2]
[1,]    1    6
[2,]    2    7
[3,]    3    8
```

```
[4,]    4    9
[5,]    5    10
```

Note the elements of the list are referred to by a double square brackets notation; so we can print the first component of the list using

```
> xylist[[1]]
 [1]  1  2  3  4  5  6  7  8  9 10
```

The components of the list can also be given names and later referred to using the list$name notation.

```
> xylist <- list(X = x, Y = y)
> xylist$X
 [1]  1  2  3  4  5  6  7  8  9 10
```

List objects can, of course, include other list objects

```
> newlist <- list(xy = xylist, z = rep(0, 10))
> newlist$xy
$X:
 [1]  1  2  3  4  5  6  7  8  9 10

$Y:
     [,1] [,2]
[1,]    1    6
[2,]    2    7
[3,]    3    8
[4,]    4    9
[5,]    5    10

> newlist$z
 [1] 0 0 0 0 0 0 0 0 0 0
```

The rows and columns of a matrix can be named using the dimnames() function and a list object.

```
> x <- matrix(seq(12), nrow = 4)
> dimnames(x) <- list(c("R1", "R2", "R3", "R4"),
+ c("C1", "C2", "C3"))
> x
   C1 C2 C3
R1  1  5  9
R2  2  6 10
R3  3  7 11
R4  4  8 12
```

The names can be created more efficiently (particularly for a large matrix) by using the `paste()` function, which combines different strings and numbers into a single string.

```
> dimnames(x) <- list(paste("row", seq(4)),
+ paste("col", seq(3)))
> x
      col 1 col 2 col 3
row 1     1     5     9
row 2     2     6    10
row 3     3     7    11
row 4     4     8    12
```

Having named the rows and columns, we can, if required, refer to elements of the matrix using these names:

```
> x["row 1", "col 3"]
[1] 9
```

1.8 Data frames

Data sets in S-PLUS are usually stored as matrices, which we have already met, or as data frames, which we shall describe in this section.

Data frames can bind vectors of different types together (for example, numeric and character), retaining the correct type of each vector. In other respects, a data frame is like a matrix so that each vector should have the same number of elements. The syntax for creating a data frame is `data.frame(vector1, vector2,···)`, and an example of how a small data frame can be created is as follows:

```
> height <- c(50, 70, 45, 80, 100)
> weight <- c(120, 140, 100, 200, 190)
> age <- c(20, 40, 41, 31, 33)
> names <- c("Bob", "Ted", "Alice", "Mary", "Sue")
> sex <- c("Male", "Male", "Female", "Female", "Female")
> data <- data.frame(names, sex, height, weight, age)
> data
   names    sex height weight age
1    Bob   Male     50    120  20
2    Ted   Male     70    140  40
3  Alice Female     45    100  41
4   Mary Female     80    200  31
5    Sue Female    100    190  33
```

Particular parts of a data frame can be extracted in the same way as for matrices.

```
> data[, c(1, 2, 5)]
  names     sex age
1   Bob    Male  20
2   Ted    Male  40
3 Alice  Female  41
4  Mary  Female  31
5   Sue  Female  33
```

Column names can also be used

```
> data[, "age"]
[1] 20 40 41 31 33
```

Variables can also be accessed as in lists:

```
> data$age
[1] 20 40 41 31 33
```

It is, however, more convenient to "attach" a data frame and work with the column names directly, for example,

```
> attach(data)
> age
[1] 20 40 41 31 33
```

Note that the attach() command places the data frame in the second position in the search path. If we assign a value to age, e.g.,

```
> age <- 10
> age
[1] 10
```

this creates a new object in the first position of the search path that 'masks' the age variable of the data frame. Variables can be removed from the first position in the search path using the rm() function:

```
> rm(age)
```

To change the value of age within the data frame, use the syntax

```
> data$age <- c(20,30,45,32,32)
```

1.9   Reading in data

S-PLUS can read data from a large number of different statistical packages and spreadsheet/database packages, including SPSS, Stata, SAS, Microsoft Excel and Microsoft Access. The diagram below shows how to read a file from another package using the GUI interface:

File
     Import Data
          From File...
               File name: *type filename*
               File of type: *select type, e.g., SPSS Files (*.sav)*
               | Open |

ASCII data can be read using the `scan()` function. For example, if the file *data.dat* in the directory `c:\users\me` contains the data

```
1 2 3
2 3 5
3 2 1
```

these can be read into a vector using the `scan()` function and then converted to a matrix using

```
> a <- matrix(scan(file = "c:\\users\\me\\data.dat"),
+ nrow = 3, byrow = T)
```

Note that the `scan()` function reads the data in lexicographical order (down the rows), so that the `byrow=T` option should be used inside the `matrix()` function.

An even more convenient way of reading in ASCII data is using the `read.table()` function. This function reads the data as a data frame. If the first row of the file contains the variable names, the `header=T` option causes these names to be used in the data frame. For example, if the data in `c:\users\me\children.dat` contain

```
age sex y
11 boy 3.2
9  boy 5.8
13 girl 1.2
```

the data can be read using

```
> child <- read.table("c:\\users\\me\\children.dat",
+ header = T)
> child
  age sex   y
1  11 boy 3.2
2   9 boy 5.8
3  13 girl 1.2
```

Only the variable `sex` is now of mode character because the data were read as a data frame.

1.10   Some commonly used S-PLUS functions for data analysis

S-PLUS contains some 3,000 functions. Here, we introduce a very small subset of these. Many other S-PLUS functions will be encountered in the rest of the book.

Suppose we wish to find the means of the numeric variables in the data frame created in Section 1.8. There are a variety of ways this could be done; for example, we can use the mean() function. (We assume that the data frame has been attached so that variables can be referred to by their names.)

```
> mean(age)
[1] 33
> mean(height)
[1] 69
> mean(weight)
[1] 150
```

Far more convenient, particularly for large data sets, is to use the apply() function. The syntax is apply(object, dim, function), where object is the name of a matrix or data frame, dim can take the value 1 or 2 depending on whether calculation is to take place on row or column elements, and function is the name of an S-PLUS function (already available or created by the user—see next section), which can be applied to numeric vectors. So to get the required three means,

```
> means <- apply(data[, c(3, 4, 5)], 2, mean)
> means
 height weight age
     69    150  33
```

We might be more interested in the medians than in the means

```
> medians <- apply(data[, c(3, 4, 5)], 2, median)
> medians
 height weight age
     70    140  33
```

Variances could be obtained similarly using the var() function.

```
> variances <- apply(data[, c(3, 4, 5)], 2, var)
> variances
 height weight  age
    505   1900 71.5
```

Standard deviations are now obtained as

```
> sqrt(variances)
    height    weight         age
 22.47221 43.58899 8.455767
```

The var() function when applied to a matrix rather than a vector gives the resulting variance-covariance matrix.

```
> var(data[, c(3, 4, 5)])
         height  weight    age
height    505.0   887.5   10.0
weight    887.5  1900.0  -45.0
   age     10.0   -45.0   71.5
```

Similarly, the cor() function can be used to find the correlation matrix of the three variables.

```
> cor(data[, c(3, 4, 5)])
             height      weight          age
height  1.00000000   0.9060369   0.05262611
weight  0.90603687   1.0000000  -0.12209073
   age  0.05262611  -0.1220907   1.00000000
```

Common mathematical functions are listed in Table 1.2. A very useful set of functions in S-PLUS are those relating to probability distributions. For most common probability distributions, S-PLUS has four functions with prefixes d, p, q and r to return the density (d), cumulative probability (p), quantile (q) or a random sample (r). For the normal distribution, the functions may be used as follows:

```
> dnorm(2, mean = 2, sd = 3)
[1] 0.1329808
> pnorm(2, mean = 2, sd = 3)
[1] 0.5
> qnorm(p = 0.025, mean = 0, sd = 1)
[1] -1.959964
> rnorm(n = 4, mean = 0, sd = 1)
[1] 0.06709 0.18382 0.07741 1.02588
```

If the mean and sd options are not specified, a standard normal distribution is assumed with mean = 0, sd = 1. Examples of other functions are pbinom(), pbeta(), pchisq(), pf() and pt() and punif(), each of which is available with the d, q and r prefixes as well.

1.11   Data manipulation

We have already discussed many tools that are useful for generating and manipulating data, e.g., the c(), rep() and seq() functions and methods of accessing variables (columns) or observations (rows) in a data frame or matrix. Here, we will describe some other tools that will be used throughout the book to manipulate data.

A vector can be sorted using the `sort()` function.

```
> x <- c(1, 5, 2)
> sort(x)
[1] 1 2 5
```

The `order()` function returns the permutation of the indices that will give the desired ordering.

```
> index <- order(x)
> index
[1] 1 3 2
> x[index]
[1] 1 2 5
```

To sort an entire data frame `data` according to `sex` and `age`, use

```
index<-order(data$sex,data$age)
data1<-data[index,]
```

(If `sex` is of mode character, the values are sorted alphabetically.)

A subset of observations can be extracted using logical expressions. To exclude observations in which the variable `age` is missing, use

```
data1<-data[!is.na(data$age),]
```

or

```
index<-(1:nrow(data))[!is.na(data$age)]
data1<-data[index,]
```

To extract observations for the *k*th group without having to know the group value, use the `unique()` function:

```
> labels <- sort(unique(data$group))
> index<-(1:nrow(data))[data$group == labels[k]]
> data1<-data[index,]
```

It is often required to compute summary measures of a number of variables within groups defined by another set of variables; i.e., to 'aggregate' or 'collapse' the data. For example, using data on patients from different hospitals, we may want to compute the hospitals' average patient characteristics:

```
> data1<-aggregate.data.frame(data, hospitals, FUN=mean)
```

Two vectors or matrices can be combined into a matrix using cbind() or rbind(), depending on whether the columns should be joined (e.g., merging different variables on the same observations) or the rows (e.g., merging different sets of observations of the same variables). These commands can also be used to combine two data frames into a single data frame. Additional vectors (variables) can be added to a data frame using the data.frame() function:

```
> data1 <- data.frame(data, age2 = data$age^2)
```

Longitudinal data can be viewed as multivariate data, in which the measurement occasions are different variables, or as univariate hierarchical data, in which the measurement occasions are different observations. Here, we show an example of how we can convert from the multivariate (wide) representation to the univariate (long) one.

```
> wide <- data.frame(id = 1:4, before = c(1, 3, 2, 4),
+ after = c(2, 1, 3, 2))
> y <- as.vector(as.matrix(wide[, 2:3]))
> subject <- rep(wide$id, 2)
> after <- c(rep(0, 4), rep(1, 4))
> long <- data.frame(subject, y, after)
> wide
  id before after
1  1      1     2
2  2      3     1
3  3      2     3
4  4      4     2
> long
  subject y after
1       1 1     0
2       2 3     0
3       3 2     0
4       4 4     0
5       1 2     1
6       2 1     1
7       3 3     1
8       4 2     1
```

Here, as.vector() stacks the columns of a matrix into a supervector. Note that we first had to convert wide[,2:3] from a data frame to a matrix using the as.matrix() function. We can use the matrix() function to convert the supervector back to a matrix.

Some functions behave differently when applied to data frames or matrices. To check whether data is a matrix or data frame, use

```
> is.matrix(data)
> is.data.frame(data)
```

TABLE 1.4. Syntax for model formulae

Expression	Meaning
$T \sim F$	T is modeled as F
$F_a + F_b$	include both F_a and F_b
$F_a - F_b$	include all F_a except what is in F_b
$F_a : F_b$	interaction between F_a and F_b
$F_a * F_b$	$F_a + F_b + F_a : F_b$
$F\hat{}m$	All terms in F crossed to order m

1.12   Modeling in S-PLUS

S-PLUS is an object-oriented language, and this feature is particularly useful for modeling. The modeling functions in S-PLUS, aov(), lm(), glm(), and so on, return objects of certain classes. Generic functions like plot(), summary() and print() are applicable to all of these objects, and their behavior (or the *method*) is determined by the class. This means that the user does not have to remember different function names for different types of modeling. For example, the plot() produces the appropriate diagnostics for generalized linear models or for analysis of variance (ANOVA) models depending on the class of object passed to it.

Another feature that is the same for all models is the *model formula*. A formula in S-PLUS is a symbolic expression that defines the structural form of the model and is interpreted by the modeling functions. Model formulas are of the form

```
Y ~ x1 + x2 + x3
```

where Y is the response variable and x1 to x3 are explanatory variables (the corresponding regression coefficients and the constant are implicit in the formula). Tabe 1.4 lists operators used in formulae (this is adapted from Chambers and Hastie, 1993) in which T denotes a term and F denotes a formula. The formula

```
Y ~ (x1 + x2 + x3)^2
```

specifies that all main effects and all pairwise interactions should be fitted. The term on the left-hand side can be an expression. For example,

```
log(Y) ~ x1*x2-1
```

means that the logarithm of Y is modeled using the main effects and interaction of x1 and x2 but no intercept. Variables on the right-hand side can also be transformed within the model formula, but because arithmetic operators have a different meaning in formulae, the expressions are enclosed in the I() function. The formula

```
Y ~ I(x1*x2)
```

means that a single explanatory variable, equal to the product `x1*x2`, is used in addition to the constant.

It is obviously important to specify whether the explanatory variables are continuous variables or discrete, possibly unordered, factors. This can be done prior to specifying the formula by defining all noncontinuous variables as factors or ordered factors.

```
> sex <- factor(c(1,0,1,1,0,0),labels=c("man","woman"))
> agegroup <- ordered(ages,
+ labels=c("18-25","26-35","36-80"))
```

By default, S-PLUS uses Helmert contrasts for unordered factors and polynomial contrasts for ordered factors. If we always prefer treatment contrasts for unordered factors (in which each level of the factor except the first is compared with the first), we can can change the defaults for the remainder of the session by issuing the command

```
> options(contrasts=c("contr.treatment","contr.poly"))
```

(The `options()` function allows many different parameters to be set—for example, to control the appearance of the output in the book, we have specified

```
> options(width = 68, digits = 4)
```

see `help(options)`.)

Contrasts can also be set in the model formula using the `C(factor, contrast)` function. To use treatment contrasts for sex, use

```
Y~C(sex,treatment)+age
```

We can also change the default contrast attribute (Helmert) of specific factors (not all factors) using the `contrats()` function:

```
> contrasts(sex)<-contr.treatment(2)
```

See Chambers and Hastie (1993) for more information on modeling in S-PLUS.

1.13   User functions

S-PLUS provides an extremely powerful method of writing functions for specific tasks of interest. Here, we give only a number of very simple examples, largely to illustrate the syntax. A detailed account of writing functions in S-PLUS is given in Venables and Ripley (2000).

Here is a function to add two numbers

```
> mysum <- function(a, b)
{
    a + b
}
> mysum(1, 3)
[1] 4
```

Here, `mysum` is the function name and `a` and `b` are names assigned to
the first and second arguments that may be passed to the function. The
command between the curly brackets defines what the function should do
with the two arguments. The result of the last command (in this case, the
only command) is returned.

Note that curly brackets are used in S-PLUS only when defining functions, curved brackets include the arguments of functions and square brackets are used to identify parts of vectors, matrices and data frames.

In addition to arguments, parameters may be defined that take on a
default value if not specified in the call to the function. For example, to
allow a power of the sum to be returned, we can alter the function as
follows:

```
> mysum <- function(a, b, p = 1)
{
    (a + b)^p
}
> mysum(1, 3)
[1] 4
> mysum(1, 3, p = 2)
[1] 16
> mysum(1, 3, 2)
[1] 16
```

Some functions in S-PLUS require the name of another function as one
of the arguments. We have already come across one such function, namely,
`apply()`. Instead of supplying one of the S-PLUS functions like `mean()` or
`var()`, we may define our function as follows:

```
> stdv <- function(y) sqrt(var(y))
> X <- matrix(1:15, ncol = 5)
> apply(X, 2, stdv)
[1] 1 1 1 1 1
```

(Note that curly brackets are only required if the function definition requires more than a single command.)

Sometimes it may be necessary to construct a loop using the syntax

```
> for(i in 1:5) {
+     print(i)
```

```
}
[1] 1
[1] 2
[1] 3
[1] 4
[1] 5
```

However, whenever possible loops should be replaced by matrix operations or the various `apply()` functions; e.g., `apply()` to loop through rows or columns of a matrix, or `sapply()` to loop through elements of a list. This is more elegant and faster than explicit looping. A very useful function to help avoid looping is the `outer()` function. Suppose we wish to compute points on a surface $f(x, y)$ for a regular grid of x and y values. Instead of using two nested loops over the values of x and y, we can use the commands

```
> f <- function(x, y)(x - 2)^2 + (y - 3)^2
> x <- seq(0, 4, 0.1)
> y <- seq(0, 6, 0.1)
> y <- outer(x, y, FUN = f)
```

All values of x are combined with all values of y, and the function is evaluated. The result, y, is a matrix containing the surface heights. Another useful function is `expand.grid()`, which forms a matrix containing all combinations of the elements of two vectors; e.g.,

```
> expand.grid(c(1, 2), c(1, 2, 3))
  Var1 Var2
1   1    1
2   2    1
3   1    2
4   2    2
5   1    3
6   2    3
```

We may wish to execute some commands only if certain conditions hold. This may be done using `if` and `else` as follows:

```
> for(i in 1:5) {
+       if(i <= 3)
+               print(i)
+       else {
+               print("hello")
+               print(i * 3)
+       }
+}
[1] 1
[1] 2
```

```
[1] 3
[1] "hello"
[1] 12
[1] "hello"
[1] 15
```

Again, braces are only needed if the 'if' or 'else' blocks have more than a single line of commands.

Functions may be defined in the **Commands** window and saved in the 'current directory' at the end of a session. However, the safest way of defining a function and not losing it is to save the required commands in a Script file.

1.14   Graphics using the command line approach

S-PLUS contains extensive graphical facilities for obtaining a variety of plots, from the simple to the sophisticated.

First, we have to specify the device to which we would like to plot. Usually, this will be a **Graphics** window. In Windows 98/2000/NT, such a window can be created using the command

```
win.graph()
```

We can now create several graphs in which each one replaces the previous one. We can also create a postscript file of a plot by setting the device as follows:

```
postscript(file = graph.ps)
```

After producing a postscript file, we must then close the file using the `dev.off()` command; otherwise, subsequent graphs will be superimposed on the first one.

To illustrate some of the simple graphical functions, we shall first generate some data from a normal distribution using the `rnorm()` function. To ensure that readers will obtain the same graph as is presented here, we first set the *seed* of the random number generator to an arbitrary value.

```
> set.seed(1234)
> x <- rnorm(100, 0, 1)
```

x contains 100 random numbers from a standard normal distribution.

We will plot a histogram using the `hist()` function and a boxplot using the `boxplot()` function

```
> hist(x)
> boxplot(x)
```

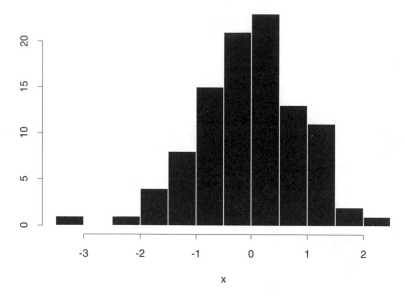

FIGURE 1.4. Histogram.

The histogram and boxplot are shown in Figures 1.4 and 1.5, respectively.
One of the most widely used graphics in statistics is the scatterplot; this
is obtained using the plot() function.

```
> y <- 5 + 2 * x + rnorm(100, 0, 1)
> plot(x, y)
```

The graph is shown in Figure 1.6.

A useful feature in S-PLUS is that we can add further elements to an
existing graph. For example, to add a line with intercept 5 and slope 2 to
the scatterplot in Figure 1.6, use the command

```
> abline(5,2)
```

giving the graph in Figure 1.7. Table 1.5 lists some of the functions available
to add further elements to an existing graph.

A large number of graphics parameters control the appearance of a graph.
Some of these are listed in Table 1.6. To find out about additional graphics
parameters, look up help for par(), for example, by typing

```
>help(par)
```

(Help files are available for all S-PLUS functions.)

We can change the default value of graphics parameters before plotting
using the par() function. One parameter we will frequently set using the
par() function is mfrow, which allows several graphs to be plotted on the
same graphics window. For example, the command

```
>par(mfrow = c(1, 2))
```

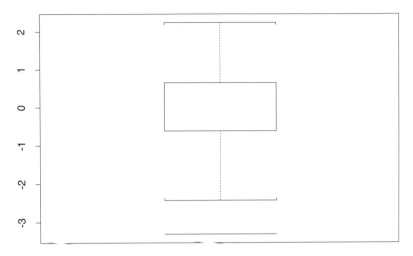

FIGURE 1.5. Box plot.

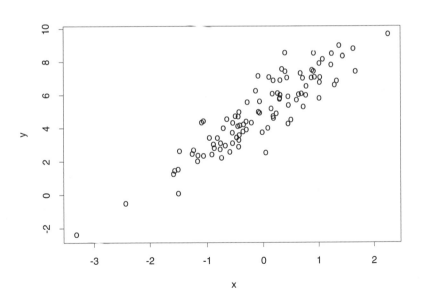

FIGURE 1.6. Scatterplot.

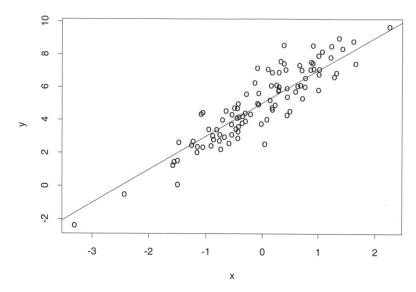

FIGURE 1.7. Scatterplot with regression line.

TABLE 1.5. Commands to add to existing graphs

Function	Description
points(x,y)	points at coordinates x and y
text(x,y,text)	text at specified coordinates
lines(x,y)	lines connecting the points given by x and y
segments(x1,y1,x2,y2)	line segments from (x1,y1) to (x2,y2)
arrows(x1,y1,x2,y2)	arrows segements from (x1,y1) to (x2,y2)
abline(a,b)	line with intercept a and slope b
legend(x,y,legend)	legend
title("title","subtitle")	title at top of figure

TABLE 1.6. Plotting parameters

Parameter	Purpose
type="p"/"l"/"h"/"s"/"n", etc.	points/lines/vertical bars/steps/nothing
axes=T/F	with/without axes
main	main title
sub	subtitle
xlab,ylab	x/y-axis label
xlim,ylim=c(min,max)	x/y-axis range
pch=1/2/3, etc. or pch="+"/"."., etc.	plot character
lty=1/2/3, etc.	line style
lwd	line width (1 default)

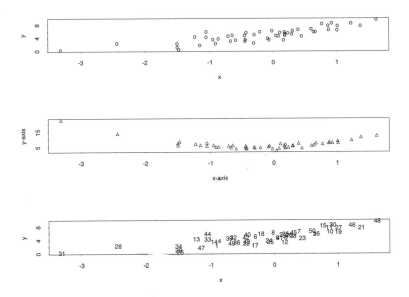

FIGURE 1.8. Three scatterplots.

splits the graphics window into two panels, layed out into one row and two columns. Subsequent graph commands will fill out the panels one by one in lexicographical order.

To illustrate the use of graphics parameters, we produce three scatterplots on a single display:

```
> x <- rnorm(50, 0, 1)
> y <- 5 + 2 * x + rnorm(50, 0, 1.3)
> z <- 5 + x + 2 * x^2 + rnorm(50, 0, 1)
> par(mfrow = c(3, 1))
> plot(x, y, xlab = "x", ylab = "y")
# xlab and ylab options used to label axes
> plot(x, z, xlab = "x-axis", ylab = "y-axis", pch = 2)
# pch changes the plotting symbol
> plot(x, y, xlab = "x", ylab = "y", type = "n")
# type = "n" suppresses the points of the scatterplot
> text(x, y, labels = 1:50)
# the text() function places labels in the positions
# specified by x, y
```

The graph is shown in Figure 1.8. (As mentioned in the previous section, the plot() function may also be used to produce 'default' plots for most analyses, by using an object returned from an analysis as the argument. Examples will appear in later chapters.)

Trellis graphics can be used to display higher dimensional data structures (see Chapter 7 for more details). A trellis device can be specified for trellis graphics using the command

```
> trellis.device(win.graph)
```

or

```
trellis.device(postscript, file = c:/users/me/graph.ps)
```

1.15   The S-PLUS GUI

S-PLUS has an extensive (GUI) that allows many statistical analyses or graphs to be produced by selecting items from menus instead of typing commands.

For example, we can produce a scatterplot for the following data set:

```
> height <- c(1.2, 1.3, 1.23, 1.45, 1.62, 1.1)
> age <- c(8, 9, 7, 11, 15, 9)
> growth <- data.frame(Height = height, Age = age)
```

as follows:

Graph
  2D Plot...
    Scatter Plot(x, y1, y2 ...)
     | OK |
      Data Set: growth
      x Column(s): Age
      x Column(s): Height
      Symbol
        Style: Box, Solid
       | OK |

The completed dialogue box is shown in Figure 1.9. Other examples are given in Appendix A.

1.16   Exercises

1.1 Use the rep() and seq() functions to produce the following three vectors:

x1: 1 2 3 4 1 2 3 4 1 2 3 4 1 2 3 4
x2: 4 4 4 4 3 3 3 3 2 2 2 2 1 1 1 1
x3: 1 2 2 3 3 3 4 4 4 4 5 5 5 5 5

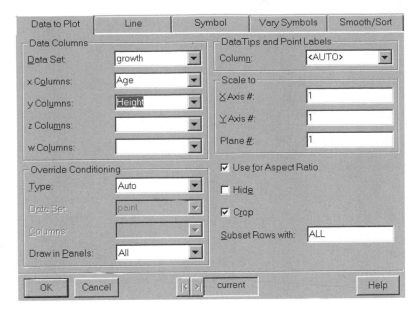

FIGURE 1.9. Dialogue box for scatterplot.

1.2 Missing values in a data set are represented in S-PLUS by NA. Generate a sample of 50 observations from a normal distribution with mean 5 and standard deviation 2, and

1. Arrange the sample as a 10×5 matrix, A.

2. Give A suitable row and column names.

3. Set the first two elements of row 2 and the third and fifth elements of row 5 of A to missing.

4. Find the mean of the nonmissing values of A.

5. Find the column and row means of the non-missing values of A.

1.3 Write a function that replaces any missing value in an $n \times p$ matrix by either the mean or the median of the nonmissing values in the same column. Allow the user of the function to select which summary measure is used. (This way of replacing missing values is *not* recommended in practice.)

1.4 The following is a hypothetical data set giving sex, ages, weights and heights of five individuals. Read the data into a data frame, Data.

Individual	Sex	Age	Weight(lbs)	Height(inches)
1	M	20	120	61
2	F	24	130	65
3	M	31	190	70
4	M	25	201	74
5	F	27	101	71

1.5 Find the covariance and correlation matrices of Age, Weight, and Height in Data.

1.6 Find the mean weight of the women in Data.

1.7 Produce a diagram containing the boxplots of Age, Weight and Height, and scatterplots of Age v Weight, Age v Height and Weight v Height.

1.8 Attach the Data data frame and then produce the same graphic as in 17 using the GUI.

1.9 Use the appropriate dialogue box to test whether the mean weight of men is different from that of women.

1.10 Use the GUI to produce a graphic including the three pairwise scatterplots of the variables in Data, each scatterplot having its least-squares regression line shown.

1.11 Write an S-PLUS function to find the position in a matrix of its maximum value.

2
Describing Data

2.1 Introduction

The first steps to understanding the general characteristics of any data set are to calculate relevant summary statistics for the data and to graph the data in some way. Which graphs and which summary statistics are most appropriate will largely depend on the type of observations and measurements that have been recorded. In this chapter, we shall illustrate the possibilities using a number of data sets containing continuous or categorical variables.

2.2 Graphing and summarizing continuous data

Table 2.1 shows the heights in centimeters of a sample of 351 elderly women, randomly selected from the community in a study of osteoporosis. Table 2.2 gives the survival times of 43 patients suffering from chronic granulocytic leukaemia, measured in days from time of diagnosis.

To begin, we shall calculate a number of summary statistics for both sets of data; these are shown in Table 2.3. For the heights data, the mean and the median have very similar values indicating the general lack of skewness of the observations. In contrast, the mean and the median of the survival times differ considerably, suggesting that these data are positively skewed.

More can be learned about the distribution of each data set by examining a number of graphical displays. Most commonly, the histogram is used, but it is not necessarily always the most informative diagram available; consideration of stem-and-leaf plots and box plots is often more interest-

TABLE 2.1. Heights of 351 elderly women

156	163	169	161	154	156	163	164	156	166	177	158
150	164	159	157	166	163	153	161	170	159	170	157
156	156	153	178	161	164	158	158	162	160	150	162
155	161	158	163	158	162	163	152	173	159	154	155
164	163	164	157	152	154	173	154	162	163	163	165
160	162	155	160	151	163	160	165	166	178	153	160
156	151	165	169	157	152	164	166	160	165	163	158
153	162	163	162	164	155	155	161	162	156	169	159
159	159	158	160	165	152	157	149	169	154	146	156
157	163	166	165	155	151	157	156	160	170	158	165
167	162	153	156	163	157	147	163	161	161	153	155
166	159	157	152	159	166	160	157	153	159	156	152
151	171	162	158	152	157	162	168	155	155	155	161
157	158	153	155	161	160	160	170	163	153	159	169
155	161	156	153	156	158	164	160	157	158	157	156
160	161	167	162	158	163	147	153	155	159	156	161
158	164	163	155	155	158	165	176	158	155	150	154
164	145	153	169	160	159	159	163	148	171	158	158
157	158	168	161	165	167	158	158	161	160	163	163
169	163	164	150	154	165	158	161	156	171	163	170
154	158	162	164	158	165	158	156	162	160	164	165
157	167	142	166	163	163	151	163	153	157	159	152
169	154	155	167	164	170	174	155	157	170	159	170
155	168	152	165	158	162	173	154	167	158	159	152
158	167	164	170	164	166	170	160	148	168	151	153
150	165	165	147	162	165	158	145	150	164	161	157
163	166	162	163	160	162	153	168	163	160	165	156
158	155	168	160	153	163	161	145	161	166	154	147
161	155	158	161	163	157	156	152	156	165	159	170
160	152	153									

TABLE 2.2. Survival times of 43 patients suffering from chronic granulocytic leukaemia, measured in days from time of diagnosis

7	47	58	74	177	232	273	285	317	429
440	445	455	468	495	497	532	571	579	581
650	702	715	779	881	900	930	968	1077	1109
1314	1334	1367	1534	1712	1784	1877	1886	2045	2056
2260	2429	2509							

TABLE 2.3. Summary statistics for heights and survival times data

```
> summary(heights)
 Min. 1st Qu. Median  Mean 3rd Qu. Max.
  142     156    160 159.8     164  178
> summary(leukaem)
 Min. 1st Qu. Median  Mean 3rd Qu. Max.
    7   442.5    702 925.1    1350 2509
```

ing. Box plots show the median, quartiles and minimum and maximum of a distribution as well as highlight possible outliers (points further than 1.5 interquartile ranges from the quartiles). Examples of histograms and box plots for both the heights and the survival times data are shown in Figure 2.1. The 'shapes' of the two data sets now become very clear; heights have a symmetric, unimodal distribution suggestive of normality; survival times, on the other hand, are positively skewed, with possibly an exponential distribution.

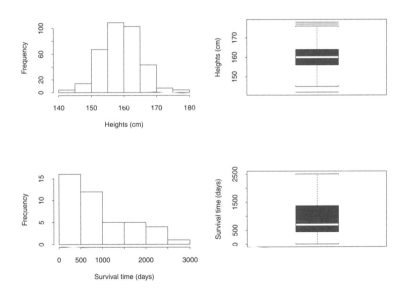

FIGURE 2.1. Histograms and box plots of heights of elderly women and survival times of patients suffering form leukaemia.

In some circumstances, more detailed investigation of the distributions of the two data sets might be merited. To assess their normality, for example, we might use *quantile-quantile plots* (Q-Q plots) as described in Display 2.1. Such plots for both the heights and the survival times are shown in Figure 2.2. That for heights is approximately linear, indicating that a normal

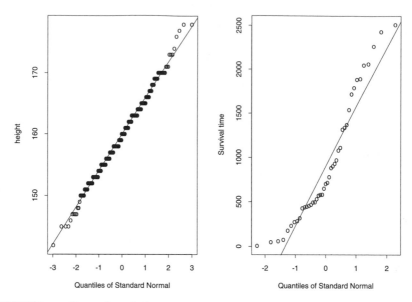

FIGURE 2.2. Normal probability plots for the heights and survival times data.

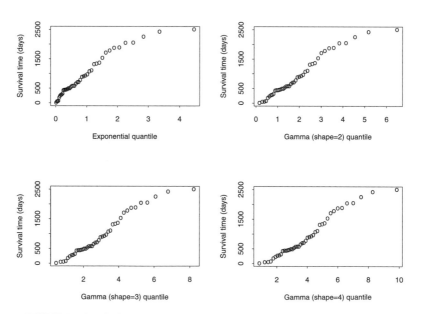

FIGURE 2.3. Q-Q plots for the survival times of leukaemia patients.

distribution is a reasonable assumption for these data. The Q-Q plot for survival times is, however, distinctly nonlinear, and the data clearly do not have a normal distribution.

Q-Q plots are not restricted to testing for normality. Figure 2.3, for example, shows four Q-Q plots of the survival times data. In Figure 2.3(a), an exponential distribution is assessed, and in the remaining three plots, gamma distributions with different shape parameters are assessed (see Display 2.2). The Q-Q plot for the exponential distribution looks approximately linear, and this may be a reasonable distribution to assume for the survival times.

It is often useful to plot the assumed theoretical probability density function of a set of data onto the sample histogram. Here, we shall use the normal distribution for heights and the exponential distribution for the survival times. (The parameters of the normal distribution μ and σ^2 are estimated by the sample mean and variance; the parameter λ of the exponential distribution is estimated as the reciprocal of the sample mean.) The resulting diagrams are shown in Figure 2.4. The assumed density functions

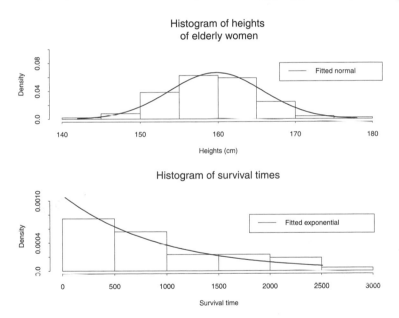

FIGURE 2.4. Histograms of heights and survival times with fitted theoretical density functions.

appear to fit reasonably well.

For many data sets, we may not be willing to assume a specific parametric form for its density function, but we would still like to find a more suitable estimate of the density than that provided by the simple histogram. There

---

Display 2.1 Probability plots

- Plots for comparing two probability distributions.
- There are two basic types, the *probability-probability plot* and the *quantile-quantile plot*. The diagram below may be used for describing each type.

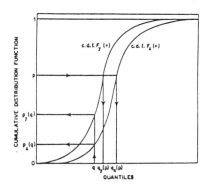

- A plot of points whose coordinates are the cumulative probabilities $\{p_x(q), p_y(q)\}$ for different values of q is a probability-probability plot, whereas a plot of the points whose coordinates are the quantiles $\{q_x(p), q_y(p)\}$ for different values of p is a quantile-quantile plot.
- As an example, a quantile-quantile plot for investigating the assumption that a set of data is from a normal distribution would involve plotting the ordered sample values $y_{(1)}, y_{(2)}, \cdots, y_{(n)}$ against the quantiles of a standard normal distribution, i.e.,

$$\Phi^{-1}[p_i] \tag{1}$$

where usually

$$p_i = \frac{i - \frac{1}{2}}{n} \quad \text{and} \quad \Phi(x) = \int_{-\infty}^{x} \frac{1}{\sqrt{2\pi}} e^{-\frac{1}{2}u^2} du \tag{2}$$

- This is usually known as a *normal probability plot*.

Display 2.2 Exponential and gamma distributions

- The exponential distribution has the form

$$f(x) = \lambda e^{-\lambda x} \tag{1}$$

Some examples with different values of λ are shown below.

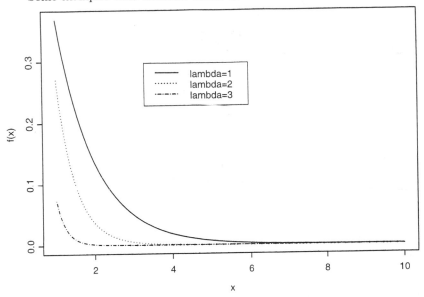

- The gamma distribution has the form

$$f(x) = \frac{x^{\gamma-1}}{\beta} \frac{\exp(-x\beta)}{\beta\Gamma(\gamma)} \quad 0 \leq x < \infty, \ \beta > 0, \ \gamma > 0 \tag{2}$$

where β is a *scale parameter* and γ is a *shape parameter*. Some examples of the distribution are shown below.

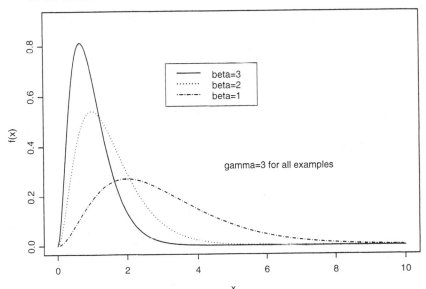

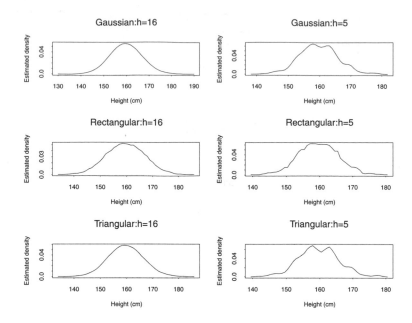

FIGURE 2.5. A variety of nonparametric density estimates for the heights of elderly women.

is now a vast amount of literature on nonparametric density estimation; see, for example, Silverman (1986). A brief description of the procedure for univariate data is given in Display 2.3.

A variety of density estimates for the heights data in which the bandwidth and the kernel are varied is shown in Figure 2.5.

2.3   Graphing and summarizing categorical data

Table 2.4 shows data collected from a survey of workers in the U.S. cotton industry. Whether they were suffering from the lung disease byssinosis is recorded along with the values of five categorical variables: the race, sex and smoking status of the worker, the length of employment and the dustiness of the work place. (Note that these data have already been partially summarized by counting the number of workers with a particular pattern of exploratory variables who do and do not have byssinosis.) Later, in the exercises of Chapter 9 we shall invite readers to explore how the incidence of byssinosis is related to the explanatory variables. Here, however, we shall simply use the data to illustrate some approaches to summarizing categorical data and displaying such data graphically.

To begin, we shall construct some simple cross classifications of the data. Tables 2.5 and 2.6, for example, show the cross classifications of the number

---

Display 2.3 Nonparametric density estimation

- Methods for estimating a probability distribution without assuming a particular parametric form. The histogram is one example.

- Perhaps the most common class of density estimators is of the form

$$\hat{f}(x) = \frac{1}{nh} \sum_{i=1}^{n} K(\frac{x - X_i}{h}) \tag{1}$$

  where h is known as *window width* or *bandwidth* and K is known as the *kernel function*, and is such that

$$\int_{-\infty}^{\infty} K(u)du = 1 \tag{2}$$

- Essentially, such *kernel estimators* sum a series of 'bumps' placed at each of the observations. The kernel function determines the shape of the bumps while h determines their width.

- Three widely used kernel functions are

- Gaussian

$$K(x) = \frac{1}{\sqrt{2\pi}} e^{-x^2/2} \tag{3}$$

- Triangular

$$K(x) = 1 - |x|, \ |x| < 1 \tag{4}$$

- Rectangular

$$K(x) = \frac{1}{2}, \ |x| < 1 \tag{5}$$

- A graphical representation of each kernel function is shown below

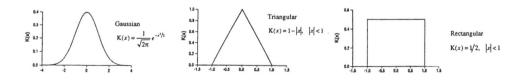

- In general, the choice of the shape of the kernel function is not usually of great importance. In contrast, the choice of bandwidth can be critical.

- There are situations in which it is satisfactory to choose the bandwidth relatively subjectively to achieve a 'smooth' estimate. More formal methods are however available. For details, see Silverman (1986).

of workers with and without byssinosis by race and dustiness of the work place.

Of more interest for these data is to classify the proportion of workers with byssinosis with respect to the other variables. In Table 2.7, for example, this proportion is shown for race against dustiness. The proportion in the 'white/high' cell appears to be out of step with the others and may indicate a race × dust interaction effect on the proportion of workers with byssinosis, a point to which we shall return in Chapter 9.

TABLE 2.4. Survey data from U.S cotton workers

Yes	No	Dust	Race	Sex	Smoking	Emp
3	37	1	1	1	1	1
0	74	2	1	1	1	1
2	258	3	1	1	1	1
25	139	1	2	1	1	1
0	88	2	2	1	1	1
3	242	3	2	1	1	1
0	5	1	1	2	1	1
1	93	2	1	2	1	1
3	180	3	1	2	1	1
2	22	1	2	2	1	1
2	145	2	2	2	1	1
3	260	3	2	2	1	1
0	16	1	1	1	2	1
0	35	2	1	1	2	1
0	134	3	1	1	2	1
6	75	1	2	1	2	1
1	47	2	2	1	2	1
1	122	3	2	1	2	1
0	4	1	1	2	2	1
1	54	2	1	2	2	1
2	169	3	1	2	2	1
1	24	1	2	2	2	1
3	142	2	2	2	2	1
4	301	3	2	2	2	1
8	21	1	1	1	1	2
1	50	2	1	1	1	2
1	187	3	1	1	1	2
8	30	1	2	1	1	2
0	5	2	2	1	1	2
0	33	3	2	1	1	2
0	0	1	1	2	1	2
1	33	2	1	2	1	2
2	94	3	1	2	1	2
0	0	1	2	2	1	2
0	4	2	2	2	1	2
0	3	3	2	2	1	2
2	8	1	1	1	2	2
1	16	2	1	1	2	2
0	58	3	1	1	2	2
1	9	1	2	1	2	2
0	0	2	2	1	2	2
0	7	3	2	1	2	2
0	0	1	1	2	2	2
0	30	2	1	2	2	2
1	90	3	1	2	2	2
0	0	1	2	2	2	2
0	4	2	2	2	2	2
0	4	3	2	2	2	2
31	77	1	1	1	1	3
1	141	2	1	1	1	3
12	495	3	1	1	1	3

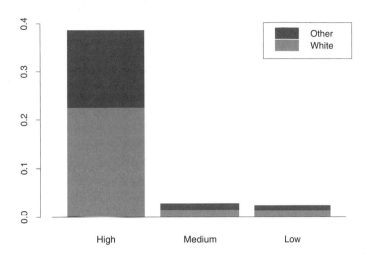

FIGURE 2.6. Barplot of the proportion of workers with byssinosis by race and dustiness of the workplace.

TABLE 2.4. Survey data from U.S cotton workers(continued)

Yes	No	Dust	Race	Sex	Smoking	Emp
10	31	1	2	1	1	3
0	1	2	2	1	1	3
0	45	3	2	1	1	3
0	1	1	1	2	1	3
3	91	2	1	2	1	3
3	176	3	1	2	1	3
0	1	1	2	2	1	3
0	0	2	2	2	1	3
0	2	3	2	2	1	3
5	47	1	1	1	2	3
0	39	2	1	1	2	3
3	182	3	1	1	2	3
3	15	1	2	1	2	3
0	1	2	2	1	2	3
0	23	3	2	1	2	3
0	2	1	1	2	2	3
3	187	2	1	2	2	3
2	340	3	1	2	2	3
0	0	1	2	2	2	3
0	2	2	2	2	2	3
0	3	3	2	2	2	3

The proportions in Table 2.7 can be displayed graphically in a *barplot*. This is shown in Figure 2.6.

TABLE 2.5. Cross classifications of the number of workers with byssinosis by race and dustiness of the workplace

```
> crosstabs(yes ~ race + dust)
Call:
crosstabs(yes ~ race + dust)
165 cases in table
+----------+
|N         |
|N/RowTotal|
|N/ColTotal|
|N/Total   |
+----------+
race   |dust
       |High    |Medium |Low     |RowTotl|
-------+-------+-------+-------+-------+
White  |49      |12     |31      |92      |
       |0.533   |0.130  |0.337   |0.56    |
       |0.467   |0.667  |0.738   |        |
       |0.297   |0.073  |0.188   |        |
-------+-------+-------+-------+-------+
Other  |56      | 6     |11      |73      |
       |0.767   |0.082  |0.151   |0.44    |
       |0.533   |0.333  |0.262   |        |
       |0.339   |0.036  |0.067   |        |
-------+-------+-------+-------+-------+
ColTotl|105     |18     |42      |165     |
       |0.64    |0.11   |0.25    |        |
-------+-------+-------+-------+-------+
Test for independence of all factors
Chi^2 = 9.934325 d.f.= 2 (p=0.006962876)
Yates' correction not used
```

TABLE 2.6. Number of workers without lung disease cross classified by race and dustiness of the workplace

```
> crosstabs(no ~ race + dust)
Call:
crosstabs(no ~ race + dust)
5254 cases in table
+----------+
|N         |
|N/RowTotal|
|N/ColTotal|
|N/Total   |
+----------+
race    |dust
        |High    |Medium |Low     |RowTotl|
--------+--------+-------+--------+-------+
White   | 218    | 843   |2363    |3424   |
        |0.064   |0.246  |0.690   |0.65   |
        |0.387   |0.658  |0.693   |       |
        |0.041   |0.160  |0.450   |       |
--------+--------+-------+--------+-------+
Other   | 346    | 439   |1045    |1830   |
        |0.189   |0.240  |0.571   |0.35   |
        |0.613   |0.342  |0.307   |       |
        |0.066   |0.084  |0.199   |       |
--------+--------+-------+--------+-------+
ColTotl|564      |1282   |3408    |5254   |
       |0.11     |0.24   |0.65    |       |
--------+--------+-------+--------+-------+
Test for independence of all factors
Chi^2 = 200.9816 d.f.= 2 (p=0)
Yates' correction not used
```

TABLE 2.7. Proportion of workers with byssinosis by race and dustiness of the workplace

	High	Medium	Low
White	0.2247706	0.01423488	0.01311892
Other	0.1618497	0.01366743	0.01052632

TABLE 2.8. Standardized mortality rate (SMR) for deaths from lung cancer and
smoking ratio for 25 occupation categories

Occupation	Smoking ratio	Lung cancer SMR
Farmers, foresters, fisherman	77	84
Miners and quarrymen	137	116
Gas, coke and chemical makers	117	123
Glass and ceramics makers	94	128
Furnace, forge, foundry, rolling mill workers	116	155
Electrical and electronic workers	102	101
Engineering and allied trades not included elsewhere	111	118
Woodworkers	93	113
Leatherworkers	88	104
Textile workers	102	88
Clothing workers	91	104
Food, drink and tobacco workers	104	129
Paper and printing workers	107	86
Makers of other products	112	96
Construction workers	113	144
Painters and decorators	110	139
Drivers of stationary engines, cranes, etc.	125	113
Labourers not included elsewhere	133	146
Transport and communications workers	115	128
Warehousemen, storekeepers, packers, bottlers	105	115
Clerical workers	87	79
Sales workers	91	85
Service, sport and recreation workers	100	120
Administrators and managers	76	60
Professional, technical workers, artists	66	51

2.4   Dotplots for classified continuous data

Many sets of data in medicine consist of one or more continuous variables
classified according to a particular categorical variable. Table 2.8, for example, shows for males in England and Wales in 1970-1972, the standardized
mortality ratio (SMR) for deaths from lung cancer for each of 25 occupation
categories or broad groups of jobs. The population used for standardization
was the male population of the whole of England and Wales. Also shown in
Table 2.8 are smoking ratios for each occupation class. The smoking ratio
is a measure of cigarette consumption for a class, again calculated using
indirect standardization. In a class with smoking ratio 100, the men would
smoke (per man per day) the same number of cigarettes that one would
expect on the basis of its age structure and national age-specific smoking
rates.

A very useful display for such data is the *dotplot*, particularly if the data are ordered before plotting. Such a plot for the SMRs is shown in Figure 2.8 and for the smoking ratio in Figure 2.7. One thing to note about the two plots is that the ordering of the job categories by SMR is considerably different from that by smoking ratio. The relationship between the two variables will be looked at in Chapter 4.

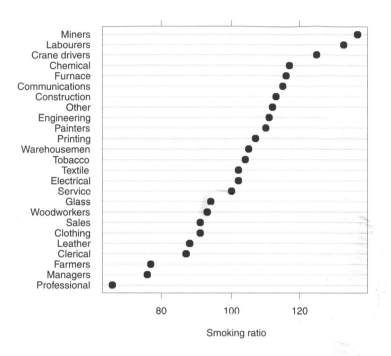

FIGURE 2.7. Dotplot of smoking ratio for 25 occupational groups.

As a further example of the use of the dotplot, we shall produce one for the data shown in Table 2.9. The data are the percentage of deaths in England and Wales in 1997 classified by sex, age and cause of death. The corresponding dotplot is shown in Figure 2.9. For many readers, the dotplot may give a clearer picture of the data than does Table 2.9. Some features that are immediately apparent from Figure 2.9 are the higher death rate due to injury and poisoning among young men (16-24) and the higher death rate from cancer among women aged 35-54.

2.5   Summary

Data analysis usually begins by calculating some appropriate summary statistics and plotting some relatively simple graphs. Using a package such

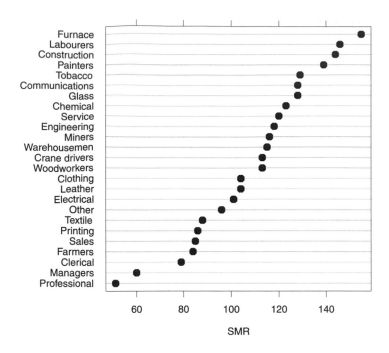

FIGURE 2.8. Dotplot of SMR for deaths from lung cancer in 25 occupational groups.

TABLE 2.9. Percentage deaths in England and Wales in 1997 by age, sex and cause of death

	<1	1–15	16-24	25–34	35–54	55–64	65–74	>74	all
Circulatory diseases	4	6	4	9	33	42	44	44	41
Cancer	1	15	7	11	27	36	34	22	27
Respiratory diseases	10	8	3	4	5	8	12	21	15
Injury and poisoning	5	31	66	53	15	3	1	1	4
Infectious diseases	9	5	2	3	2	1	1	–	1
Other causes	71	36	19	21	18	10	8	11	11
All males(=100%)									
(thousands)	2.4	1.2	2.7	4.6	22.4	33.7	77.9	155.6	300.4
Circulatory diseases	3	5	7	10	17	28	38	46	41
Cancer	2	19	14	30	51	49	36	15	23
Respiratory diseases	14	8	6	5	6	9	13	20	17
Injury and poisoning	5	22	41	28	8	2	1	1	2
Infectious diseases	10	7	6	4	1	1	1	–	1
Other causes	67	40	26	24	18	12	11	18	16
All females(=100%)									
(thousands)	1.9	0.9	1.0	2.0	14.7	21.0	55.7	232.2	329.3

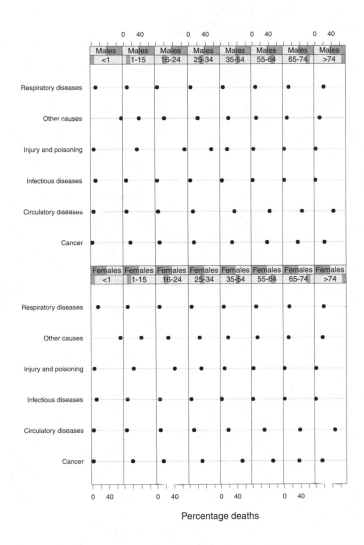

FIGURE 2.9. Dotplot of percentage deaths in England and Wales in 1997 by age, sex and cause of death.

as S-PLUS makes the production of such summaries and graphs very straightforward. In this chapter, only simple data sets have been considered, but as we shall see in later chapters, even when the data and the necessary analyses become more complex, the methods outlined in this chapter remain important in the initial stage of an investigation in which researchers are attempting to understand the main characteristics of their observations.

2.6   Using S-PLUS

Section 2.2

The code for this section includes the use of the `hist()`, `boxplot()` and `qqnorm()` functions for graphing histograms, boxplots and probability plots. The normal density function is computed using the `dnorm()` function, and the exponential using `dexp()`. The `locator()` function is used to allow legends to be placed on diagrams interactively. Nonparametric density estimates are obtained using the `density()` function. The `rug()` function is used to add a frequency distribution to the plotted densities after using the `jitter()` function to add a small amount of random variation to the data before plotting. This often helps in giving a clearer picture. (Jittering is more fully described in Chapter 4.)

Script for Section 2.2

```
# Use scan() to read in the heights and survival times
heights<-scan("elderly.dat")
leukaem<-scan("leukaem.dat")

# Get summary statistics using the summary() function
summary(heights)
summary(leukaem)                                 ⟹  Table 2.3

# Set up graphical window with four plotting areas
win.graph()
par(mfrow=c(2,2))

# Plot histograms and boxplots
hist(heights,xlab="Heights (cm)",ylab="Frequency",col=0)
boxplot(heights,ylab="Heights (cm)")
hist(leukaem,xlab="Survival time (days)",ylab="Frequency",col=0)
boxplot(leukaem,ylab="Survival time (days)")     ⟹  Figure 2.1

# Split graphical window into two plotting areas
par(mfrow=c(1,2))

# Plot normal Q-Q plot of each set of data using qqnorm()
qqnorm(heights,ylab="height")
qqline(heights)
# adds a line
qqnorm(leukaem,ylab="Survival time")
qqline(leukaem)                                  ⟹  Figure 2.2
```

```
# Split graphical window into four plotting areas
par(mfrow=c(2,2))

# Plot Q-Q plot of survival times for an exponential distribution
# and three gamma distributions with different shape parameters
plot(qexp(ppoints(leukaem)),sort(leukaem),
    ylab="Survival time (days)",xlab="Exponential quantile")
plot(qgamma(ppoints(leukaem),2),sort(leukaem),
    ylab="Survival time (days)",xlab="Gamma (shape=2) quantile")
plot(qgamma(ppoints(leukaem),3),sort(leukaem),
    ylab="Survival time (days)",xlab="Gamma (shape=3) quantile")
plot(qgamma(ppoints(leukaem),4),sort(leukaem),
    ylab="Survival time (days)",xlab="Gamma (shape=4) quantile")
```

$\Longrightarrow$ Figure 2.3

```
# Add distribution to histograms of heights and survival times
par(mfrow=c(2,1))
mw<-mean(heights)
sdw<-sqrt(var(heights))
# Calculates sample mean and standard deviation

ranm<-range(heights)
# vector with minimum and maximum value
x<-seq(ranm[1],ranm[2],length=100)
# Sets up 100 values at which to calculate the normal density

# Calculate normal density using dnorm()
y<-dnorm(x,mw,sdw)

hist(heights,xlab="Heights (cm)",ylab="Density",col=0,
    probability=T,ylim=c(0,0.10))
# The probability=T option scales the histogram as a density

# Add a title
title("Histogram of heights\n of elderly women")
# \n puts a new line in a title

lines(x,y,lwd=2)
# Adds the fitted density to the histogram
# lwd=2 gives a thicker line

legend(locator(1),c("Fitted normal"),lty=1)
# Adds a figure legend at a place chosen interactively
# by clicking into the graph

# Construct same plot for survival times, fitting
```

```
# an exponential distribution
mc<-mean(leukaem)
mc<-1/mc
x<-seq(range(leukaem)[1],range(leukaem)[2],length=100)

# Calculate exponential density using function dexp()
y<-dexp(x,mc)

hist(leukaem,xlab="Survival time",ylab="Density",col=0,
    probability=T,ylim=c(0,0.001))
title("Histogram of survival times")
lines(x,y,lwd=2)
legend(locator(1),c("Fitted exponential"),lty=1)
```
$\implies$ Figure 2.4

```
# Calculate a variety of nonparametric (kernel) density
# estimates for heights using the density() function.
# Both bandwidth and kernel shape are altered.

par(mfrow=c(3,2))
iqd<-summary(heights)[5]-summary(heights)[2]
# find the interquartile range
# (2*iqd gives a reasonable bandwidth)

plot(density(heights,width=2*iqd),type="l",xlab="Height (cm)",
    ylab="Estimated density")
rug(jitter(heights))
title("Gaussian:h=16")
plot(density(heights,width=5),type="l",xlab="Height (cm)",
    ylab="Estimated density")
rug(jitter(heights))
title("Gaussian:h=5")
plot(density(heights,window="r",width=2*iqd),type="l",
    xlab="Height (cm)",ylab="Estimated density")
rug(jitter(heights))
title("Rectangular:h=16")
plot(density(heights,window="r",width=5),type="l",
    xlab="Height (cm)",ylab="Estimated density")
rug(jitter(heights))
title("Rectangular:h=5")
plot(density(heights,window="t",width=2*iqd),type="l",
    xlab="Height (cm)",ylab="Estimated density")
rug(jitter(heights))
title("Triangular:h=16")
plot(density(heights,window="t",width=5),type="l",
    xlab="Height (cm)",ylab="Estimated density")
rug(jitter(heights))
title("Triangular:h=5")
```
$\implies$ Figure 2.5

Section 2.3

The byssinosis data are stored as a data frame object using the function `as.data.frame()`, after being read in using the `scan()` function. The `crosstabs()` function is used to construct various tables, and the `barplot()` function allows barplots of various quantities to be constructed.

Script for Section 2.3

```
# Read byssinosis data using scan() and convert to a matrix
# with seven columns---data are stored by row.
lung<-matrix(scan("lung.dat"),ncol=7,byrow=T)
dimnames(lung)<-list(NULL,c("yes","no","dust","race",
   "sex","smoking","emp"))
# Assigns names to columns using the dimnames function

# Convenient to store data as data frame
lung<-as.data.frame(lung)

# Convert some of the variables to factors
lung$dust<-factor(lung$dust,levels=1:3,
   labels=c("High","Medium","Low"))
lung$race<-factor(lung$race,levels=1:2,
   labels=c("White","Other"))
lung$sex<-factor(lung$sex,levels=1:2,
   labels=c("Male","Female"))
lung$smoking<-factor(lung$smoking,levels=1:2,
   labels=c("smoker","non-smoker"))
lung$emp<-factor(lung$emp,levels=1:3,
   labels=c("<10 years","10-20 years","> 20 years"))

# Attach data frame
attach(lung)

# Find crosstabulations
crosstabs(yes~race+dust)                         ⟹  Tables 2.5

crosstabs(no~race+dust)                          ⟹  Tables 2.6


# Find the proportions with lung disease by race and dust
prop<-tapply(yes,list(race,dust),sum)/
   tapply(no,list(race,dust),sum)
prop                                             ⟹  Table 2.7

# Display proportions graphically in a barplot
par(mfrow=c(1,1))
barplot(prop,names=c("High","Medium","Low"),
   legend=c("White","Other"))
                                                 ⟹  Figure 2.6
```

Section 2.4

In the code for this section, dotplots are produced using the dotplot()
function. Note that values and labels have to be reordered before plotting
using the order() function to get a more useful graphic. The unlabeled
U.K. deaths rate data are read in using the scan() function and then
appropriate labels are added, making use of the rep() function. The dotplot
is an example of a trellis graph. A large number of options are available to
improve the appearance of the graphs. These can be found under help for
trellis.args.

Script for Section 2.4

```
# Read in lung cancer data and convert to a matrix
cancer<-matrix(scan("cancer.dat"),ncol=2,byrow=T)
occup<-c("Farmers","Miners","Chemical","Glass","Furnace",
    "Electrical","Engineering","Woodworkers","Leather",
    "Textile","Clothing","Tobacco","Printing","Other",
    "Construction","Painters","Crane drivers","Labourers",
    "Communications","Warehousemen","Clerical","Sales",
    "Service","Managers","Professional")
dimnames(cancer)<-list(occup,c("Ratio","SMR"))
# Assigns occupation labels and variable labels

# Store as data frame
cancer<-as.data.frame(cancer)
attach(cancer)

# Produce dotplots of each of the two variables
# ordered by variable value
index<-order(SMR)
labs<-occup[index]
occup.fac<-factor(1:25,labels=labs)
trellis.device(win.graph)
dotplot(occup.fac~SMR[index],aspect=1,cex=1.5,xlab="SMR")
```
⟹ Figures 2.7

```
trellis.device(win.graph)
index<-order(Ratio)
labs<-occup[index]
occup.fac<-factor(1:25,labels=labs)
dotplot(occup.fac~Ratio[index],aspect=1,cex=1.5,
    xlab="Smoking ratio")
```
⟹ Figures 2.8

```
# Read in U.K. death rates data.
death<-scan("ukdeath.dat")
```

```
# Assign cause of death labels, etc., to appropriate data
type<-c("Circulatory diseases","Cancer","Respiratory diseases",
    "Injury and poisoning","Infectious diseases","Other causes")
type<-factor(rep(rep(type,2),8))
sex<-c("Males","Females")
sex<-factor(rep(rep(sex,c(6,6)),8))
age<-factor(1:8,labels=
    c("<1","1-15","16-24","25-34","35-54","55-64","65-74",">74"))
# define age as a factor with 8 levels and correct labels

age<-factor(rep(age,rep(12,8)))

# Store data as data frame
deaths<-data.frame(age,sex,type,death)

# Plot dotplot
trellis.device(win.graph)
attach(deaths)
dotplot(type~death|age*sex,xlab="Percentage deaths",
par.strip.text=list(cex=0.8),scales=list(draw=T,cex=0.7))
# here we used the par.strip.text() and scales() options
# to increase the size of the text of the strips and
# axis labels, respecively, see help(trellis.args)
```

$\implies$ Figure 2.9

2.7 Exercises

2.1 Use the stem() function to find stem-and-leaf plots of both the heights and survival times data.

2.2 Find the number of women who have heights between 156 and 162.

2.3 Write a general S-PLUS function that will determine the number of observations in a specified range for a data set. Use it on the survival times data to determine the number of patients with survival times between 400 and 500 days.

2.4 Construct a histogram of the heights data that contains an indication of the height of each individual in the sample. (The rug() and jitter() functions are useful here—use the appropriate help file to examine what they do.)

2.5 For the bysinnosis data, construct a bar chart of the proportion of people with lung disease in each category of the dust × smoking cross classification.

2.6 Find the proportion of people with lung disease in each category of the dust × sex × race cross classification.

2.7 Construct dotplots for each variable in the lung cancer data in which the occupations in each diagram are ordered by the SMR values.

3
Basic Inference

3.1   Introduction

Inference—the process of drawing conclusions about a population on the basis of measurements or observations made on a sample of individuals from the population—is central to statistics in general, and medical statistics in particular. In this chapter, we shall look at some basic inferential methods, beginning with those most suitable for continuous variables having, approximately at least, a normal distribution.

3.2   Simple inference for continuous data

3.2.1   The independent samples t-test

The data set in Table 3.1 gives the recorded birthweights of 50 infants who displayed severe idiopathic respiratory distress syndrome (SIRDS). This is a serious condition that can result in death and did so in the case of 27 of these children. One of the questions of interest about the data is whether the babies who died differed in birthweight from those who survived.

As a first step to answering this question, we shall examine box plots of birthweight for each group. The birthweight box plots are shown in Figures 3.1. The figure makes it pretty clear that the babies who survived had on average higher birthweights. But most investigators would not be willing to accept this informal evidence of a difference and would apply an appropriate significance test, in this case, the two sample t-test. They might also

TABLE 3.1. Birthweights (kg) of infants with severe idiopathic respiratory distress syndrome

Children who survived							
1.130	1.575	1.680	1.760	1.930	2.015	2.090	2.600
2.700	2.950	3.160	3.400	3.640	2.830	1.410	1.715
1.720	2.040	2.200	2.400	2.550	2.570	3.005	
Children who died							
1.050	1.175	1.230	1.310	1.500	1.600	1.720	1.750
1.770	2.275	2.500	1.030	1.100	1.185	1.225	1.262
1.295	1.300	1.550	1.820	1.890	1.940	2.200	2.270
2.440	2.560	2.730					

want to construct a confidence interval for the difference in birthweight of babies who survived and those who died. Display 3.1 describes both the two sample t-test and the calculation of the relevant confidence interval. Because one of the assumptions of the t-test is the normality of the observations in each group, Figure 3.2 shows normal probability plots of children who survived and those who died. There is perhaps some evidence of departure from normality, but here this will be conveniently ignored, and we shall put our trust in the robutness of the t-test!

The results of both the significance test and the calculation of a confidence interval, with and without the assumption that the populations have the same variance, are given in Table 3.2. These results indicate that there is clearly a significant difference in the average birthweights of the two groups with those who died having a smaller value than those who survived. The 95% confidence intervals indicate that the true difference in means is somewhere between a third to one kilogram.

The box plots and probability plots of the birthweight data show that it is reasonably well behaved in respect of the assumptions of the t-test (normality, homogeneity of variance).

Unfortunately, things are not always so straightforward. Consider, for example, the data given in Table 3.3, which were collected by the Western Collaborative Group Study carried out in California in 1960-1961. In this study, 3,154 middle-aged men were used to investigate the relationship between behaviour pattern and the risk of coronary heart disease. The particular data appearing in Table 3.3 were obtained from the 40 heaviest men in the study (all weighing at least 225 pounds). Cholesterol measurements (mg per 100 ml) and behaviour type are recorded; type A is characterized by urgency, aggression and ambition, and type B behaviour is relaxed, noncompetitive and less hurried. The question of interest is whether, in heavy middle-aged men, cholesterol level is related to behaviour type.

Let's begin by examining the box plots of cholesterol level for each group—see Figure 3.3. Immediately, a problem becomes apparent—there is a very distinct outlier in the type B group. For the moment, we shall ignore the problem and proceed with the usual independent samples t-test,

---

Display 3.1 Independent samples t-test

- The independent samples t-test is used to test the null hypothesis that the means of two populations are the same, $H_0 : \mu_1 = \mu_2$, when a sample of observations from each population is available. The subjects must all be independent of each other. For example, subjects of one population must not be individually matched with subjects from the other population and the subjects within each group should not be related to each other.

- The variable to be compared is assumed to have a normal distribution with the same standard deviation in both populations.

- The test-statistic is

$$t = \frac{\bar{y}_1 - \bar{y}_2}{s\sqrt{\frac{1}{n_1} + \frac{1}{n_2}}} \tag{1}$$

where $\bar{y}_1$ and $\bar{y}_2$ are the means in groups 1 and 2, n_1 and n_2 are the sample sizes and s is the pooled standard deviation defined by

$$s = \sqrt{\frac{(n_1 - 1)s_1^2 + (n_2 - 1)s_2^2}{n_1 + n_2 - 2}} \tag{2}$$

where s_1 and s_2 are the standard deviation in the two groups.

- Under the null hypothesis, the t-statistic has a student's t-distribution with $n_1 + n_2 - 2$ degrees of freedom.

- A $100(1 - \alpha)\%$ confidence interval for the difference between two means can be constructed as follows:

$$\bar{y}_1 - \bar{y}_2 \pm t_{\alpha,n_1+n_2-2} s\sqrt{\frac{1}{n_1} + \frac{1}{n_2}} \tag{3}$$

where t_{α,n_1+n_2-2} is a percentage point of the t-distribution such that the cumulative distribution function, $P(t < t_{\alpha,n_1+n_2-2})$, equals $1 - \alpha/2$.

- If the two populations are suspected of having different variances, a modified form of the t-statistic may be used, namely

$$t = \frac{\bar{y}_1 - \bar{y}_2}{\sqrt{\frac{s_1^2}{n_1} + \frac{s_2^2}{n_2}}} \tag{4}$$

In this case, t has a student's t-distribution with ν degrees of freedom, where

$$\nu = \left[\frac{c}{n_1 - 1} + \frac{(1 - c)^2}{n_2 - 1} \right]^{-1} \tag{5}$$

with

$$c = \frac{s_1^2/n_1}{s_1^2/n_1 + s_2^2/n_2} \tag{6}$$

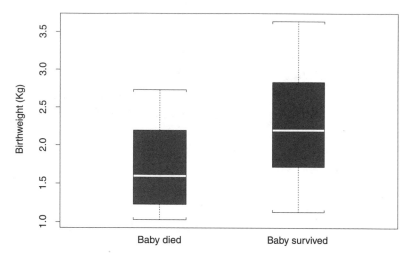

FIGURE 3.1. Box plots of birthweight by group.

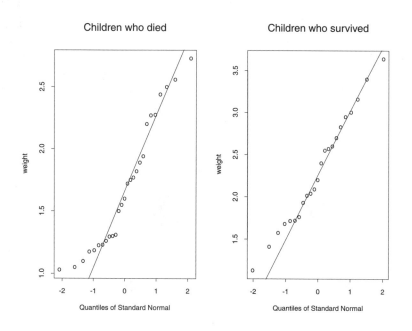

FIGURE 3.2. Normal probability plots of birthweight for each group.

TABLE 3.2. Results of *t*-test on SIRDS data in Table 3.1. Here, `sirdsd` and `sirdsa` are the vectors of birhtweights of the children who died and survived, respectively.

```
          Standard Two-Sample t-Test

data:  sirdsd and sirdsa
t = -3.6797, df = 48, p-value = 0.0006
alternative hypothesis: true difference in means is not equal to 0
95 percent confidence interval:
 -0.9520466 -0.2792545
sample estimates:
 mean of x mean of y
  1.691741  2.307391
```

```
       Welch Modified Two-Sample t-Test

data:  sirdsd and sirdsa
t = -3.607, df = 41.28, p-value = 0.0008
alternative hypothesis: true difference in means is not equal to 0
95 percent confidence interval:
 -0.9603 -0.2710
sample estimates:
 mean of x mean of y
     1.692     2.307
```

TABLE 3.3. Cholesterol and behaviour type

				Type A behaviour					
233	291	312	250	246	197	268	224	329	
239	254	276	234	181	248	252	202	218	325
				Type B behaviour					
420	185	263	246	224	212	188	250	148	169
226	175	242	153	183	137	202	194	213	

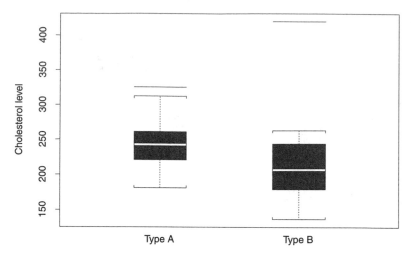

FIGURE 3.3. Box plots of cholesterol levels by group.

TABLE 3.4. Results of *t*-test on cholesterol data in Table 3.3

```
            Standard Two-Sample t-Test

data:  behA and behB
t = 1.9501, df = 38, p-value = 0.0586
alternative hypothesis: true difference in means is not equal to 0
95 percent confidence interval:
 -1.178332  63.078332
sample estimates:
 mean of x mean of y
    245.05     214.1
```

the results of which are given in Table 3.4. The p-value suggests that we should conclude that there is no significant difference in mean cholesterol level in the two types, although the confidence interval, while containing the value zero, seems perhaps to be suggesting a higher level in type A. (Using the form of the t-test that does not assume equal variances also leads to a nonsignificant result.)

What happens if we remove the outlier and repeat the t-test? The resulting box plots are given in Figure 3.4 and the t-test results in Table 3.5. Now the test is highly significant and the confidence interval suggests that average cholesterol level in the type A behaviour is between 18 and 66 mg per 100 ml higher than in type B. So which result should be accepted? Here, the suspect measurement is so extreme that it is probably safe to leave it out of the analysis and conclude that there is a difference in cholesterol level in the two types. An alternative approach will be outlined in Section 3.3.

TABLE 3.5. Results of t-test for cholesterol data in Table 2.3 after removal of outlier

```
        Standard Two-Sample t-Test

data:  behA and behB
t = 3.5103, df = 37, p-value = 0.0012
alternative hypothesis: true difference in means is not equal to 0
95 percent confidence interval:
 17.66703 65.90666
sample estimates:
 mean of x mean of y
    245.05   203.2632
```

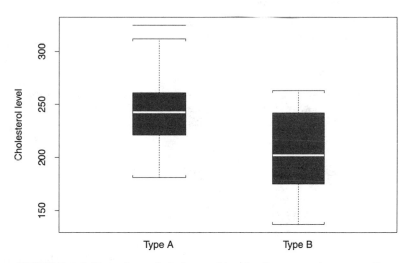

FIGURE 3.4. Box plots of cholesterol levels after removing an outlier.

3.2.2   Paired t-tests

The data in Table 3.6 come from a study of the *Stillman diet* reported in Rickman *et al.* (1974). This diet consists primarily of protein and animal fats, restricting carbohydrate intake. In Table 3.6, triglyceride values (mg/100 ml) are given for 16 participants both before beginning the diet and at the end of a period of time following the diet. Here, interest is on whether there has been a change in triglyceride level that might be attributed to the diet. As measurements on the same subjects on two occasions are to be compared, it is inappropriate to use an independent samples *t*-test because the observations are likely to be correlated rather than independent. Instead, a paired samples test is used. Details of the test are given in Display 3.2. But before applying the test, we might examine a

---

Display 3.2 Paired *t*-test

- A paired *t*-test is used to compare the means of two populations when samples from the populations are available, in which each individual in one sample is paired with an individual in the other sample. Examples are anorexic girls and their healthy sisters or the same patients before and after treatment.

- If the values of the variable of interest y for the members of the ith pair in groups 1 and 2 are denoted as y_{1i} and y_{2i}, then the differences $d_i = y_{1i} - y_{2i}$ are assumed to have a normal distribution.

- The null hypothesis here is that the mean difference is zero, i.e., $H_0 : \mu_d = 0$.

- The paired *t*-statistic is

$$t = \frac{\overline{d_i}}{s_d/n} \tag{1}$$

where $\overline{d_i}$ is the mean difference between the paired groups and s_d is the standard deviation of the differences d_i. Under the null hypothesis, the test-statistic has a *t*-distribution with $n-1$ degrees of freedom.

- A $100(1 - \alpha)\%$ confidence interval can be constructed as follows:

$$\overline{d_i} \pm t_{\alpha,n-1} s_d/n \tag{2}$$

where $P(t < t_{\alpha,n-1}) = 1 - \alpha/2$.

---

probability plot of the differences between the measurements before and after following the diet—see Figure 3.5. This plot gives no evidence that the assumption of the *t*-test (normality of the differences) is violated by these data, and so the test can be safely applied. The results are shown in Table 3.7. The data give no evidence that the diet has had an effect on triglyceride level.

TABLE 3.6. Triglyceride values (mg/100 ml) for 16 participants on the Stillman diet

Subject	Baseline	Final
1	159	194
2	93	122
3	130	158
4	174	154
5	148	93
6	148	90
7	85	101
8	180	99
9	92	183
10	89	82
11	204	100
12	182	104
13	110	72
14	88	108
15	134	110
16	84	81

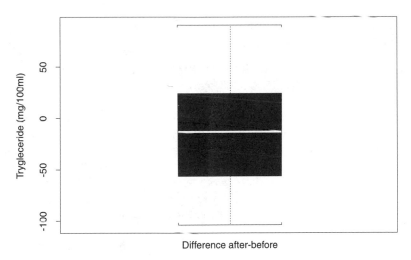

FIGURE 3.5. Probability plot of change in triglycerine values.

TABLE 3.7. Results of paired t-test on triglyceride data in Table 3.6. Here, the two columns of `tryg` correspond to the baseline and final values

```
Paired t-Test

data:  tryg[, 1] and tryg[, 2]
t = 1.2019, df = 15, p-value = 0.248
alternative hypothesis: true mean of differences is not equal to 0
95 percent confidence interval:
 -12.0368  43.1618
sample estimates:
 mean of x - y
      15.5625
```

3.3   Distribution free tests

An alternative to the appropriate t-test to assess differences between independent or paired samples is to use the analogous *distribution-free tests*. Such tests have properties that hold under relatively mild assumptions regarding the underlying populations from which the data are obtained. In particular, distribution-free methods forgo the traditional assumption that the underlying populations are normal. A vast range of distribution-free tests are now available (see Hollander and Wolfe, 1999), although here we shall be concerned only with those that are most commonly used in place of the independent samples and paired samples t-tests.

3.3.1   A distribution-free rank sum test—Wilcoxon/ Mann-Whitney test

The data on cholesterol level in overweight middle-aged men discussed in the previous section (see Table 3.3) caused problems for the independent samples t-test because of the presence of an outlier. With the outlier included, there was no evidence of a difference between the two groups, but with the outlying observation excluded, the difference was significant. The distribution-free analogue of this type of t-test is the Wilcoxon Mann-Whitney rank sum test. The test is outlined in Display 3.3.

Because here the test-statistic is based on the ranks of the observations rather than on the observations, it will not be as vulnerable to outliers as the t-test. The results of applying the test to the cholesterol data both with and without the extreme observation are as follows.

All data: Normal approximation $z = 2.5$, p-value $= 0.012$.

Data with outlier removed: Normal approximation $z = 2.88$, p-value $= 0.004$.

Here, the result in both cases indicates a significant difference in location of the two groups. This implies a difference between the population medians.

Display 3.3 Wilcoxon Mann-Whitney rank sum test

- The null hypothesis to be tested is that the two populations being compared have identical distributions. (For two normally distributed populations with common variance, this would be equivalent to the hypothesis that the means of the two populations are the same.)

- The alternative hypothesis is that the population distributions differ in location (the median).

- Samples of observations are available from each of the two populations being compared.

- The test is based on the joint ranking of the observations from the two samples (as if they were from a single sample). If there are ties, the tied observations are given the average of the ranks for which the observations are competing.

- The test-statistic is the sum of the ranks of one sample (the lower of the two rank sums is generally used).

- For small samples, p-values for the test-statistic can be assigned relatively simply.

- A large sample approximation is available that is suitable when the two sample sizes n_1 and n_2 are both greater than 15, and there are no ties. The test-statistic Z is given by

$$Z = \frac{S - n_1(n_1 + n_2 + 1)/2}{\sqrt{n_1 n_2 (n_1 + n_2 + 1)/12}}$$

  where S is the test-statistic based on the sample with n_1 observations. Under the null hypothesis, Z has approximately a standard normal distribution.

- A modified z-statistic is available when there are ties; see Hollander and Wolfe (1999).

TABLE 3.8. Hamilton depression scale scores

Subject	Occasion 1	Occasion 2
1	1.83	0.878
2	0.50	0.647
3	1.62	0.598
4	2.48	2.05
5	1.68	1.06
6	1.88	1.29
7	1.55	1.06
8	3.06	3.14
9	1.30	1.29

3.3.2 A distribution-free signed rank test—Wilcoxon test

The data shown in Table 3.8 are part of the data reported in Salsburg (1970). The nine patients, all diagnosed as having mixed anxiety and depression, each had a recording on the Hamilton depression scale on two occasions; the first a short time after initiation of therapy with a particular tranquilizer, the second some weeks later. The question is whether there has been a reduction in depression consistent with an improvement due to treatment with the tranquilizer. A paired samples *t*-test *could* be applied to the observations, but with so few observations, it is not possible to gather any evidence that the assumption of normality is reasonable. The distribution-free alternative in this case is the Wilcoxon signed rank test—see Display 3.4. The results of applying the test to the Hamilton depression scale data are as follows.

Signed rank statistic: $V = 40$, $n = 9$, *p*-value $= 0.039$.

There is some evidence of an improvement as measured by a reduction in the Hamilton scale.

3.4   Simple inference for categorical data

3.4.1   Test for contingency table data

The data in Table 3.9 come from a clinical trial and show the effect of the drug sulplinpyrazole on deaths after myocardial infarction; this is an example of a 2×2 contingency table. The question of interest is whether the drug reduces mortality. The appropriate test is a chi-squared test for a difference in the proportion of deaths in the populations of patients treated with the drug and the placebo—see Display 3.5. The results of the test are $X^2 = 3.59$, $df = 1$, $p = 0.058$. The test fails to reach significance at the 5% level, and the conclusion is that there is no convincing evidence that treatment of these patients with sulplinpyrazole reduces mortality.

Display 3.4 Wilcoxon signed rank test

- Assume, we have two observations, x_i and y_i, on each of n subjects in our sample, e.g., before and after treatment. We first calculate the differences, $z_i = x_i - y_i$, between each pair of observations.

- To compute the Wilcoxon signed-rank statistic T^+, form the absolute values of the differences z_i and then order them from least to greatest.

- If there are ties among the calculated differences, assign each of the observations in a tied group the average of the integer ranks that are associated with the tied group.

- Now assign a positive or negative sign to the ranks of the differences according to whether the corresponding difference was postive or negative. (Zero values are discarded, and the sample size n altered accordingly.)

- The statistic T^+ is the sum of the positive ranks. Tables are available for assigning p-values—See Table A.4 in Hollander and Wolfe (1999).

- A large sample approximation involves testing the statistic Z as a standard normal:

$$Z = \frac{T^+ - n(n+1)/4}{\sqrt{n(n+1)(2n+1)/24}}$$

TABLE 3.9. Sulplinpyrazone and heart attacks

	Deaths	Survivors
Sulplinpyrazone	41	692
Placebo	60	682

Display 3.5 Chi-squared test for a 2 × 2 contingency table

- The general 2 × 2 contingency table can be written as

		Variable 2		
		1	2	
Variable 1	1	a	b	a+b
	2	c	d	c+d
		a+c	b+d	a+b+c+d=N

- The null hypothesis is that the two variables are independent.

- The test statistic is

$$X^2 = \frac{N(ad - bc)^2}{(a+b)(c+d)(a+c)(b+d)}$$

- Under the null hypothesis of independence, the statistic has a chi-squared distribution with a single degree of freedom.

The test for a difference in two proportions in a 2×2 contingency table is also a test that the row and column classifications are independent. The test of independence is also important in contingency tables with more than two rows and two columns. Details of the test are given in Display 3.6. Consider, for example, Table 3.10, which shows the subjective assessments of personal health by respondents in five regional health and lifestyle surveys. The chi-squared test for independence gives $X^2 = 18.45, df = 8, p = 0.02$. Clearly, region and subjective assessment of health are not independent. (See Exercise 3.4 for how the lack of independence might be investigated in more detail.)

Display 3.6 Testing for independence in an $r \times c$ contingency table

- The general $r \times c$ contingency table can be written as

		Column variable			
		1	$\cdots$	c	
Row variable	1	n_{11}	$\cdots$	n_{1c}	$n_{1.}$
	2	n_{21}	$\cdots$	n_{2c}	$n_{2.}$
	$\vdots$	$\vdots$	$\vdots$	$\vdots$	$\vdots$
	r	n_{r1}	$\cdots$	n_{rc}	$n_{2.}$
		$n_{.1}$	$\cdots$	$n_{.2}$	N

- Under the null hypothesis that the row and column classifications are independent, estimated expected values, E_{ij}, for the ijth cell can be found as

$$E_{ij} = \frac{n_{i.}n_{.j}}{N} \qquad (1)$$

- The test-statistic for assessing independence is

$$X^2 = \sum_{i=1}^{r} \sum_{j=1}^{c} \frac{(n_{ij} - E_{ij})^2}{E_{ij}} \qquad (2)$$

- Under the null hypothesis of independence, X^2 has a chi-squared distribution with $(r-1)(c-1)$ degrees of freedom.

TABLE 3.10. Subjective health assessment in five regions of the U.K.

Region	Good	Fairly Good	Not Good
Southampton	954	444	78
Swindon	985	504	87
Jersey	459	175	43
Guernsey	377	176	35
West Dorset	926	503	109

Display 3.7 Fisher's exact test for a 2×2 table

- The probability of any particular arrangement of the frequencies a, b, c and d in a 2×2 contingency table, when the marginal totals are fixed and the two variables are independent, is

$$P = \frac{(a+b)!(a+c)!(c+d)!(b+d)!}{a!b!c!d!N!}$$

- This is a hypergeometric distribution.

- Fisher's exact test employs this distribution to find the probability of the observed arrangement of frequencies and of every arrangement giving as much or more evidence of a departure from independence, when the marginal totals are fixed.

3.4.2 Fisher's exact test

One of the requirements of the chi-squared test used in the examples above is that the expected values are not too small. Historically, this has been interpreted as being greater than 5. Although there is some evidence that this recommendation is rather too conservative, very sparse contingency tables can be a problem for the usual chi-squared test. For a 2×2 table, the usual alternative suggested is Fisher's exact test. A brief account of this test is given in Display 3.7. The test can be illustrated on the data shown in Table 3.11, which came from a study comparing the health of juvenile delinquent boys with a nondelinquent control group. They relate to the subset of the boys who failed a vision test and show the numbers who did and did not wear glasses. The question of interest is whether delinquents with poor eyesight are more or less likely to wear glasses than are nondelinquents with poor eyesight. Applying Fisher's test to these data gives a p-value of 0.035. There is some evidence of a difference in spectacle wearing between juvenile delinquents and nonjuvenile delinquents with poor eyesight. A lower proportion of the delinquents wear spectacles. (For interest, the chi-squared test in this case gives a p-value of 0.051.)

TABLE 3.11. Spectacle wearing and delinquency

		Juvenile delinquents	Nondelinquents	Total
Spectacle wearers				
	Yes	1	5	6
	No	8	2	10
	Total	9	7	16

Although in the past Fisher's test has been largely applied to sparse 2×2 tables, it can also be applied to larger tables when there is concern about small values in some cells. The last decade has seen a large amount of work on exact tests for contingency tables in which the counts are small (see, for example, Mehta and Patel, 1986). To illustrate this use of Fisher's exact test, we shall use the data shown in Table 3.12, which give the distribution of the oral lesion site found in house-to-house surveys in three geographic regions of rural India. Application of Fisher's test to the data gives a p-value of 0.019 indicating a strong association between site of lesion and geographic region. For comparison, the chi-square statistic for these data takes the value 20.70, which with 14 degrees of freedom has an associated p-value of 0.11 suggesting no association. Here, the contingency table is so sparse that the usual chi-squared asymptotic distribution with 14 df is unlikely to yield accurate p-values.

TABLE 3.12. Oral lesions data set

Site of lesion	Kerala	Gujarat	Andhra
Buccal mucosa	8	1	8
Commissure	0	1	0
Gingiva	0	1	0
Hard palate	0	1	0
Soft palate	0	1	0
Tongue	0	1	0
Floor of mouth	1	0	1
Alveolar ridge	1	0	1

3.4.3 The Mantel-Haenszel test

A commonly occurring form of data in medical studies is a set of 2×2 contingency tables. Table 3.13 gives an example from a study involving cases of bronchitis by level of organic particulates in the air and by age (Somes and O'Brien, 1985). Three 2×2 tables are available, one from each of three age groups. The data could be collapsed over age and the aggregate 2×2 table analysed as described previously. But the dangers of this are well documented (see, for example, Everitt, 1993). In particular, such pooling of tables can generate an association when in the separate tables there is none. A more appropriate test of association in this situation is the *Mantel-Haenszel* test described in Display 3.8.

Applying the Mantel-Haenszel test for the bronchitis data leads to a value of $X^2 = 0.11$ with an associated p-value of 0.74, indicating a lack of association between bronchitis and level of organic particulates in the air.

3.4.4 McNemar's test for correlated proportions

The tests on categorical data described previously have assumed that the observations are independent. Often, however, categorical data arise from *paired observations*, for example, cases matched with controls on variables

---

Display 3.8 Mantel-Haenszel test

- For a series of k 2×2 contingency tables, the Mantel-Haenszel statistic for testing the hypothesis of no association is

$$X^2 = \frac{[\sum_{i=1}^{k} a_i - \sum_{i=1}^{k} \frac{(a_i+b_i)(a_i+c_i)}{N_i}]^2}{\sum_{i=1}^{k} \frac{(a_i+b_i)(c_i+d_i)(a_i+c_i)(b_i+d_i)}{N_i^2(N_i-1)}}$$

  where a_i, b_i, c_i, d_i represent the counts in the four cells of the ith table and N_i is the total number of observations in the ith table.

- Under the null hypothesis, this statistic has a chi-squared distribution with a single degree of freedom.

- The test is only appropriate if the degree and direction of the association between the two variables is the same in each stratum. A possible test of this assumption is that due to Breslow and Day (see Agresti, 1996).

TABLE 3.13. Number of cases of bronchitis by level of organic particulates in the air and by age

	Particulates level	Age yes	Organic no	Bronchitis total
15-24	High	20	382	402
	Low	9	214	223
23-30	High	10	172	182
	Low	7	120	127
40+	High	12	327	339
	Low	6	183	189

TABLE 3.14. Post oral contraceptive use in 175 pairs of married women

Oral contraceptive use	Number of pairs
Used by both members of the pair	10
Used by the case only	57
Used by the control only	13
Used by neither the case or the control	95

TABLE 3.15. Distance vision

		Left eye grade (1 = high)			
		1	2	3	4
Right eye	1	1520	266	124	66
	2	234	1512	432	78
grade	3	117	362	1772	205
	4	36	82	179	492

such as sex, age, and so on, or observations made on the same subjects on two occasions (cf. paired t-test). A set of such data is shown in Table 3.14. Here, the cases were 175 women of reproductive age (15-44) discharged alive from 43 hospitals in five cities after initial attacks of idiopathic thrombo-plebities, pulmonary embolism or cerebral thrombosis or embolism. The controls were matched with their cases for hospital, residence, time of hos-pitalisation, race, age, marital status, and a number of other variables. The history of oral contraceptive use by the women was then determined.

For this type of paired data, the required procedure is McNemar's test—see Display 3.9. Here, the value of the test-statistic is 27.66 and the asso-ciated p-value is very small. There is a statistically significant association between thromboembolism and oral contraceptive use. The proportion of pairs in which only the case has used oral contraceptives is greater than the porportion in which only the control has used the pill.

Although the McNemar test is most commonly used on 2×2 tables, it can be extended to larger tables to test the hypothesis of symmetry, namely, that the probability of an observation being classified into cell i, j is the same as the probability of being classified into cell j, i. To illustrate the use of the test in this context, we shall use the data shown in Table 3.15, which give the unaided distance vision of the left and right eyes of 7,477 women aged 30–39 rated on a four-point scale. The result of applying McNemar's test to these data is $X^2 = 19.11$, $df = 6$, p-value $= 0.004$. Clearly, more women have superior vision in the right eye compared with the left than vice versa.

Display 3.9 McNemar's test for grouped data

- The frequencies in a matched samples data set can be written as

		Sample 1	
		present	absent
Sample 2	present	a	b
	absent	c	d

- Under the hypothesis that the two populations do not differ in their probability of having the characteristic present, the test-statistic

$$X^2 = \frac{(a-d)^2}{a+d}$$

has a chi-squared distribution with a single degree of freedom.

3.5 An introduction to the bootstrap

The bootstrap is a data-based method for statistical inference. Its introduction into statistics is relatively recent because the method is computationally intensive. In essence, the bootstrap approach provides a general method for obtaining standard deviations of estimators and confidence intervals for parameters without requiring a tractable mathematical expression for the asymptotic variance of the estimator. The technique overcomes the mathematical intractability hurdle by relying on computer power. The technique is described in a series of papers—Efron (1979), Efron and Gong (1983) and Efron and Tibshirani (1993). The essential stages in the bootstrap approach are

1. Choose a test-statistic S.

2. Calculate S for the original set of observations.

3. Obtain the *bootstrap distribution* of S by repeatedly sampling from the observations and computing S for each bootstrap sample. Sampling is with replacement.

4. Construct a confidence interval for the parameter of interest using the bootstrap distribution.

For example, for the data set in Table 3.3, we could use bootstrapping to obtain a confidence interval for the difference in median cholesterol levels between the two groups of men. Because we have two populations of men with different behavioral patterns, resampling has to be done within each population. The bootstrap distribution of the difference between the medians based on 1,000 bootstrap samples is shown in Figure 3.6. The approximate limits of the 95% confidence interval can be obtained from the 2.5 and 95.5 percentiles of this distribution. Better estimates are the *accelerated bias-corrected percentile limits* (see Efron and Tibshirani, 1993), giving values of 0.54 and 62. The type A personality group had a higher median cholesterol level than did the type B group (difference in medians = 35.5, 95% confidence interval from 0.54 to 62).

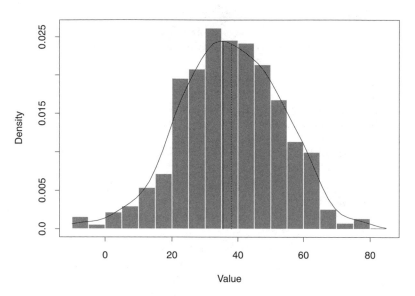

FIGURE 3.6. Bootstrap distribution of difference between median cholesterol levels for type A and type B personalities.

3.6 Summary

Basic significance tests such as the *t*-test and the chi-squared test are the most frequently used of all statistical techniques. They can be applied extremely simply using any statistical package, including S-PLUS. But users need to remember that the tests are based on underlying assumptions that need to be considered before they are used. When such assumptions are violated, alternative procedures such as nonparametric tests or bootstrap can be used. Both are easy to apply in S-PLUS.

3.7   Using S-PLUS

Section 3.2

The code for Section 3.2 contains little that is new. The scan() function is used to read in a data set, the boxplot() function is used generate useful box plots of the data, and the t.test() function used to perform both an independent sample and a paired t-test using the paired=T/F option to specify which.

Script for Section 3.2

```
# Read in data on SIRDS using the scan() function
sirds<-scan("sirds.dat")

# Creae separate vectors for children who survived and children
# who died
sirdsd<-sirds[1:27]
sirdsa<-sirds[28:50]
boxplot(sirdsd,sirdsa,ylab="Birthweight (Kg)",
   names=c("Baby died","Baby Survived"))
```
⟹ Figure 3.1

```
# Probability plots
par(mfrow=c(1,2))
qqnorm(sirdsd,ylab="weight")
title("Children who died")
qqline(sirdsd)
qqnorm(sirdsa,ylab="weight")
title("Children who survived")
qqline(sirdsa)
```
⟹ Figure 3.2

```
# Perform t-test using function t.test
t.test(sirdsd,sirdsa)
t.test(sirdsd,sirdsa,var.equal=F)
```
⟹ Table 3.2

```
# Read in cholesterol data of two behavioural types
behave<-scan("behave.dat")
behA<-behave[1:20]
behB<-behave[21:40]

# Box plot data and perform $t$-test
boxplot(behA,behB,ylab="Cholesterol level",
   names=c("Type A","Type B"))
```
⟹ Figure 3.3

```
t.test(behA,behB)
```
⟹ Table 3.4

```
# Remove outlier, replot box plot and perform t-test again
behA<-behB[-1]
boxplot(behA,behB,ylab="Cholesterol level",
    names=c("Type A","Type B"))
```
$\implies$ | Figure 3.4 |

```
t.test(behA,behB)
```
$\implies$ | Table 3.5 |

```
# Read in triglyceride data
tryg<-matrix(scan("tryg.dat"),ncol=2,byrow=T)
```

```
# Box plot of differences and paired t-test
boxplot(tryg[,2]-tryg[,1],names=c("Difference after-before"),
    ylab="Trygleceride (mg/100 ml)")
```
$\implies$ | Figure 3.5 |

```
t.test(tryg[,1],tryg[,2],paired=T)
```
$\implies$ | Table 3.7 |

Section 3.3

The code for Section 3.3 introduces the `wilcox.test()` function to perform the Wilcoxon test as a nonparametric alternative to the independent samples and paired t-test.

Script for Section 3.3

```
# Perform Wilcoxon test using wilcox.test function
wilcox.test(behA,behB)

# Enter data on Hamilton depressions scores
ham1<-c(1.83,0.50,1.62,2.48,1.68,1.88,1.55,3.06,1.3)
ham2<-c(0.88,0.65,0.60,2.05,1.06,1.29,1.06,3.14,1.29)

# Perform Wilcoxon signed rank test
wilcox.test(ham1,ham2,paired=T)
```

Section 3.4

In the script for Section 3.4, the `chisq.test()` and `fisher.test()` functions are used to test independence in contingency tables. The `array()` function is used to put data for the Mantel-Haenszel test into the correct form; the test is applied using the `mantelhaen.test()` function. Lastly, `mcnemar.test()` is used for McNemar's test.

Script for Section 3.4

```
# Enter myocardial infarction data
mci<-matrix(c(41,692,60,682),ncol=2,byrow=T)

# Perform chi-square test of independence using
# the function chisq.test()
chisq.test(mci, correct=F)
#apply chi-square test
#without Yates's correction
#which is not considered
#useful these days

# Enter data on health assessment
health<-matrix(c(954,444,78,985,504,87,459,175,
    43,377,176,35,926,503,109),ncol=3,byrow=T)
chisq.test(health)

# Enter data on eyesight and juvenile delequency
eye<-matrix(c(1,5,8,2),ncol=2,byrow=T)

# Perform Fisher's exact test
fisher.test(eye)

# Enter oral lesions data
lesion<-matrix(c(8,1,8,0,1,0,0,1,0,0,1,0,0,1,0,
    0,1,0,1,0,1,1,0,1),ncol=3,byrow=T)
fisher.test(lesion)

# Perform chi-square test for comparison
chisq.test(lesion)

# Enter data on bronchitis
bron<-c(20,382,9,214,10,172,7,120,12,327,6,183)

# Set up data as an array of three 2 x 2 tables using
# the array() function
bron<-array(bron,c(2,2,3))

# Perform Mantel-Haenszel test
mantelhaen.test(bron)

# Enter data for oral contraceptive study
oral<-matrix(c(10,57,13,95),ncol=2,byrow=T)
# Perform McNemar's test
mcnemar.test(oral)

# Enter eyesight data
```

```
vision<-matrix(c(1520,266,124,66,234,1512,432,78,117,
    362,1772,205,36,82,179,492),ncol=4,byrow=T)
mcnemar.test(vision)
```

Section 3.5

The `bootstrap()` function is used to generate bootstrap samples of the difference between medians and to compute percentiles and accelerated bias-corrected percentile limits. The `group` option allows the resampling to be stratified by group. We also use the `plot()` function to obtain the appropriate plot for the objects returned by the `bootstrap()` function.

Script for Section 3.5

```
# Read data and construct data frame
chol<-scan("behave.dat")
group<-c(rep(1,20),rep(2,20))
cholest<-data.frame(chol=chol, group=group)

# Carry out bootstrapping
set.seed(143211)
# Sets random number seed so that same results
# are obtained each time
boot<-bootstrap(cholest, B=1000,
    median(chol[group==1])-median(chol[group==2]),
    group=group)
# The third argument specifies the statistic
boot

# Percentiles of bootstrap distribution
limits.emp(boot)

# accelerated bias-corrected percentile limits
limits.bca(boot)

# plot bootstrap distribution
plot(boot)
```
$\implies$ Figure 3.6

3.8 Exercises

3.1 Compare the cumulative distribution functions of birthweights of the babies who died and those who survived in the SIRDS data using the `cdf.compare()` function. Test whether they differ using the Kolmogorov-Smirnoff test (use the `ks.gof()` function). Use the appropriate help files to find out about the new functions.

3.2 Again, use the `cdf.compare()` function to assess if the birth-weights of babies who died and babies who survived have normal distributions.

3.3 Repeat 3.1 and 3.2 for the cholesterol data from men with type A and type B behaviour.

3.4 A procedure that is often useful in identifying the cells of a contingency table responsible for a significant overall chi-square value is inspection of some form of residual. Two that have been suggested for contingency tables are as follows.

Standardised: (Observed-Expected)/sqrt(Expected).

Adjusted: Standardised/Adjustment,

where the 'Adjustment' term is

Adjustment
= sqrt[(1-row total/sample size)(1-column total/sample size)]

Write a general S-PLUS function to calculate each of these for a general $r \times c$ contingency table and then apply it to the subjective assessment of health data.

3.5 For a series of 2×2 contingency tables, the Mantel-Haenszel estimator of the assumed common odds ratio is

$$\omega = \frac{\sum_{i=1}^{k} a_i d_i / N_i}{\sum_{i=1}^{k} b_i c_i / n_i} \tag{3.1}$$

Write a general S-PLUS function to calculate ω and then apply it to the bronchitis data.

3.6 Use bootstrapping to construct a confidence interval for the ratio of the medians of the two groups of men.

4

Scatterplots, Simple Regression and Smoothing

4.1   Introduction

Often, the data collected in medical investigations consist of observations on a pair of variables, and several issues may be of interest. For example, are the variables correlated? Can one variable be predicted from another? What form of equation links the two variables? Such questions will be addressed in this chapter.

4.2   The scatterplot

The simple xy scatterplot has been in use since at least the 18th century and has many virtues—indeed, according to Tufte (1983):

> The relational graphic—in its barest form the scatterplot and its variants—is the greatest of all graphical designs. It links at least two variables encouraging and even imploring the viewer to assess the possible causal relationship between the plotted variables. It confronts causal theories that x causes y with empirical evidence as to the actual relationship between x and y.

The use of the scatterplot will first be illustrated on the two sets of data given in Tables 4.1 and 4.2. The first gives the heights and resting pulse measurements of a sample of hospital patients, and the second gives

TABLE 4.1. Heights and resting pulse rates for hospital patients

Height	Pulse	Height	Pulse
160	68	167	80
162	84	175	80
185	80	162	80
173	92	167	92
170	80	170	80
163	80	158	80
157	80	160	78
170	90	177	80
166	72	170	80
148	82	175	76
160	84	153	70
185	80	165	82
165	84	160	68
185	80	163	95
177	80	165	76
182	100	162	88
172	90	177	90
168	90	178	80
182	76	167	80
170	84	160	80
182	80	168	80
155	80	175	104
168	80	180	68
175	84	145	64
170	84	175	72

the oxygen uptake and the expired ventilation of a number of subjects performing a standard exercise task.

The basic scatterplots of each data set appear in Figures 4.1 and 4.2. The diagrams have very different stories to tell about each data set. The first suggests that increasing height is associated with an increase in resting pulse and that the relationship between the two variables is, approximately at least, linear. Figure 4.2, on the other hand, gives very strong evidence that the relationship between oxygen uptake and expired ventilation is nonlinear. The correlation between height and resting pulse is 0.22, and that between oxygen uptake and expired volume is 0.95 (using the correlation coefficient in the latter case is problematic because the relationship between the two variables is clearly nonlinear).

As a further example of a simple scatterplot, Figure 4.3 shows the smoking ratio and SMR data for the 25 occupations met in Chapter 2. Here, a unique label identifying each occupation is plotted. The correlation is strong but far from perfect.

TABLE 4.2. Oxygen uptake and expired ventilation of a number of subjects performing a standard exercise task

Oxygen	Ventilation	Oxygen	Ventilation
574	21.9		
592	18.6	664	18.6
667	19.1	718	19.2
770	16.9	927	18.3
947	17.2	1020	19.0
1096	19.0	1277	18.6
1323	22.8	1330	24.6
1599	24.9	1639	29.2
1787	32.0	1790	27.9
1794	31.0	1874	30.7
2049	35.4	2132	36.1
2160	39.1	2292	42.6
2312	39.9	2475	46.2
2489	50.9	2490	46.5
2577	46.3	2766	55.8
2812	54.5	2893	63.5
2957	60.3	3052	64.8
3151	69.2	3161	74.7
3266	72.9	3386	80.4
3452	83.0	3521	86.0
3543	88.9	3676	96.8
3741	89.1	3844	100.9
3878	103.0	4002	113.4
4114	111.4	4152	119.9
4252	127.2	4290	126.4
4331	135.5	4332	138.9
4390	143.7	4393	144.8

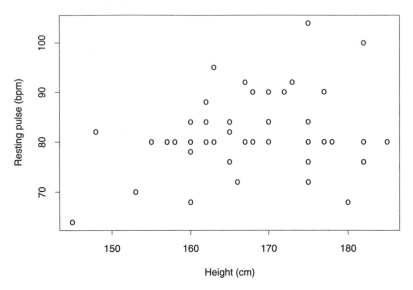

FIGURE 4.1. Scatterplot of heights and resting pulse data.

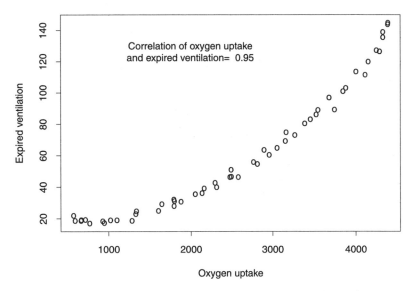

FIGURE 4.2. Scatterplot of oxygen uptake and expired ventilation.

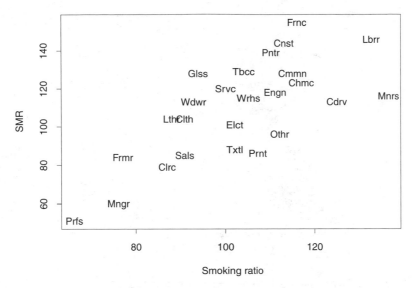

FIGURE 4.3. Scatterplot of smoking ratio and SMR.

4.2.1 Jittering a scatterplot

Because of the nature of the data, some scatterplots will include a multiplicity of points at many of the plotting locations. In such cases, the diagram can often be made more informative if the data are 'jittered' before plotting. *Jittering* is a procedure in which a small amount of random variation is added to the observations (see Cleveland, 1979, for more details). To illustrate jittering, we shall use some data generated during an fMRI investigation. Two measures of the intensity of each of 2836 voxels in an image were available, PD and T2. The data to be plotted here consist of the measurements for a sample of 1,000 voxels. A small part of the data is shown in Table 4.3. The scatterplots of both the original observations and the 'jittered' observations are shown in Figure 4.4. In this case, noise has been added to the measurements of both variables; for each variable, the noise was generated from a uniform distribution on an interval that is centred on zero and that is small compared with the range of measurements. The jittered scatterplot shows the structure of the data somewhat better than does the scatterplot of the raw data.

4.2.2 Including information about marginal distributions on a scatterplot

It is often useful to include on a scatterplot of bivariate data information about the marginal distributions of each variable. Jointly plotting bivariate and marginal distributions is usually good data analysis practice. This marginal information can be supplied in a variety of ways. In Figure 4.5, for

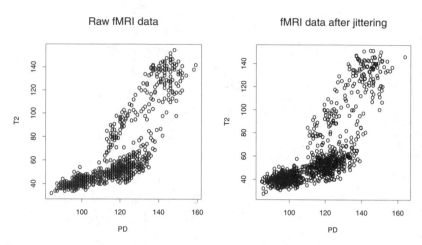

FIGURE 4.4. Scatterplot and jittered scatterplot of T2 and PD in an fMRI image.

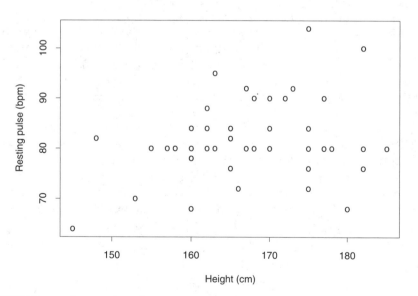

FIGURE 4.5. Scatterplot of heights and resting pulse rate with rug plots indicating the distribution of the separate variables.

TABLE 4.3. A sample of the fMRI data

Voxel	PD	T2
1	105	51
2	109	53
3	115	60
4	120	62
5	123	60
6	122	60
7	108	53
8	110	57
9	117	60
10	120	58

example, simple 'rug plots' of height and resting pulse have been added to the scatterplot of the two variables. In Figure 4.6, the scatterplot of height and resting pulse is enhanced by the addition of nonparametric density estimates of the separate variables, and in Figure 4.7, a histogram and a box plot are used to display the marginal distributions.

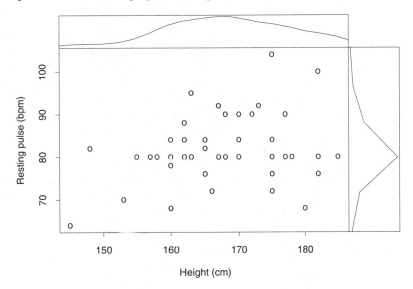

FIGURE 4.6. Scatterplot of heights and resting pulse rate with nonparametric estimates of marginal distributions shown.

4.2.3   Convex hull trimming of bivariate data

Outliers can often distort the value of a correlation coefficient. A procedure that can often be usefully applied to a set of bivariate data to allow robust

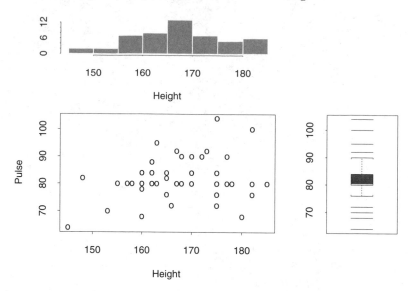

FIGURE 4.7. Scatterplot of heights and resting pulse rate with histogram and box plot indicating marginal distributions.

estimation of the correlation is *convex hull trimming*. In this approach, the points defining the convex hull of the observations are deleted before the correlation coefficient is calculated. (The convex hull of a set of bivariate data consists of the vertices of the smallest convex polyhedron in variable space within which or on which all data points lie.) The major attraction of this method is that it eliminates isolated outliers without disturbing the general shape of the bivariate distribution.

To illustrate the use of convex hull trimming, we shall again use a sample of observations from the fMRI data. The convex hull of the observations for the selected 25 voxels is shown on the scatterplot of the data in Figure 4.8. The correlation of the original data is 0.78. When the points defining the convex hull are removed, this correlation becomes 0.93.

4.2.4   The aspect ratio of a scatterplot

An important parameter of a scatterplot that can greatly influence our ability to recognise patterns is the *aspect ratio*, the physical length of the vertical axis divided by that of the horizontal axis. Most computer packages produce plots with an aspect ratio near 1, but this is not always the best value. To illustrate how changing this characteristic of a scatterplot can help understand what the data are trying to tell us, we shall use the example given by Cook and Weisberg (1994) involving the monthly U.S. births, per thousand population for the years 1940-1948. The data are given in Table 4.4, and a scatterplot of the birthrates against month with an aspect ratio of one is shown in Figure 4.9. The plot shows that the U.S. birthrate

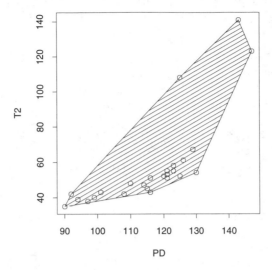

FIGURE 4.8. Convex hull of fMRI data.

was increasing between 1940 and 1943, decreasing between 1943 and 1946, rapidly increasing during 1946, and then decreasing again during 1947-1948. As Cook and Weisberg comment:

TABLE 4.4. U.S. monthly birthrates between 1940 and 1943 (read along rows for temporal sequence)

1890	1957	1925	1885	1896	1934	2036	2069	2060
1922	1854	1852	1952	2011	2015	1971	1883	2070
2221	2173	2105	1962	1951	1975	2092	2148	2114
2013	1986	2088	2218	2312	2462	2455	2357	2309
2398	2400	2331	2222	2156	2256	2352	2371	2356
2211	2108	2069	2123	2147	2050	1977	1993	2134
2275	2262	2194	2109	2114	2086	2089	2097	2036
1957	1953	2039	2116	2134	2142	2023	1972	1942
1931	1980	1977	1972	2017	2161	2468	2691	2890
2913	2940	2870	2911	2832	2774	2568	2574	2641
2691	2698	2701	2596	2503	2424			

These trends seem to deliver an interesting history lesson since the U.S. involvement in World War II started in 1942 and troops began returning home during the first part of 1945, about nine months before the rapid increase in the birth rate.

Now, let us see what happens when the data are replotted with an aspect ratio of 0.3; the result appears in Figure 4.10. The new plot displays many

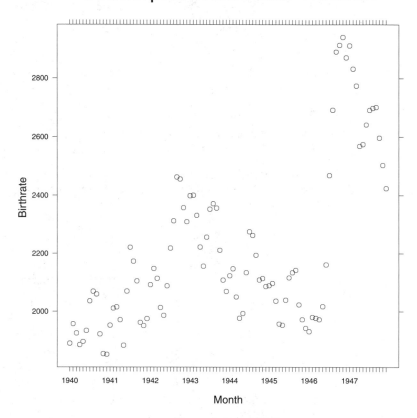

FIGURE 4.9. U.S. birthrate against year plotted with aspect ratio = 1.0.

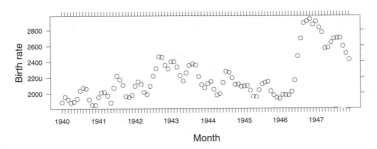

FIGURE 4.10. U.S. birthrate aginst year with aspect ratio = 0.3.

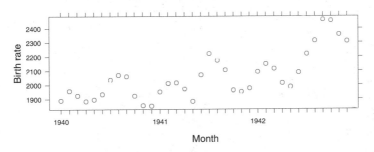

FIGURE 4.11. U.S. birthrate against year (1940-1943) with aspect ratio = 0.3.

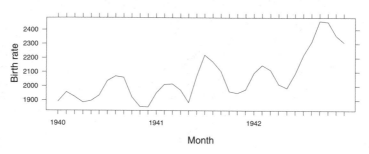

FIGURE 4.12. U.S. birthrate against year (1940-1943) with observations joined and aspect ratio = 0.3.

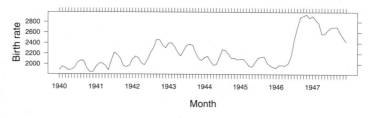

FIGURE 4.13. U.S. birthrate against year with aspect ratio 0.2 and observations joined.

TABLE 4.5. Birthrates and death rates for 69 countries

Country	Birth	Death	Country	Birth	Death
alg	36.4	14.6	con	37.3	8.0
egy	42.1	15.3	gha	55.8	25.6
ict	56.1	33.1	mag	41.8	15.8
mor	46.1	18.7	tun	41.7	10.1
cam	41.4	19.7	cey	35.8	8.5
chi	34.0	11.0	tai	36.3	6.1
hkg	32.1	5.5	ind	20.9	8.8
ids	27.7	10.2	irq	20.5	3.9
isr	25.0	6.2	jap	17.3	7.0
jor	46.3	6.4	kor	14.8	5.7
mal	33.5	6.4	mog	39.2	11.2
phl	28.4	7.1	syr	26.2	4.3
tha	34.8	7.9	vit	23.4	5.1
can	24.8	7.8	cra	49.9	8.5
dmr	33.0	8.4	gut	47.7	17.3
hon	46.6	9.7	mex	45.1	10.5
nic	42.9	7.1	pan	40.1	8.0
usa	21.7	9.6	arg	21.8	8.1
bol	17.4	5.8	bra	45.0	13.5
chl	33.6	11.8	clo	44.0	11.7
ecu	44.2	13.5	per	27.7	8.2
urg	22.5	7.8	ven	42.8	6.7
aus	18.8	12.8	bel	17.1	12.7
brt	18.2	12.2	bul	16.4	8.2
cze	16.9	9.5	dem	17.6	19.8
fin	18.1	9.2	fra	18.2	11.7
gmy	18.0	12.5	gre	17.4	7.8
hun	13.1	9.9	irl	22.3	11.9
ity	19.0	10.2	net	20.9	8.0
now	17.5	10.0	pol	19.0	7.5
pog	23.5	10.8	rom	15.7	8.3
spa	21.5	9.1	swe	14.8	10.1
swz	18.9	9.6	rus	21.2	7.2
yug	21.4	8.9	ast	21.6	8.7
nzl	25.5	8.8			

peaks and troughs and suggests perhaps some minor within-year trends in addition to the global trends apparent in Figure 4.9. A clearer picture is obtained by plotting only a part of the data, as is done in Figure 4.11 for the years 1940-1943. Now, a within-year cycle is clearly apparent with the lowest within-year birthrate at the beginning of the summer and the highest occurring in the autumn. This pattern is made clearer by connecting adjacent points in the plot with a line— see Figure 4.12. By reducing the aspect ratio to 0.2, replotting all 96 observations and again joining adjacent points with a line, both the within-year and global trends become clearly visible—see Figure 4.13.

4.3   Estimating bivariate densities

Examination of scatterplots often centres on assessing density patterns such as clusters, gaps or outliers. But humans are not particularly good at visually examining point density, and some type of density estimate added to the scatterplot will frequently be very helpful. There is now a vast literature on density estimation (see, for example, Silverman, 1986), and its use in association with univariate data has already been described in Chapter 2. The estimation of bivariate densities is briefly described in Display 4.1.

Display 4.1 Estimating bivariate density functions

- The data set whose underlying density is to be estimated is $\mathbf{X}_1, \mathbf{X}_2, \cdots, \mathbf{X}_n$.

- The bivariate kernel density estimator with kernel K and window width h is defined by

$$\hat{f}(\mathbf{x}) = \frac{1}{nh^2} \sum_{i=1}^{n} K\{\frac{1}{h}(\mathbf{x} - \mathbf{X}_i\} \tag{1}$$

- The kernel function $K(\mathbf{x})$ is a function, defined for bivariate $\mathbf{x}$, satisfying

$$\int K(\mathbf{x})d\mathbf{x} = 1 \tag{2}$$

- Usually $K(\mathbf{x})$ will be a radially symmetric unimodal probability density function, for example, the standard bivariate normal density function:

$$K(\mathbf{x}) = \frac{1}{2\pi} \exp(-\frac{1}{2}\mathbf{x}'\mathbf{x}) \tag{3}$$

- Another possibility is the bivariate Epanechnikov kernel

$$K(\mathbf{x}) = \begin{cases} \frac{2}{\pi}(1 - \mathbf{x}'\mathbf{x}) & \text{if } \mathbf{x}'\mathbf{x} < 1 \\ 0 & \text{otherwise} \end{cases} \tag{4}$$

To illustrate how bivariate density estimation can be used to enhance a scatterplot, we shall use the data on birthrates and death rates for 69 countries given in Table 4.5. In Figure 4.14(a), the scatterplot of the data is shown enhanced with a contour plot of the estimated bivariate density of birthrates and death rates; here, a Gaussian kernel was used with bandwidth equal to $\frac{1}{69^{0.2}} = 0.43$. Figure 4.14(b) shows the scatterplot with a contour plot of the density estimate given by using the Epanechnikov kernel and again a bandwidth of 0.43. Both plots give some evidence of two modes in the data, perhaps indicating the presence of 'clusters' of countries, a possibility that will be investigated further in Chapter 19.

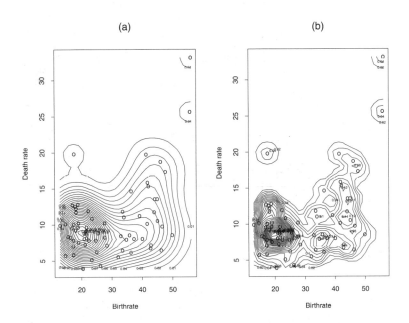

FIGURE 4.14. Contour plots of estimated bivariate density for birthrate/death rate data: (a) Gaussian kernel and (b) Epanechnikov kernel.

The density estimates can also be presented in the form of perspective plots as shown in Figure 4.15(a) and (b). Also shown in Figure 4.15(c) is a perspective plot of the two-dimensional histogram of the data. The latter is far less informative about the structure in the data than are the other two perspective plots. The density estimate provided by the histogram is just too rough to be useful.

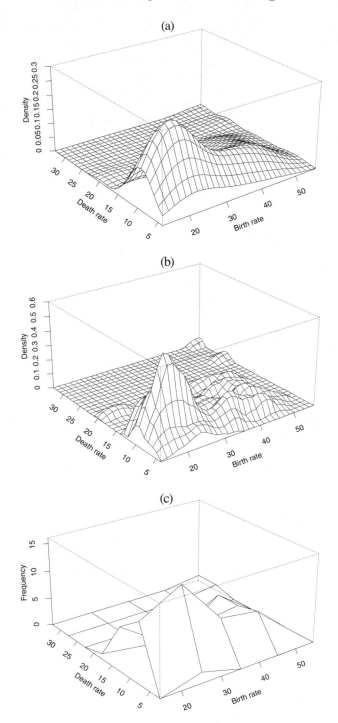

FIGURE 4.15. Perspective plots of estimated densities for birthrate/death rate data: (a) Gaussian kernel, (b) Epanechnikov, and (c) two-dimensional histogram.

4.4 Simple regression and locally weighted regression

To investigate further the relationships between the pairs of variables in the data sets given in Tables 4.1 and 4.2, we might fit simple and perhaps not-so-simple regression models. The fitted regression lines can then be added to the scatterplots. In Figures 4.16 and 4.17, for example, the least-squares regression line (see Display 4.2) is shown on the scatterplots introduced in Section 4.2. As we might have expected, the fitted linear regression for the oxygen uptake data represents the observations very poorly.

Display 4.2 Simple linear regression

- Assume y_i represents the value of the response variable on the ith individual (plotted on the vertical axis), and that x_i represents the individual's values on an explanatory variable (plotted on the horizontal axis).

- The simple regression model is

$$y_i = \beta_0 + \beta_1 x_i + \epsilon_i$$

  where β_0 is the intercept and β_1 is the slope of the linear relationship and ϵ_i is an error term or residual.

- The residuals are assumed to be independent random variables having a normal distribution with mean zero and constant variance σ^2.

- The *regression coefficients*, β_0 and β_1 may be estimated as $\hat{\beta}_0$ and $\hat{\beta}_1$ using *least squares*. Here, the sum of squared differences between the observed values of the response variable y_i and the values 'predicted' by the regression equation, $\hat{y}_i = \hat{\beta}_0 + \hat{\beta}_1 x_i$ is minimised, leading to the estimates

$$\hat{\beta}_0 = \overline{y} - \hat{\beta}_1 \overline{x}$$

$$\hat{\beta}_1 = \frac{\sum (y_i - \overline{y})(x_i - \overline{x})}{\sum (x_i - \overline{x})^2}$$

Parametric regression models are very useful, but not adequate for all data sets. The patterns in many bivariate relationships are too complex to be described by a simple parametric family. An alternative approach to dealing with such data is to fit a curve to the observations *locally*, so that at any point the curve at that point depends only on the observations at that point and some specified neighbouring points. Because such a fit produces an estimate of the response that is less variable than the original observed response, the result is often called a *smooth* and procedures for producing such fits are called *scatterplot smoothers*. A brief description of one such technique is given in Display 4.3.

To illustrate the ideas of smoothing, we shall use the data shown in Table 4.6. These arise from simulated motorcycle accidents used to test

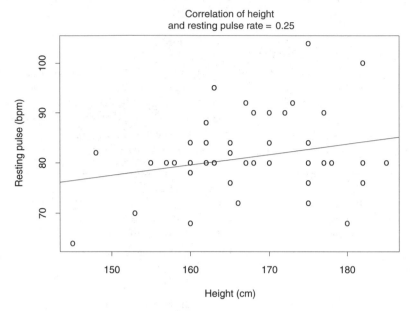

FIGURE 4.16. Scatterplot of pulse against height with regression line.

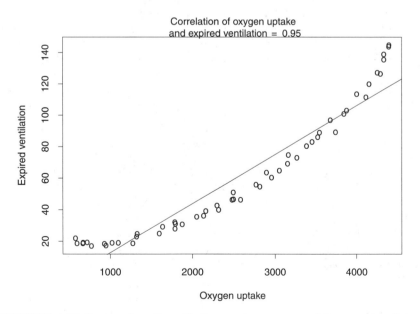

FIGURE 4.17. Scatterplot of ventilation against oxygen with regression line.

Display 4.3 Local regression models (lowess)

- We assume we have observations on a response variable y and an explanatory variable x.

- We assume that y and x are related by

$$y_i = g(x_i) + \epsilon_i \tag{1}$$

where g is a 'smooth' function and the ϵ_i are random variables with mean zero and constant scale.

- Fixed values $\hat{y}_i$ are used to estimate the y_i at each x_i by fitting polynomials using weighted least squares with large weights for points near to x_i and small otherwise.

- Two parameters need to be chosen to fit a lowess curve; the first is a smoothing parameter with larger values leading to smoother curves, and the second is the degree of certain polynomials that are fitted by the method.

---

crash helmets. The data are plotted with two types of smooth curves in Figure 4.18. Both appear to give a very good representation of the data.

4.5 Summary

The scatterplot is the basic tool for exploring bivariate data. From it the form of the relationship between the two variables is often apparent, and this will often indicate what is and what is not a sensible model to fit to the data. Other information such as an estimate of the bivariate density or a fitted regression line can often be added to the scatterplot to increase its usefulness. As we shall see in Chapter 7, the scatterplot also forms the basis of other more ambitious graphic procedures for exploring complex data sets.

TABLE 4.6. Motorcycle accidents used to test crash helmets

Time	Accel	Time	Accel
2.4	0	2.6	−1.3
3.2	−2.7	3.6	0
4	−2.7	6.2	−2.7
6.6	−2.7	6.8	−1.3
7.8	−2.7	8.2	−2.7
8.8	−1.3	8.8	−2.7
9.6	−2.7	10	−2.7
10.2	−5.4	10.6	−2.7
11	−5.4	11.4	0
13.2	−2.7	13.6	−2.7
13.8	0	14.6	−13.3
14.6	−5.4	14.6	−5.4
14.6	−9.3	14.6	−16
14.6	−22.8	14.8	−2.7
15.4	−22.8	15.4	−32.1
15.4	−53.5	15.4	−54.9
15.6	−40.2	15.6	−21.5
15.8	−21.5	15.8	−50.8
16	−42.9	16	−26.8
16.2	−21.5	16.2	−50.8
16.2	−61.7	16.4	−5.4
16.4	−80.4	16.6	−59
16.8	−71	16.8	−91.1
16.8	−77.7	17.6	−37.5
17.6	−85.6	17.6	−123.1
17.6	−101.9	17.8	−99.1
17.8	−104.4	18.6	−112.5
18.6	−50.8	19.2	−123.1
19.4	−85.6	19.4	−72.3
19.6	−127.2	20.2	−123.1
20.4	−117.9	21.2	−134
21.4	−101.9	21.8	−108.4
22	−123.1	23.2	−123.1
23.4	−128.5	24	−112.5
24.2	−95.1	24.2	−81.8
24.6	−53.5	25	−64.4
25	−57.6	25.4	−72.3
25.4	−44.3	25.6	−26.8
26	−5.4	26.2	−107.1
26.2	−21.5	26.4	−65.6
27	−16	27.2	−45.6
27.2	−24.2	27.2	9.5
27.6	4	28.2	12
28.4	−21.5	28.4	37.5
28.6	46.9	29.4	−17.4
30.2	36.2	31	75
31.2	8.1	32	54.9
32	48.2	32.8	46.9
33.4	16	33.8	45.6
34.4	1.3	34.8	75
35.2	−16	35.2	−54.9
35.4	69.6	35.6	34.8
35.6	32.1	36.2	−37.5
36.2	22.8	38	46.9
38	10.7	39.2	5.4
39.4	−1.3	40	−21.5
40.4	−13.3	41.6	30.8
41.6	−10.7	42.4	29.4
42.8	0	42.8	−10.7
43	14.7	44	−1.3
44.4	0	45	10.7
46.6	10.7	47.8	−26.8
47.8	−14.7	48.8	−13.3
50.6	0	52	10.7
53.2	−14.7	55	−2.7
55	10.7	55.4	−2.7
57.6	10.7		

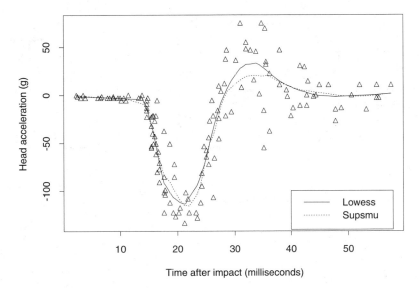

FIGURE 4.18. Time after impact and acceleration in simulated motorcycle accidents with two fitted 'smooths'.

4.6   Using S-PLUS

Section 4.2

In this section, the `read.table()` function is used to read in data as a data frame object. The `plot()` function is used to construct scatterplots. The `rug()` and `jitter()` functions are used to enhance the plots. The `type="n"` option is used with the `plot()` function to produce a graph without points. Labels are then superimposed using the `text()` function. Here, the `abbreviate()` function is used to get unique, abbreviated labels for the occupations when producing Figure 4.3. The `subplot()` function is introduced. This allows several graphs to be plotted on the same diagram. The `usr` parameter is used to ensure that different graphs using the same variables use the same scales. The `hull()` and `polygon()` functions are used to construct and then draw the convex hull of a data set. An example of trellis graphics is given, and the trellis graphics scatterplot function `xyplot()` is employed that allows the aspect ratio to be changed. A model formula is used to specify the variables to be plotted. The `frame()` function is used to clear the graph window.

Script for Section 4.2

```
# Read in data on resting pulse rate and height as a data frame
# using the read.table function. The header=T specifies that
# variables are named in data file. Names are Height and Pulse
# (note capital letter)
rest<-read.table("resting.dat",header=T)

# Produce scatterplot using the plot() function
win.graph()
attach(rest)
plot(Height,Pulse,xlab="Height (cm)",ylab="Resting pulse (bpm)")
```
$\Longrightarrow$ ⟦ Figure 4.1 ⟧

```
# Read in data on oxygen uptake
uptake<-read.table("anaerob.dat",header=T)
attach(uptake)

# Plot oxygen uptake against expired ventilation
plot(Oxygen,Ventilation,xlab="Oxygen uptake",
   ylab="Expired ventilation")
text(locator(1),paste("Correlation of oxygen uptake and
   expired ventilation= ",round(cor(Oxygen,Ventilation),
   digits=2)))
# locator() allows the user to determine the position
# by clicking in the graph window.
```
$\Longrightarrow$ ⟦ Figure 4.2 ⟧

```
# Use cancer data from Chapter 1
cancer<-matrix(scan("cancer.dat"),ncol=2,byrow=T)
occup<-c("Farmers","Miners","Chemical","Glass","Furnace",
    "Electrical","Engineering","Woodworkers","Leather",
    "Textile","Clothing","Tobacco","Printing","Other",
    "Construction","Painters","Crane drivers","Labourers",
    "Communications","Warehousemen","Clerical","Sales",
    "Service","Managers","Professional")
dimnames(cancer)<-list(occup,c("Ratio","SMR"))

# Store as data frame
cancer<-as.data.frame(cancer)
attach(cancer)

plot(Ratio,SMR,xlab="Smoking ratio",ylab="SMR",type="n")
text(Ratio,SMR,labels=abbreviate(occup))
```
$\Longrightarrow$ Figure 4.3

```
# Read in image data
image<-read.table("image.dat", header=T)
attach(image)

# Plot a sample of 1,000 observations from the data
par(pty="s")
index<-sample(1:length(PD),size=1000)
plot(PD[index],T2[index],xlab="PD",ylab="T2")
title("Raw fMRI data")
plot(jitter(cbind(PD[index],T2[index]),factor=2),
    xlab="PD",ylab="T2")
title("fMRI data after jittering")
```
$\Longrightarrow$ Figure 4.4

```
# Replot scatterplot of height and pulse, and add
# rug plots for each variable
attach(rest)
plot(Height,Pulse,xlab="Height (cm)",ylab="Resting pulse (bpm)")
rug(jitter(Height),side=1)
rug(jitter(Pulse),side=2)
```
$\Longrightarrow$ Figure 4.5

```
# Add information about marginal distributions of Height and
# Pulse using the subplot function and the density function
win.graph()
# Set user coordinates for ranges of x and y axes within
# plotting area
par(usr=c(0,1,0,1))
# now locations of subplots can be set in relation to these
# coordinates
```

```
# Plot first subplot, and save associated plotting parameters
# as rest.par. The x and y axes are specified as spanning
# from the bottom left corner to 85% of the full range.
rest.par<-subplot(x=c(0,0.85),y=c(0,0.85),
fun=plot(Height,Pulse,xlab="Height (cm)",
    ylab="Resting pulse (bpm)"))
rest.usr<-rest.par$usr
# rest.par$usr contains ranges of x and y-values in the
# units of the plotted variables, Height and Pulse. We
# need to use this later to ensure that the same scales
# are used in the other subplots.

# Compute nonparametric probability densities of Height
# and Pulse
Height.den<-density(Height,2*(summary(Height)[5]
    -summary(Height)[2]))
Pulse.den<-density(Pulse,2*(summary(Pulse)[5]
    -summary(Pulse)[2]))

# Plot second subplot: use same x-axis range as first
# subplot, and use top 15% of space for y-axis
subplot(x=c(0,0.85),y=c(0.85,1),
fun={par(usr=c(rest.usr[1:2],0,1.04*max(Height.den$y)))
     lines(Height.den)
     box()})
# Here, the par(usr=...) option is used to specify the
# ranges of the x and y axes in the units of the plotted
# variables.

# Plot third subplot: use top 15% of space for x-axis
# and same y-axis space, and scale as first subplot
subplot(x=c(0.85,1),y=c(0,0.85),
fun={par(usr=c(0,1.04*max(Pulse.den$y),rest.usr[3:4]))
     lines(Pulse.den$y,Pulse.den$x)
     box()})
# Note that the x- and y-values are interchanged
# so that Pulse.x is plotted on the vertical axis.
```

$\implies$ Figure 4.6

```
# A simple way of showing marignal distributions on
# scatterplot
frame()
# Clears the graph window
par(fig=c(0,0.7,0,0.7))
# This sets plotting area to be occupied by next plot
plot(Height,Pulse)
par(fig=c(0,0.7,0.65,1))
```

```
hist(Height)
par(fig=c(0.65,1,0,0.7))
boxplot(Pulse)
```
⟹ Figure 4.7

```
# Produce convex hull on sample of fMRI data
# from data on fMRI
index<-sample(1:length(PD),size=25)
win.graph()
par(pty="s")
PD<-PD[index]
T2<-T2[index]
hull<-chull(PD,T2)
plot(PD,T2,pch=1)
polygon(PD[hull],T2[hull],density=15,angle=30)
```
⟹ Figure 4.8

```
# Find correlation of two variables
cor(PD,T2)

# Find correlation after removal of points defining convex hull
cor(PD[-hull],T2[-hull])


# Read in data on birthrates in the U.S. in the 1940s
births<-scan("usbirths.dat")

# Make suitable labels for the months that observations are made
y<-rep(" ",11)
y<-c("1940",y,"1941",y,"1942",y,"1943",y,"1944",y,"1945",y,
  "1946",y,"1947",y)

# Set up trellis graphics window for plotting
Y<-1:96
trellis.device(win.graph)
xyplot(births~Y,xlab="Month",ylab="Birth rate",type="p",
   main=list("Scatterplot of Birthrate v Month",cex=2),
   sub=list("Data from USA",cex=1.5),
   scales=list(cex=0.7,x=list(tick.number=5,at=1:96,labels=y)),
     aspect=1.0)
```
⟹ Figure 4.9

```
# Replot data with aspect ratio changed to 0.3

xyplot(births~Y,xlab="Month",ylab="Birth rate",type="p",
   main=list("Scatterplot of Birthrate v Month",cex=2),
   sub=list("Data from USA",cex=1.5),
   scales=list(cex=0.7,x=list(tick.number=5,at=1:96,labels=y)),
     aspect=0.3)
```

⟹ Figure 4.10

```
# Now plot only years 1940-1943
trellis.device(win.graph)
xyplot(births[1:36]~Y[1:36],xlab="Month",ylab="Birth rate",
    type="p",
    main=list("Scatterplot of Birthrate v Month",cex=2),
    sub=list("Data from USA",cex=1.5),
    scales=list(cex=0.7,x=list(tick.number=5,at=1:36,
        labels=y[1:36])),
  aspect=0.3)
```

⟹ Figure 4.11

```
# Now join points with a line usint the type="l" option
trellis.device(win.graph)
xyplot(births[1:36]~Y[1:36],xlab="Month",ylab="Birth rate",
    type="l",
    main=list("Scatterplot of Birthrate v Month",cex=2),
    sub=list("Data from USA",cex=1.5),
    scales=list(cex=0.7,x=list(tick.number=5,at=1:36,
        labels=y[1:36])),
    aspect=0.3)
```

⟹ Figure 4.12

```
# Finally replot all data with smaller aspect ratio and
# joining points with a line
trellis.device(win.graph)
xyplot(births~Y,xlab="Month",ylab="Birth rate",type="l",
    main=list("Scatterplot of Birthrate v Month",cex=2),
    sub=list("Data from USA",cex=1.5),
    scales=list(cex=0.7,x=list(tick.number=5,at=1:96,
        labels=y)),
    aspect=0.2)
```

⟹ Figure 4.13

Section 4.3

In this section, code for a function, tdden1(), is included. This function computes bivariate density estimates using either a normal or an Epanechikov kernel. The important aspect of this function is the use of the outer() function to evaluate the estimated density for a single data point over a user-specified grid. These estimates are then accumulated for all data using a for loop. The outer() function essentially replaces two more possible for loops in the function, which, if used, would make the density estimation extremely slow. The contour() and persp() functions are used to get two graphical displays of the estimated densities.

Script for Section 4.3

```
# Function for finding density estimates as outlined in Display 4.1
# Outer() function is used for efficient computation
tdden1<-function(x,y,ngridx=30,ngridy=30,constant.x=1,
  constant.y=1,K="normal") {
    # x and y are vectors containing the bivariate data
    # ngridx and ngridy are the number of x-values and
    # y-values in the grid
    mx<-mean(x)
    sdx<-sqrt(var(x))
    my<-mean(y)
    sdy<-sqrt(var(y))
    # scale x and y before estimation
    x<-scale(x)
    y<-scale(y)
    den<-matrix(0,ngridx,ngridy)

    # Find possible value for bandwidth
    n<-length(x)
    hx<-constant.x*n^(-0.2)
    hy<-constant.y*n^(-0.2)
    h<-hx*hy
    hsqrt<-sqrt(h)
    seqx< seq(range(x)[1],range(x)[2],length=ngridx)
    seqy<-seq(range(y)[1],range(y)[2],length=ngridy)
    for(i in 1:n) {
        X<-x[i]
        Y<-y[i]
        xx<-(seqx-X)/hsqrt
        yy<-(seqy-Y)/hsqrt
        if(K=="normal")
            den<-den+outer(xx,yy,function(x,y)exp(-0.5*(x^2+y^2)))
        if(K=="Epan")
            den<-den+outer(xx,yy,
                    function(x,y) {
                      test<-x^2+y^2
                      xxx<-x
                      yyy<-y
                      xxx[test>=1]<-1/sqrt(2)
                      yyy[test>=1]<-1/sqrt(2)
                      xxx[test<1]<-x[test<1]
                      yyy[test<1]<-y[test<1]
                      1-xxx^2-yyy^2
                    } )
    }
    if(K=="normal") den<-den/(n*2*pi*h)
    if(K=="Epan") den<-2*den/(n*h*pi)
```

```
    seqx<-sdx*seqx+mx
    seqy<-sdy*seqy+my
    result<-list(seqx=seqx,seqy=seqy,den=den)
    result
}


# Read in birthrates and death rates for 69 countries
birdea<-read.table("birdea.dat",header=T)
attach(birdea)

# Use the function tdden1() to calculate bivariate density
# estimates for data using both a Gaussian and
# Epachnekov kernel
density<-tdden1(birth,death)
density1<-tdden1(birth,death,K="Epan")

# Set up plotting area to take contour plots
win.graph()
par(mfrow=c(1,2))

# Plot data and add contour plot
plot(birth,death,xlab="Birth rate",ylab="Death rate")
contour(density$seqx,density$seqy,density$den,add=T,
    nlevels=25,labex=0.5)
title("(a)")
plot(birth,death,xlab="Birth rate",ylab="Death rate")
contour(density1$seqx,density1$seqy,density1$den,add=T,
    nlevels=25,labex=0.5)
title("(b)")
```

$\implies$ Figure 4.14

```
# Get perspective plots
par(mfrow=c(1,3))
h2d<-hist2d(birth,death)
persp(density$seqx,density$seqy,density$den,
    xlab="Birth rate",
    ylab="Death rate",zlab="Density")
title("(a)")
persp(density1$seqx,density1$seqy,density1$den,
    xlab="Birth rate",
    ylab="Death rate",zlab="Density")
title("(b)")
persp(h2d,xlab="Birth rate",ylab="Death rate",
    zlab="Frequency")
title("(c)")
```

$\implies$ Figure 4.15

Section 4.4

In the code for this section, various 'smoothers' are used, for example, the functions lowess() and supsmu(). The results from these functions can be graphed to a scatterplot using the lines() function. The lm() function for linear regression is also used here to find the least-squares estimates of the parameters in a simple regression. Regression lines are superimposed on the scatterplot using the abline() function. The function will be examined in more detail in Chapter 7.

Script for Section 4.4

```
# Replot height and pulse-rate data and add regression line
attach(rest)
plot(Height,Pulse,xlab="Height (cm)",ylab="Resting pulse (bpm)")

# Put test on plot indicating the correlation between
# the two variables using the cor() and paste() function.
# Use only two decimal places.
text(locator(1),paste("Correlation of height\n and
   resting pulse rate= ",round(cor(Height,Pulse),digits=2)))

# Add least-squares regression line
# The function lm() will be described in detail in Chapter 6
# The function abline() uses the coefficients calculated by
# lm() to plot line
abline(lm(Pulse~Height))                          ⟹ Figure 4.16

# Replot oxygen and ventilation data and add regression line
attach(uptake)
plot(Oxygen,Ventilation,xlab="Oxygen uptake",
   ylab="Expired ventilation")
text(2500,160,paste("Correlation of oxygen uptake and expired
   ventilation= ",round(cor(Oxygen,Ventilation),digits=2)))
abline(lm(Ventilation~Oxygen))                    ⟹ Figure 4.17

# Read in data on testing crash helmets
helmets<-read.table("helmets.dat",header=T)
attach(helmets)

# Set up plotting window plot scatter diagram and
# add two type of smoothing curve
plot(Time,Accel,xlab="Time after impact (milliseconds)",
ylab="Head acceleration (g)",pch=2)
lines(lowess(Time,Accel,f=0.2))
lines(supsmu(Time,Accel),lty=2)
legend(locator(1),c("Lowess","Supsmu"),lty=1:2)  ⟹ Figure 4.18
```

4.7 Exercises

4.1 Using the method described in Display 4.1, estimate the bivariate density of the height and resting pulse data in Table 4.1. Using the `contour()` function, construct a contour plot of the estimated bivariate density.

4.2 For the data in Table 4.2, construct a scatterplot of log-expired volume against oxygen uptake that includes the value of the correlation of the two variables, the fitted regression line, and nonparametric density estimates of the marginal distributions of each variable. Does the resulting diagram give any evidence that fitting a linear relationship between log-expired volume and oxygen uptake may not be adequate for these data?

4.3 For the oxygen uptake and expired ventilation data, consider fitting a curve of the form:

$$E(\text{expired volume}) = \beta_1 \exp(\beta_2 \times \text{oxygen uptake})$$

How could the coefficients β_1 and β_2 be estimated? Use the estimated coefficients to add the fitted exponential curve to the original scatterplot, and add two types of 'smoothed' curves to the data. Use different line types for each curve, and add an informative legend and title.

4.4 The data below in Table 4.7 give monthly deaths from bronchitis, emphysema and asthma in the U.K. from 1974 to 1979 for both men and women. Investigate plotting the data with different aspect ratios. Also, try different smoothing procedures for fitting a curve through the observations.

4.5 Produce a scatterplot of the birthrate and death rate data in Table 4.5, which identifies each country by a suitable label and includes both the linear and locally weighted regressions of death rate on birthrate.

TABLE 4.7. Deaths from bronchitis data

Year	Month					
	1	2	3	4	5	6
1974	3035	2552	2704	2554	2014	1655
1975	2933	2889	2938	2497	1870	1726
1976	2787	3891	3179	2011	1636	1580
1977	2996	2523	2540	2520	1994	1641
1978	2899	2990	2890	2379	1933	1734
1979	2841	3535	3010	2091	1667	1589

Year	Month					
	7	8	9	10	11	12
1974	1721	1524	1596	2074	2199	2512
1975	1607	1545	1396	1787	2076	2837
1976	1489	1300	1356	1653	2013	2823
1977	1691	1479	1596	1877	2032	2484
1978	1617	1495	1440	1777	1970	2745
1979	1518	1349	1392	1619	1954	2633

5
Analysis of Variance and Covariance

5.1 Introduction

This chapter will be concerned with the analysis of designed experiments in medical investigations. Typically, such experiments involve a numeric response variable and one or more categorical variables (*factors*) that are typically under the control of the experimenter, although this is not always so. In addition, it is often the case that other continuous variables need to be included in the analysis. The relevant procedures for handling such studies are *analysis of variance* (ANOVA) and *analysis of covariance* (ANCOVA), and it is these that will be discussed in this chapter.

5.2 A simple one-way example

Twenty-two patients undergoing cardiac bypass surgery were randomized to one of three ventilation groups:

- (Group I): Patients received a 50% nitrous oxide and 50% oxygen mixture continuously for 24 hours.

- (Group II): Patients received a 50% nitrous oxide and 50% oxygen mixture only during the operation.

- (Group III): Patients received no nitrous oxide but received 35-50% oxygen for 24 hours.

Table 5.1 shows red cell foliate levels for the three groups after 24 hours ventilation. The question of interest is whether the three ventilation methods result in a different mean red cell foliate level. The question can be addressed by a one-way analysis of variance, as described in Display 5.1. Before carrying out the analysis, however, some graphical examination of the data is in order to check for departures from normality, any obvious signs of heterogeneity, outliers, and so on.

TABLE 5.1. Red cell foliate levels of patients undergoing cardiac bypass surgery randomized to one of three ventilation groups

Group 1	Group 2	Group 3
243	206	241
251	210	258
275	226	270
291	249	293
347	255	328
354	273	
380	285	
392	295	
309		

The first plot, shown in Figure 5.1, gives the means and medians of red cell foliate levels in each ventilation group. The means and medians are relatively similar, giving some reassurance that non-normality is probably not a problem. The box plots of the observations in each ventilation group shown in Figure 5.2 also indicate that there are no outliers in the data to be concerned about and that the distributions of foliate levels are approximately symmetric.

The analysis of variance table for the data is shown in Table 5.2. The significant F-value indicates that the three ventilation methods do appear to differ in average red cell foliate level.

Having decided that there *is* evidence of a difference between the three ventilation groups in their foliate levels, the question arises as to whether all of the groups differ from each other. Answering this more specific question is the topic to be discussed in the next section.

TABLE 5.2. Analysis of variance table for red foliate levels in different treatment groups

	Df	Sum of Sq	Mean Sq	F-Value	Pr(F)
Group	2	15516	7758	3.711	0.04359
Residuals	19	39716	2090		

Display 5.1 One way analysis of variance

- Let y_{ij} be the jth observation in the ith group. The model assumed is

$$y_{ij} = \mu + \alpha_i + \epsilon_{ij} \tag{1}$$

where μ is the overall mean, α_i is the group effect and ϵ_{ij} is a random error term, assumed to be normally distributed with mean zero and variance σ^2

- Because the model is overparameterized, the group effects need to be constrained in some way, most usually by requiring that $\sum_{i=1}^{k} \alpha_i = 0$, where k is the number of groups.

- The hypothesis of the equality of group means can be written in terms of the group effects as

$$H_0 : \alpha_1 = \alpha_2 = \cdots = \alpha_k = 0 \tag{2}$$

- The total variation in the observations is partitioned into that due to differences in the group means and that due to differences among observations within groups. Under the hypothesis of the equality of group means, both the between-group variance and the within-group variance are estimates of σ^2. Thus, an F-test of the equality of the two variances provides a test of H_0.

- The necessary terms for the F-test are usually arranged in an analysis of variance table as follows (N is the total number of observations):

Source	DF	SS	MS	MSR
Between groups	$k - 1$	$\sum_{i=1}^{k} n_i(\bar{y}_i - \bar{y})^2$	SS/DF (1)	(1)/(2)
Within groups	$N - k$	$\sum_{i=1}^{k} \sum_{j=1}^{n_i}(y_{ij} - \bar{y}_i)^2$	SS/DF (2)	
Total	$N - 1$	$\sum_{i=1}^{k} \sum_{j=1}^{n_i}(y_{ij} - \bar{y})^2$		

- If H_0 is true and the assumptions below are valid, then MSR has an F-distribution with $k - 1$ and $N - k$ degrees of freedom.

- The assumptions made in a one-way analysis of variance are as follows:

    - The observations in each group come from a normal distribution.
    - The population variances of each group are the same.
    - The observations are independent of one another.

- In some studies, the interest is not in testing the equality of means but in testing the significance of one or more linear combinations of means, known as *contrasts*, i.e. (where the c_k are given constants with $\sum c_k = 0$),

$$H_0 : c_1\alpha_1 + c_2\alpha_2 + \cdots + c_k\alpha_k = 0. \tag{3}$$

- The sum of squares for a contrast is given by

$$SS_c = \sum_{i=1}^{k}(c_i\bar{y}_i)^2 / \left(N \sum_{i=1}^{k} c_i^2 \right) \tag{4}$$

with 1 degree of freedom, and the F-statistic is obtained by dividing this by the within-groups sum of squares.

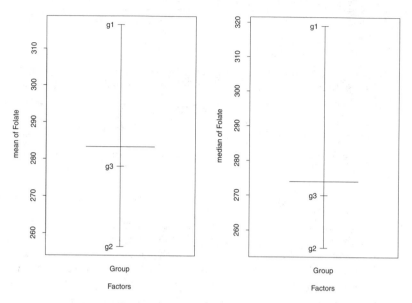

FIGURE 5.1. Means and medians of red foliate levels in each ventilation group.

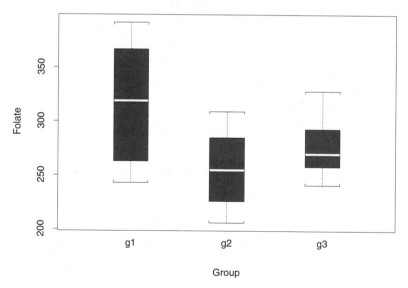

FIGURE 5.2. Box plots of red foliate levels for each ventilation group.

5.3   Multiple comparison procedures

When the the F-test in an analysis of variance produces evidence of a difference between the levels of a factor, the analysis usually needs to proceed further to determine both the details of the differences and how large they are. There are two different approaches. One is to carry out a small number of planned comparisons to test a set of specific hypotheses via *contrasts*. In the example considered in the previous section, an obvious possibility is to compare the low oxygen group, group III, with the two groups receiving higher doses of oxygen and then to compare groups I and II with each other. The contrasts coefficients are $-1, -1, 2$ and and $1, -1, 0$, respectively. These contrasts are orthogonal and are an example of *Helmert* contrasts, in which each of the groups except the first is compared with the mean of the preceding groups. Splitting the group sums of squares into these two contrasts gives $F_{1,19} = 7.29, p = 0.014$ for the difference between groups I and II, and $F_{1,19} = 0.14, p = 0,72$ for the difference between groups III and the other two groups.

The alternative approach is compare all pairs of groups. Because this results in a large number of tests if the number of groups is large, the probability of finding at least one pairwise difference when there are no true differences between the groups can become large. One way of safegarding against such false-positive findings is to carry out the pairwise test only if the F-test of the ANOVA is significant. In addition, the significance level of the individual pairwise comparisons is reduced. There are many different ways of adjusting the significance levels, resulting in many different *multiple comparison* procedures.

All of these procedures produce intervals or bounds for the difference in (usually) one pair of means of the form (estimate) ± (critical point) × (standard error of estimate). The critical point used depends on the specified multiple comparison method. One of the most commonly used is that due to Scheffé (1953); this is described briefly in Display 5.2.

The results of applying the Scheffé procedure to the ventilation experiment described in the previous section are shown in Table 5.3. The results are plotted in Figure 5.3. It appears that there is only a difference in average red cell foliate level between groups I and II.

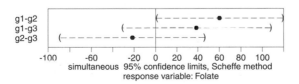

FIGURE 5.3. Graphical display of multiple comparison of ventilation groups.

Display 5.2 Scheffé's multiple comparison procedure

- The t-statistic used is

$$t = \frac{\text{mean difference}}{s(1/n_1 + 1/n_2)^{1/2}} \tag{1}$$

where s^2 is the error mean square and n_1 and n_2 are the number of observations in the two groups being compared.

- Each test-statistic is compared with the critical value

$$[(k-1)F_{k-1,N-k}(\alpha)]^{1/2},$$

where $F_{k-1,N-k}(\alpha)$ is the F-value with $k-1, N-k$ degrees of freedom, corresponding to a significance level α. (Details are given by Maxwell and Delaney, 1990.)

- The confidence interval for two means is in this case

$$\text{mean difference} \pm \text{critical value} \times s \left(\frac{1}{n_1} + \frac{1}{n_2} \right)^{\frac{1}{2}} \tag{2}$$

where the critical value is as described above.

TABLE 5.3. Multiple comparison of ventilation groups

```
95 % simultaneous confidence intervals for specified
linear combinations, by the Scheffe method

critical point: 2.654
response variable: Folate
rank used for Scheffe method: 2

intervals excluding 0 are flagged by '****'
```

	Estimate	Std.Error	Lower Bound	Upper Bound	
g1-g2	60.2	22.2	1.22	119.0	****
g1-g3	38.6	26.1	-30.60	108.0	
g2-g3	-21.6	25.5	-89.20	46.1	

We will return to a further application of multiple comparisons later in this chapter.

5.4   A factorial experiment

Maxwell and Delaney (1990) report a study designed to investigate the effects of three possible treatments on hypertension. The three treatments were as follows:

1. *drug medication*: drug X, drug Y, drug Z.

2. *biofeed*: physiological feedback, present or absent

3. *diet*: present, absent

All 12 combinations of treatments were included in the study. So here we are dealing with a $3 \times 2 \times 2$ design. Six subjects were randomly allocated to each cell of the design, and the response variable measured was blood pressure. The data are given in Table 5.4. As always, before carrying out any formal analysis, it is worth examining the data graphically. One procedure that is often useful in highlighting whether the data should be transformed before analysis is to plot both cell standard deviations against cell means and cell variances against cell means. (The variance should be constant, i.e., independent of the mean.) Both plots are shown in Figure 5.4. Here, there appears to be no obvious relationship between the means and the standard deviations or the means and variances that would indicate the need for a transformation. In Figure 5.5, box plots of blood pressure for each of the levels of each treatment are given. The distributions appear to be symmetric, and there is no suggestion of any outliers.

A suitable model on which to base the analysis of these data is described in Display 5.3. The analysis of variance table corresponding to this model is shown in Table 5.5. Several of the main effects are highly significant, but it is the significant second-order interaction term drug $\times$ biofeed $\times$ diet that first requires interpretation. Perhaps the simplest approach to trying to understanding the meaning of this interaction is to examine the plots of the cell means shown in Figure 5.6. For drug X, there is a large difference in means between biofeedback being present and absent, when the diet is not given, but a far smaller difference when the diet is given. For drug Y, the reverse is the case, and for drug Z, the two differences are approximately equal.

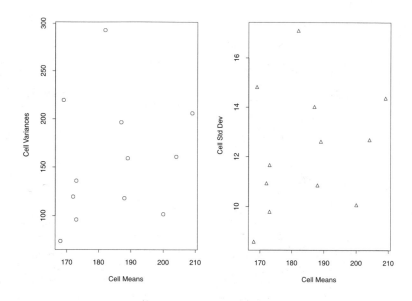

FIGURE 5.4. Plots of blood pressure means against variance and against standard deviations for the biofeedback data.

TABLE 5.4. Data in bp.raw

	Biofeedback		No Biofeedback		
drug X	drug Y	drug Z	drug X	drug Y	drug Z
Diet absent					
170	186	180	173	189	202
175	194	187	194	194	228
165	201	199	197	217	190
180	215	170	190	206	206
160	219	204	176	199	224
158	209	194	198	195	204
Diet present					
161	164	162	164	171	205
173	166	184	190	173	199
157	159	183	169	196	170
152	182	156	164	199	160
181	187	180	176	180	179
190	174	173	175	203	179

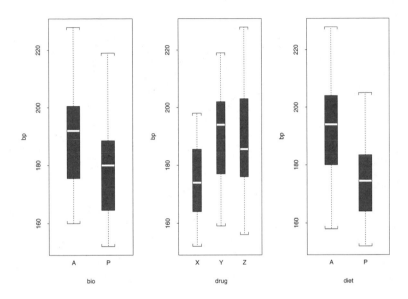

FIGURE 5.5. Box plots of blood pressure levels for each of the three factors in the biofeedback data.

TABLE 5.5. Analysis of variance of biofeedback data

	Df	Sum of Sq	Mean Sq	F Value	Pr(F)
drug	2	3675	1837	11.73	0.0001
bio	1	2048	2048	13.07	0.0006
diet	1	5202	5202	33.20	0.0000
drug:bio	2	259	129	0.83	0.4425
drug:diet	2	903	451	2.88	0.0638
bio:diet	1	32	32	0.20	0.6529
drug:bio:diet	2	1075	537	3.43	0.0388
Residuals	60	9400	157		

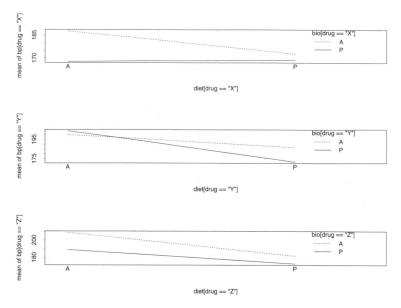

FIGURE 5.6. Interaction diagrams.

5.5   Unbalanced designs

The data shown in Table 5.6 are from a study reported in Rifland *et al.* (1976) concerned with antipyrine clearance of people suffering from β-thalassemia, a chronic type of anaemia. In this disease, abnormally thin red blood cells are produced. The treatment of the disease has undesirable side effects, including liver damage. Antipyrine is a drug used to assess liver function with a high clearance rate, indicating satisfactory liver function. The main questions of interest is whether there is any difference in clearance rate, among the pubertal stages (1 = infant; 3 = adult) or between the sexes.

TABLE 5.6. Antipyrine clearance (half-life in hours)

	1			2			3
Males	7.4	5.6	3.7	10.9	11.3	13.3	
	6.6	6.0		12.2	10.0		
Females	9.1	6.3	7.1	11.0	8.3		
	11.3	9.4	7.9		4.3		

The data in Table 5.6 involve two factors, sex and pubertal stage, but the unbalanced nature of the observations present considerably more problems for analysis than would a balanced 2×3 design. The main difficulty is that when the data are unbalanced, there is no unique way of finding a 'sum of

---

Display 5.3 Model for three factor design

- The model for the observations is

$$y_{ijkl} = \mu + \alpha_i + \beta_j + \gamma_k + \delta_{ij} + \tau_{ik} + \omega_{jk} + \theta_{ijk} + \epsilon_{ijkl} \qquad (1)$$

where α_i, β_j and γ_k represent main effects, δ_{ij}, τ_{ik} and ω_{jk} represent first-order interactions, θ_{ijk} represents the second-order interaction and ϵ_{ijkl} are random error terms assumed to be normally distributed with zero mean and variance σ^2. (Once again, the parameters have to be constrained in some way; for details, see Maxwell and Delaney, 1990.)

- The hypothesis of interest can be written in terms of the parameters of the model as

$$
\begin{array}{llllllllll}
H_0^{(1)} & : & \alpha_1 & = & \alpha_2 & = & \cdots & = & \alpha_a & = & 0 \\
H_0^{(2)} & : & \beta_1 & = & \beta_2 & = & \cdots & = & \beta_b & = & 0 \\
H_0^{(3)} & : & \gamma_1 & = & \gamma_2 & = & \cdots & = & \gamma_c & = & 0 \\
H_0^{(4)} & : & \delta_{11} & = & \delta_{12} & = & \cdots & = & \delta_{ab} & = & 0 \\
H_0^{(5)} & : & \tau_{11} & = & \tau_{12} & = & \cdots & = & \tau_{ac} & = & 0 \\
H_0^{(6)} & : & \omega_{11} & = & \omega_{12} & = & \cdots & = & \omega_{bc} & = & 0 \\
H_0^{(7)} & : & \theta_{111} & = & \theta_{112} & = & \cdots & = & \theta_{abc} & = & 0
\end{array}
\qquad (2)
$$

where a, b and c are the numbers of levels of the three factors.

- The analysis of variance table is as follows:

Source	SS	DF	MS
A	ASS	$a-1$	$ASS/a-1)$
B	BSS	$b-1$	$BSS/b-1)$
C	CSS	$c-1$	$CSS/a-1)$
A×B	ABSS	$(a-1)(b-1)$	$ABSS/(a-1)(b-1)$
A×C	ACSS	$(a-1)(c-1)$	$ACSS/(a-1)(c-1)$
B×C	BBSS	$(b-1)(c-1)$	$ABSS/(a-1)(b-1)$
A×B×C	ABCSS	$(a-1)(b-1)(c-1)$	$ABSS/(a-1)(b-1)(c-1)$
Within cell (error)	WCSS	$abc(n-1)$	$WCSS/abc(n-1)$

For each term, the F-statistic is the ratio of the MS divided by the Error MS.

squares' corresponding to each main effect and their interaction, because these effects are no longer independent of one another. (When the data are balanced, the among-cells sums of squares partitions orthogonally into the three component sums of squares.) Several methods have been suggested for dealing with this problem, each leading to a different type of sums of squares. There have been numerous discussions over which type is most appropriate in the analysis of unbalanced designs; see, for example, Nelder (1977) and Aitkin (1978). Both of these authors give compelling arguments for using what are known as *Type I sums of squares*. These represent the effect of adding a term to an existing model, in one particular order. So, for example, a set of Type I sums of squares such as

Source	Type I SS
A	SSA
B	SSB|A
AB	SSAB|A,B

essentially represent a comparison of the following models:

- SSAB|A,B model including an interaction and main effects with one including only main effects.

- SSB|A model including both main effects, but no interaction, with one including only the main effect of factor A.

- SSA model containing only the A main effect with one containing only the overall mean.

The use of these sums of squares in a series of tables in which the effects are considered in different orders will often provide the most appropriate analysis for an unbalanced design.

The results of the analysis for the data in Table 5.6 are shown in Table 5.7. First, the main effects are considered in the order Stage, Sex and then in the reverse order. Both the main effect of Stage and the Stage × Sex interaction are highly significant. The plot of means given in Figure 5.7 shows that males have a lower average half-life in infancy than have women, whereas in adulthood, the reverse is the case.

5.6 Analysis of covariance

Analysis of covariance is essentially analysis of variance in which differences between levels of a factor are tested, after controlling for other variables, termed covariates. The response variable and the covariate are assumed to be related in some way, and from the estimated relationship, the subject's response values are adjusted in an attempt to account for factor level

TABLE 5.7. Type I sums of squares for analysis of variance of antipyrine clearance data

	Df	Sum of Sq	Mean Sq	F Value	Pr(F)
Stage	2	44.67	22.34	7.599	0.0065
Sex	1	0.08	0.08	0.027	0.8731
Stage:Sex	2	52.24	26.12	8.886	0.0037
Residuals	13	38.21	2.94		

	Df	Sum of Sq	Mean Sq	F Value	Pr(F)
Sex	1	0.76	0.76	0.258	0.6201
Stage	2	43.99	22.00	7.483	0.0069
Stage:Sex	2	52.24	26.12	8.886	0.0037
Residuals	13	38.21	2.94		

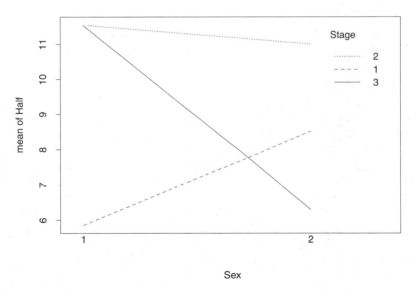

FIGURE 5.7. Interaction diagram for antipyrine clearance data.

differences in the covariates. Following this adjustment, the usual analysis-of-variance tests are applied to see whether there remain any difference in average response in the different factor levels. For a single factor design and a single covariate, the usual model is described in Display 5.4.

Display 5.4 Analysis of covariance

- The model assumed is

$$y_{ij} = \mu + \alpha_i + \beta(x_{ij} - \bar{x}) + \epsilon_{ij} \tag{1}$$

where β is the regression coefficient linking response variable and covariate and $\bar{x}$ is the grand mean of the covariate values.

- NB: The regression coefficient is assumed to be the same in each group.

- The means of the response variable adjusted for the covariate are obtained simply as

$$\text{adjusted group mean} = \text{group mean} + \hat{\beta}(\bar{x}_i - \bar{x}) \tag{2}$$

where $\bar{x}_i$ is the mean of the ith group.

As an illustration of analysis of covariance, it will be applied to the data shown in Table 5.8, which come from an investigation of young girls suffering from anorexia. A number of such patients were randomly assigned to receive one of the following three treatments:

- (Treatment 1): Cognitive behavioural treatment.

- (Treatment 2): Standard treatment.

- (Treatment 3): Family therapy.

The weight of each patient was recorded both before treatment began and after a fixed period of time on the treatment regimen.

Before applying analysis of covariance, it will be helpful to examine the data graphically in a variety of ways. First, we can look at the scatterplot of the weights before and after treatment, identifying the treatment group of each patient. Adding the line corresponding to equal before and after weight is helpful in identifying those patients who lost weight and those who gained weight. We might also include the regression line of weight after treatment on weight before treatment calculated separately for each treatment group to the scatterplot. This will help in assessing whether the assumption that the lines are parallel is justified. The resulting diagram is shown in Figure 5.8. Clearly, the regression lines for the three groups are *not* parallel. Here, however, this problem will be conveniently ignored (but see Exercise 4.3), and we shall carry out an analysis of covariance on the data, with the results shown in Table 5.9.

There is strong evidence that after allowing for initial weight, there is a difference in final weight in the three groups. In an effort to identify which

TABLE 5.8. Young girls and anorexia

Group	Before	After	Group	Before	After	Group	Before	After
g1	80.5	82.2	g2	80.7	80.2	g3	83.8	95.2
g1	84.9	85.6	g2	89.4	80.1	g3	83.3	94.3
g1	81.5	81.4	g2	91.8	86.4	g3	86.0	91.5
g1	82.6	81.9	g2	74.0	86.3	g3	82.5	91.9
g1	79.9	76.4	g2	78.1	76.1	g3	86.7	100.3
g1	88.7	103.6	g2	88.3	78.1	g3	79.6	76.7
g1	94.9	98.4	g2	87.3	75.1	g3	76.9	76.8
g1	76.3	93.4	g2	75.1	86.7	g3	94.2	101.6
g1	81.0	73.4	g2	80.6	73.5	g3	73.4	94.9
g1	80.5	82.1	g2	78.4	84.6	g3	80.5	75.2
g1	85.0	96.7	g2	77.6	77.4	g3	81.6	77.8
g1	89.2	95.3	g2	88.7	79.5	g3	82.1	95.5
g1	81.3	82.4	g2	81.3	89.6	g3	77.6	90.7
g1	76.5	72.5	g2	78.1	81.4	g3	83.5	92.5
g1	70.0	90.9	g2	70.5	81.8	g3	89.9	93.8
g1	80.4	71.3	g2	77.3	77.3	g3	86.0	91.7
g1	83.3	85.4	g2	85.2	84.2	g3	87.3	98.0
g1	83.0	81.6	g2	86.0	75.4			
g1	87.7	89.1	g2	84.1	79.5			
g1	84.2	83.9	g2	79.7	73.0			
g1	86.4	82.7	g2	85.5	88.3			
g1	76.5	75.7	g2	84.4	84.7			
g1	80.2	82.6	g2	79.6	81.4			
g1	87.8	100.4	g2	77.5	81.2			
g1	83.3	85.2	g2	72.3	88.2			
g1	79.7	83.6	g2	89.0	78.8			
g1	84.5	84.6						
g1	80.8	96.2						
g1	87.4	86.7						

TABLE 5.9. Analysis of variance of anorexia data

	Df	Sum of Sq	Mean Sq	F Value	Pr(F)
Before	1	507	506.5	10.40	0.001936
Group	2	766	383.1	7.87	0.000844
Residuals	68	3311	48.7		

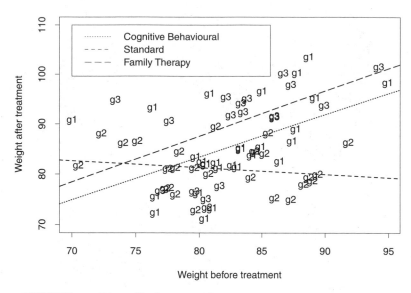

FIGURE 5.8. Plot of before and after weights for anorexia patients.

particular treatments differ, we can again use the multiple comparison approach described in Section 5.3. The results for the means of weight after treatment *adjusted* for initial weight are shown in Table 5.10 and in diagrammatic form in Figure 5.9. It appears that family therapy achieves a higher final weight than does standard treatment.

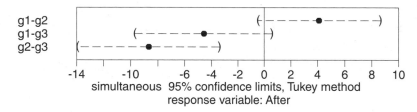

FIGURE 5.9. Graphical display of multiple comparison results of anorexia data.

5.7   Summary

In this chapter, we have described a number of simple analysis of variance procedures. As we shall see later in Chapter 8, analysis of variance models can be formulated in linear regression terms and are further subsumed under a more general approach, known as generalized linear models, to be discussed in Chapter 9.

TABLE 5.10. Multiple comparison of anorexia data

95 % simultaneous confidence intervals for specified
linear combinations, by the Tukey method

critical point: 2.3961
response variable: After

intervals excluding 0 are flagged by '****'

	Estimate	Std.Error	Lower Bound	Upper Bound	
g1-g2	4.10	1.89	-0.44	8.630	
g1-g3	-4.56	2.13	-9.67	0.549	
g2-g3	-8.66	2.19	-13.90	-3.410	****

5.8   Using S-PLUS

Section 5.2

The `aov()` function is used in this section's code to give the analysis of variance table for the red cell data. Some special analysis of variance plot functions `plot.design()` and `plot.factor()` are also used to get various useful graphics.

Script for Section 5.2

```
# Read in data on treatment of patients undergoing cardiac
# bypass surgery
redcell<-read.table("redf.dat",header=T)
attach(redcell)

# Produce some preliminary graphs of the data
win.graph()
par(mfrow=c(1,2))
plot.design(redcell)
plot.design(redcell,fun=median)
```
$\implies$ $\boxed{\text{Figure 5.1}}$

```
# Reset plotting window and produce box plots for each group
win.graph()
plot.factor(redcell)
```
$\implies$ $\boxed{\text{Figure 5.2}}$

```
# Carry out analysis of variance using the aov function
redcell.aov<-aov(Folate~Group)
summary(redcell.aov)
```
$\implies$ $\boxed{\text{Table 5.2}}$

Section 5.3

The `split` option is used in the `summary()` function applied to an `aov` object to obtain a sums of squares table in which the sums of squares for groups is split into the contributions from the two contrasts. A multiple comparison test is applied using the `multicomp()` function and useful plots for interpreting an interaction in a factorial design obtained using the function `interaction.plot()`.

Script for Section 5.3

```
# Test contrasts
redcell.aov<-aov(Folate~Group,
    contrasts = list(Group = contr.helmert))
# contrast option not necessary here because
```

```
# Helmert is the default

summary(redcell.aov, split=list(Group=list(O=1,T=2)))
# The group sums of squares is split into two components,
# one for each contrast. The contrasts are given arbitrary names
# O and T


# Proceed to multiple comparison tests using multicomp function
redcell.mca<-multicomp(redcell.aov,focus="Group",
    method="scheffe")
par(mgp=c(3,0.5,0))
# specifies position of axis title, label and line
plot(redcell.mca)

redcell.mca

dettach(redcell)
```

$\Longrightarrow$ $\boxed{\text{Figure 5.3}}$

$\Longrightarrow$ $\boxed{\text{Table 5.3}}$

Section 5.4

Here, the blood pressure values are read in using scan(), and then appropriate factor variables are defined using the rep() function. Data and
factors are then combined into a data frame object. The tapply() function is used to obtain means and variances for the cells defined by drug,
diet and bio. The plot.factor() function is used to plot box plots of the
dependent variable for the levels of each factor, and the aov() function is
used to fit an ANOVA model.

Script for Section 5.4

```
# Read in biofeed data
bp<-scan("biofeed.dat")


# Now set data up as a data frame with appropriate levels of
# each of the three factors
bio<-factor(rep(c("P","A"),c(36,36)))


# The first 36 observations are for biofeedback present,
# and the last 36 have biofeedback absent
drug<-factor(rep(rep(c("X","Y","Z"),c(12,12,12)),2))
# assigns the correct drug label to the observations

diet<-factor(rep(rep(c("A","P"),c(6,6)),6))
# Finally the diet labels are assigned

biofeed<-data.frame(bio,drug,diet,bp)
biofeed
attach(biofeed)
```

```
# Plots of variances against means and sds against means
# use the tapply() function to get the required cell means
means<-tapply(bp,list(drug,diet,bio),mean)
vars<-tapply(bp,list(drug,diet,bio),var)
sd<-sqrt(vars)
par(mfrow=c(1,2))
plot(means,vars,xlab="Cell Means",ylab="Cell Variances",pch=1)
plot(means,sd,xlab="Cell Means",ylab="Cell Std Dev",pch=2)
```
$\Longrightarrow$ | Figure 5.4 |

```
# Box plots for separate factors
par(mfrow=c(1,3))
plot.factor(biofeed)
```
$\Longrightarrow$ | Figure 5.5 |

```
# Analysis of variance
biofeed.aov<-aov(bp~drug*bio*diet)
summary(aov(biofeed.aov))
```
$\Longrightarrow$ | Table 5.5 |

```
# Interaction plots
par(mfrow=c(3,1))
interaction.plot(diet[drug=="X"],bio[drug=="X"],bp[drug=="X"])
interaction.plot(diet[drug=="Y"],bio[drug=="Y"],bp[drug=="Y"])
interaction.plot(diet[drug=="Z"],bio[drug=="Z"],bp[drug=="Z"])
```
$\Longrightarrow$ | Figure 5.6 |

```
dettach(biofeed)
```

Section 5.5

For the antipyrine data, Stage and Sex are converted to factor variables
after they have been read in. Note how the original parts of the data frame
are replaced by the newly defined factor variables.

Script for Section 5.5

```
# Read in data on antipyrine clearance
antip<-read.table("antip.dat",header=T)
antip$Stage<-as.factor(antip$Stage)
antip$Sex<-as.factor(antip$Sex)
attach(antip)

# Carry out two anovas with different orders of main effects
summary(aov(Half~Stage+Sex+Stage:Sex))
summary(aov(Half~Sex+Stage+Stage:Sex))
```
$\Longrightarrow$ | Table 5.7 |

```
interaction.plot(Sex,Stage,Half,
    ylab="mean of half life in hours")
```
$\Longrightarrow$ | Figure 5.7 |

Section 5.6

Here, the lm() function is used to fit simple least-squares regression lines for the observations from each group in the anorexia data. The abline() function is used to add the regression lines to an existing graph. The multicomp() function is again used to perform a multiple comparison test.

Script for Section 5.6

```
# Read in anorexia data as data frame. The group label and before
# and after weights are given
anorexia<-read.table("anorexia.dat",header=T)
attach(anorexia)

# Plot data
win.graph()
plot(Before,After,type="n",xlab="Weight before treatment",
   ylab="Weight after treatment",ylim=c(70,110))
# extend y-axis to allow space for legend
text(Before,After,labels=as.character(Group),lwd=2)
abline(lm(After[Group=="g1"]~Before[Group=="g1"]),lwd=2,lty=2)
abline(lm(After[Group=="g2"]~Before[Group=="g2"]),lty=3,lwd=2)
abline(lm(After[Group=="g3"]~Before[Group=="g3"]),lty=4,lwd=2)
legend(locator(1),c("Cognitive Behavioural","Standard",
   "Family Therapy"),lty=2:4)
```
$\implies$ Figure 5.8

```
# Analysis of covariance with the preweight as covariate
anorexia.fit<-aov(After~Before+Group)
summary(anorexia.fit)
```
$\implies$ Table 5.9

```
# Carry out multiple comparison test
anorexia.mca<-multicomp(anorexia.fit,focus="Group")
anorexia.mca
```
$\implies$ Table 5.10

```
par(mgp=c(3,0.5,0))
# determines positions of tick labels and title
plot(anorexia.mca)
```
$\implies$ Figure 5.9

5.9 Exercises

5.1 Use the mca() function to apply some alternative multiple comparison procedures to the one used in the text to the red foliate level data.

5.2 In the biofeedback data, apply analysis of variance separately to the observations for each drug. If appropriate, use a multiple comparison analysis to determine where any differences lie.

5.3 The usual analysis of covariance assumption of parallel regression lines in the different groups is clearly not met by the data on anorexic patients. Suggest and carry out an alternative analysis that does not make this assumption.

5.4 Reanalyze the biofeedback data after taking a log transformation of blood pressure.

5.5 Examine the residuals from fitting a main effects model only to the biofeedback data first with blood pressure as dependent variable and then with log blood pressure as dependent variable.

6
The Analysis of Longitudinal Data

6.1   Introduction

Studies in which patients are observed on several occasions over a period of time are particularly common in medical research. Most clinical trials, for example, are of this format. The characteristic feature of such studies is that multiple measurements of a response variable are obtained at a set of time points for each participant in the study. There are two main difficulties in the analysis of data from such longitudinal studies:

- The analysis is complicated by the dependence among repeated observations made on the same experimental unit.

- There may be a substantial proportion of missing values due to participants not attending at all scheduled visits or perhaps dropping out of the study altogether.

In this chapter, a number of relatively simple methods for analysing such data will be described. More complex analyses using a variety of modeling techniques will be discussed in Chapters 11 and 12.

6.2   Graphical displays of longitudinal data

Gregoire *et al.* (1996) give details of a double-blind, placebo-controlled study of the use of estrogen given transdermally in the treatment of postnatal depression. In the study, 61 women with major depression that began within 3 months of childbirth and persisted for up to 18 months postnatally were allocated randomly to active treatment ($n = 34$: 3 months of transdermal 17β-oestradiol 200 mg daily alone, then 3 months with added cyclical dydrogesterone 10 mg daily for 12 days each month) or placebo ($n = 27$: placebo patches and tablets according to the same regime). The women were assessed by self-ratings of depressive scale (EPDS); higher scores imply more depressed. These assessments were made on six, two-monthly visits for a year after treatment began. In addition, two assessments were made prior to the start of treatment. Only 45 of the women had a complete set of eight ratings on the EPDS. The data are given in Table 6.1; a '-9' indicates a missing value.

TABLE 6.1: Data from clinical trial of estrogen patches in the treatment of postnatal depression Treatment Group: 0 = placebo, 1 = active

Group	Pre 1	Pre 2	Post 1	Post 2	Post 3	Post 4	Post 5	Post 6
0	18	18	17	18	15	17	14	15
0	25	27	26	23	18	17	12	10
0	19	16	17	14	-9	-9	-9	-9
0	24	17	14	23	17	13	12	12
0	19	15	12	10	8	4	5	5
0	22	20	19	11	9	8	6	5
0	28	16	13	13	9	7	8	7
0	24	28	26	27	-9	-9	-9	-9
0	27	28	26	24	19	13	11	9
0	18	25	9	12	15	12	13	20
0	23	24	14	-9	-9	-9	-9	-9
0	21	16	19	13	14	23	15	11
0	23	26	13	22	-9	-9	-9	-9
0	21	21	7	13	-9	-9	-9	-9
0	22	21	18	-9	-9	-9	-9	-9
0	23	22	18	-9	-9	-9	-9	-9
0	26	26	19	13	22	12	18	13
0	20	19	19	7	8	2	5	6
0	20	22	20	15	20	17	15	13
0	15	16	7	8	12	10	10	12
0	22	21	19	18	16	13	16	15
0	24	20	16	21	17	21	16	18
0	-9	17	15	-9	-9	-9	-9	-9
0	24	22	20	21	17	14	14	10
0	24	19	16	19	-9	-9	-9	-9
0	22	21	7	4	4	4	3	3
0	16	18	19	-9	-9	-9	-9	-9
1	21	21	13	12	9	9	13	6
1	27	27	8	17	15	7	5	7
1	24	15	8	12	10	10	6	5
1	28	24	14	14	13	12	18	15
1	19	15	15	16	11	14	12	8
1	17	17	9	5	3	6	0	2
1	21	20	7	7	7	12	9	6
1	18	18	8	1	1	2	0	1

TABLE 6.1. Data from clinical trial of estrogen patches (continued)

Group	Pre 1	Pre 2	Post 1	Post 2	Post 3	Post 4	Post 5	Post 6
1	24	28	11	7	3	2	2	2
1	21	21	7	8	6	6	4	4
1	19	18	8	6	4	11	7	6
1	28	27	22	27	24	22	24	23
1	23	19	14	12	15	12	9	6
1	21	20	13	10	7	9	11	11
1	18	16	17	26	−9	−9	−9	−9
1	22	21	19	9	9	12	5	7
1	24	23	11	7	5	8	2	3
1	23	23	16	13	−9	−9	−9	−9
1	24	24	16	15	11	11	11	11
1	25	25	20	18	16	9	10	6
1	15	22	15	17	12	9	8	6
1	26	20	7	2	1	0	0	2
1	22	20	12	8	6	3	2	3
1	24	25	15	24	18	15	13	12
1	22	18	17	6	2	2	0	1
1	27	26	1	18	10	13	12	10
1	22	20	27	13	9	8	4	5
1	20	17	20	10	8	8	7	6
1	22	22	12	−9	−9	−9	−9	−9
1	20	22	15	2	4	6	3	3
1	21	23	11	9	10	8	7	4
1	17	17	15	−9	−9	−9	−9	−9
1	18	22	7	12	15	−9	−9	−9
1	23	26	24	9	−9	−9	−9	−9

As in most areas of statistics, it is wise to graph longitudinal data before undertaking any formal analyses. The following are some simple but useful guidelines:

- Show as much of the relevant data as possible rather than data summaries.

- Highlight aggregate patterns of potential scientific interest.

- Make easy the identification of unusual individuals or unusual observations.

An initial plot showing each women's profile of EPDS ratings is shown in Figure 6.1. The profiles belonging to each treatment group are identified by having different line types.
A number of points to note about Figure 6.1 are:

- Some profiles contain fewer than eight observations; these correspond to the women with missing values.

- There is a general decline in EPDS values over time.

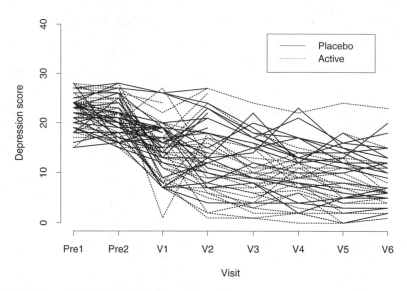

FIGURE 6.1. Individual EPDS profiles of the 61 women in the clinical trial of estrogen patches for postnatal depression.

- There is considerable variation in the response profiles.

- Women who are most depressed at the beginning of the study tend to be most depressed throughout. This phenomenon is known as *tracking*.

Tracking in a longitudinal study is usually more clearly seen if standardized values are plotted, i.e., the values obtained by subtracting the visit mean from the original observation and then dividing by the corresponding visit standard deviation. The resulting plot is given in Figure 6.2.

As well as the plots of individual profiles that are 'messy', we may want to produce some type of summary plot or plots. One that is often helpful is to construct box plots of the observations made on each visit separately for each treatment group. The resulting diagram is shown in Figure 6.3.

Once again, the series of box plots indicates a general decline in depression in both groups; it also indicates a possible outlying observation in the active treatment group on visits 3 to 6.

A more commonly used summary graph is that involving the mean profiles of each group, perhaps with some information about variability in each visit. Two possibilities are shown in Figures 6.4 and 6.5.

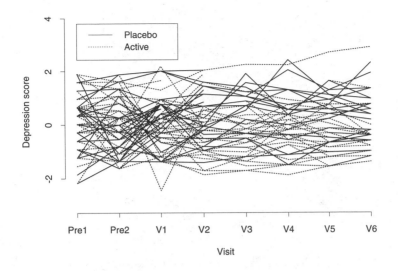

FIGURE 6.2. Plot of standardized EPDS values.

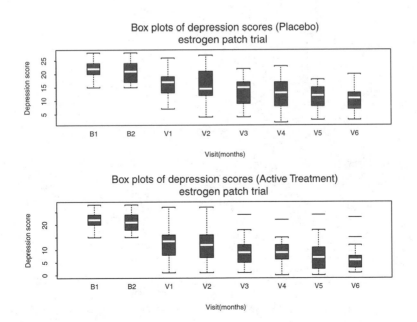

FIGURE 6.3. Box plots for each treatment group for the estrogen patch data.

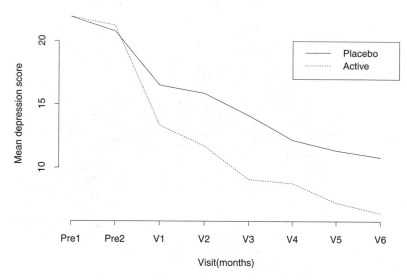

FIGURE 6.4. Treatment mean profiles for the estrogen patch data.

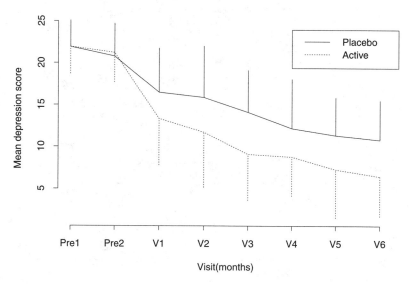

FIGURE 6.5. Treatment mean profiles for the estrogen patch data with visit standard deviations indicated.

6.3 Summary measure analysis of longitudinal data

A relatively straightforward approach to the analysis of longitudinal data is to first transform the T repeated measurements for each subject into a single number considered to 'capture' some important aspect of a subject's response profile; i.e., for each subject, calculate s given by

$$s = f(\mathbf{x}) \tag{6.1}$$

where $\mathbf{x}' = [x_1, x_2, \cdots, x_T]$ contains the set of T response values for the subject.

The summary measure to be used needs to be decided on before the analysis of the data begins and should, of course, be relevant to the particular questions that are of interest in the study. Commonly used summary measures are:

1. Overall mean

2. Maximum (minimum) value

3. Time to maximum (minimum) response

4. Regression slope

5. Time to reach a particular value (e.g., a fixed percentage of baseline)

Having identified a suitable summary measure, the analysis of treatment differences is reduced to a simple t-test (two groups) or analysis of variance (more than two groups). Alternatively, the nonparametric equivalents of these methods might be used if there is evidence of a departure from normality in the chosen summary measure.

To apply the summary measure approach to the postnatal depression data, we first need to consider how to deal with two possible complications:

• Missing values

• Two pretreatment assessments of the EPDS

To begin with we shall consider only the post-treatment measures and shall use the mean as our chosen summary statistic. And to deal with the missing values problem, we shall simply take the mean of the EPDS values a woman actually has.

The resulting summary measures are shown in Table 6.2. Before using these to look for any treatment difference, we can examine their distributional properties with a number of the simple plots discussed in Chapter 2. Figure 6.6, for example, shows Q-Q plots of the means in each treatment group. There is no compelling evidence of a departure from linearity in either plot, and so we will now apply an independent samples t-test to

TABLE 6.2. Mean summary measures of post-treatment EPDS ratings in estrogen patch trial

Placebo group

[1] 16.000	17.667	15.500	15.167	7.333	9.667	9.500	26.500	17.000	13.500
[11] 14.000	15.833	17.500	10.000	18.000	18.000	16.167	7.833	16.667	9.833
[21] 16.167	18.167	15.000	16.000	17.500	4.167	19.000			

Active group

[1] 10.333	9.833	8.500	14.333	12.667	4.167	8.000	2.167	4.500	5.917
[11] 7.000	23.667	11.333	10.167	21.500	10.167	6.000	14.500	12.500	13.167
[21] 11.167	2.000	5.667	16.167	4.667	10.667	11.000	9.833	12.000	5.500
[31] 8.167	15.000	11.333	24.000						

TABLE 6.3. *t*-test results on mean summary measures of estrogen patch data

```
Standard Two-Sample t-Test

data:  estrogen.rmp and estrogen.rma
t = 3.242, df = 59, p-value = 0.002
alternative hypothesis: true difference in means is not equal to 0
95 percent confidence interval:
 1.612 6.810
sample estimates:
 mean of x mean of y
     14.73     10.52
```

the summary measures for each treatment group. The results are shown in Table 6.3; they clearly indicate a difference between the two treatment groups. (There are a number of other ways to deal with the missing values; see Exercise 6.1.)

The pretreatment values available for each woman could be used in an analysis of the data in at least two ways:

- Calculation of change scores

- As covariates in an analysis of covariance

The results of both analyses are shown in Table 6.4. Again, a clear treatment difference is indicated in each case.

A number of authors have discussed the competing claims of change score analysis and analysis of covariance in the analysis of longitudinal data. All find in favour of analysis of covariance because it is more powerful than using change scores in all but pathological situations. For detailed discussions, see Frison and Pocock (1992) and Senn (1997).

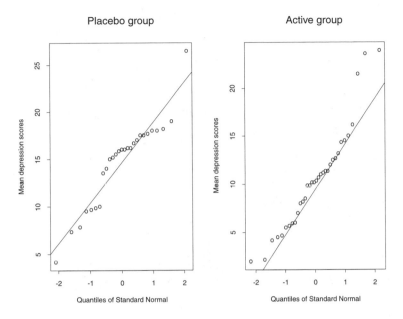

FIGURE 6.6. Q-Q normal plots for profile means in each treatment group of the estrogen patch data.

TABLE 6.4. Change score analysis using a t-test and ANCOVA
t-test

Standard Two-Sample t-Test

data: estrogen.pc and estrogen.ac
t = 3.489, df = 59, p-value = 0.0009
alternative hypothesis: true difference in means
    is not equal to 0
95 percent confidence interval:
 1.937 7.144
sample estimates:
 mean of x mean of y
    -6.531   -11.07

Analysis of covariance

	Df	Sum of Sq	Mean Sq	F Value	Pr(F)
group	1	267	266.9	11.38	0.00133
covar	1	138	137.5	5.86	0.01861
Residuals	58	1360	23.5		

6.4   Summary

The summary measure approach to the analysis of longitudinal data has the considerable advantage of being relatively simple and easy to understand by medical researchers who are not trained statisticians. Missing values can be handled without difficulty as can pretreatment baseline measures of the response variable. But the user of this approach needs to be aware that there are a number of questions that need to be considered.

- When there are missing values, the summary measure will be based on differing numbers of observations for each subject and, consequently, will have different precisions for each subject. This is conveniently forgotten in the use of a t-test, as described in this chapter. Mathews *et al.* (1990) describe a more refined summary measure approach that attempts to deal with this difficulty.

- The summary measure approach can introduce biases when there are missing values. For example, if there is a decreasing trend in depression and some subjects drops out early, the mean of all *available* data is likely to be an overestimate for those subjects.

- The summary measure approach does not always answer questions about how the response evolves over time; this would depend on the chosen summary measure.

So the summary measure approach to longitudinal data, while providing a simple and convenient first step in the analysis of such data, will, in general, need to be supplemented by other more complex analyses. Some possibilities will be discussed in Chapters 11 and 12 (see also exercises of these two chapters).

6.5   Using S-PLUS

Section 6.2

In this section of code the `matplot()` function is used to plot each individual's profile of depression scores on the same diagram. The `axis()` function is used to specify non-numeric axis labels. The `locator()` function is used to place appropriate legends interactively. Error bars are plotted using the `segments()` function.

Script for Section 6.2

```
estrogen<-matrix(scan("estrogen.dat"),ncol=9,byrow=T)
estrogen[estrogen==-9]<-NA
# -9 is used to code missing values. These values are
# replaced by the S-PLUS notation for missing values, NA

# individual profile plots
matplot(1:8,t(estrogen[,2:9]),type="l",
    lty=c(rep(1,27),rep(2,34)),lwd=2,axes=F,
    ylim=c(0,40),xlab="Visit",ylab="Depression score")
# axis=F stops the axes being plotted

axis(1,at=1:8,
    labels=c("Pre1","Pre2","V1","V2","V3","V4","V5","V6"))
axis(2)
legend(locator(1),c("Placebo","Active"),lty=1:2)
# a legend can be inserted; space was left by setting ylim
# larger than necessary to accommodate the data
```
⟹ Figure 6.1

```
# profiles plots of standardized values
mn<-apply(estrogen[,2:9],2,mean,na.rm=T)
sd<-sqrt(apply(estrogen[,2:9],2,var,na.method="omit"))
X<-sweep(estrogen[,2:9],2,mn)
X<-sweep(X,2,sd,FUN="/")
matplot(1:8,t(X),type="l",lty=c(rep(1,27),rep(2,34)),
    lwd=2,axes=F,
    ylim=c(-3,4),xlab="Visit",ylab="Depression score")
axis(1,at=1:8,
    labels=c("Pre1","Pre2","V1","V2","V3","V4","V5","V6"))
axis(2)
legend(locator(1),c("Placebo","Active"),lty=1:2)
```
⟹ Figure 6.2

```
#boxplots by group
estrogen.p<-estrogen[estrogen[,1]==0,-1]
```

```
estrogen.a<-estrogen[estrogen[,1]==1,-1]
# separates the data for the placebo and active groups

par(mfrow=c(2,1))
boxplot(estrogen.p[,1],estrogen.p[,2],estrogen.p[,3],
    estrogen.p[,4],estrogen.p[,5],estrogen.p[,6],
    estrogen.p[,7],estrogen.p[,8],
    names=c("B1","B2","V1","V2","V3","V4","V5","V6"),
    xlab="Visit(months)",
    ylab="Depression score",lwd=2)
# Produces the boxplots of each visit's observations
# for the placebo group

title("Box plots of depression scores (Placebo)\n
    estrogen patch trial",lwd=2)
boxplot(estrogen.a[,1],estrogen.a[,2],estrogen.a[,3],
    estrogen.a[,4],estrogen.a[,5],estrogen.a[,6],
    estrogen.a[,7],estrogen.a[,8],
    names=c("B1","B2","V1","V2","V3","V4","V5","V6"),
    xlab="Visit(months)",
    ylab="Depression score",lwd=2)
title("Box plots of depression scores (Active Treatment)\n
    estrogen patch trial",lwd=2)
```
⟹ Figure 6.3

```
# mean profile plot by group
par(mfrow=c(1,1))
meanp<-apply(estrogen.p,2,mean,na.rm=T)
meana<-apply(estrogen.a,2,mean,na.rm=T)
# the na.rm=T argument removes missing values before
# applying the mean
ylim<-range(c(meana,meanp))
# find a suitable range for the y-axis
plot(1:8,meanp,xlab="Visit(months)",
    ylab="Mean depression score",ylim=ylim,
    type="l",axes=F)
# plots mean profile for placebo without axes
axis(1,at=1:8,
    labels=c("Pre1","Pre2","V1","V2","V3","V4","V5","V6"))
axis(2)
lines(1:8,meana,lty=2)
legend(locator(1),c("Placebo","Active"),lty=1:2)
```
⟹ Figure 6.4

```
# Same plot with add error bars
sdp<-sqrt(apply(estrogen.p,2,var,na.method="avail"))
sda<-sqrt(apply(estrogen.a,2,var,na.method="avail"))

ylim<-c(min(min(meana-sda),min(meanp)),
```

```
      max(max(meana),max(meanp+sdp)))
plot(1:8,meanp,xlab="Visit(months)",
     ylab="Mean depression score",ylim=ylim,
     type="l",axes=F)
# Plots mean profile for placebo without axes
axis(1,at=1:8,
     labels=c("Pre1","Pre2","V1","V2","V3","V4","V5","V6"))
axis(2)
lines(1:8,meana,lty=2)
x<-1:8
segments(x, meanp+sdp, x, meanp)
# Draws line segments from (x[i],meanp[i]+sdp[i])
# to (x[i],meanp[i])
segments(x, meana, x, meana - sda,lty=2)
legend(locator(1),c("Placebo","Active"),lty=1:2)
```

$\Longrightarrow$ Figure 6.5

Section 6.3

Here, the `apply()` function is used to get the mean summary measure for
each individual. The functions `qqnorm()` and `qqline()` are used to plot
Q-Q plots, and `t.test()` and `aov()` are used for a *t*-test and ANCOVA.

Script for Section 6.3

```
# Summary measure analysis
estrogen.rmp<-apply(estrogen.p[,3:8],1,mean,na.rm=T)
estrogen.rma<-apply(estrogen.a[,3:8],1,mean,na.rm=T)
```

$\Longrightarrow$ Table 6.2

```
# Q-Q plot of means by group
par(mfrow=c(1,2))
qqnorm(estrogen.rmp,ylab="Mean depression scores")
qqline(estrogen.rmp)
title("Placebo group")
qqnorm(estrogen.rma,ylab="Mean depression scores")
qqline(estrogen.rma)
title("Active group")
```

$\Longrightarrow$ Figure 6.6

```
# We now have the required post-treatment summary measures
# for the two groups (means of usable values).
t.test(estrogen.rmp,estrogen.rma)
```

$\Longrightarrow$ Table 6.3

```
# Change score approach
estrogen.rmpp<-apply(estrogen.p[,1:2],1,mean,na.rm=T)
estrogen.rmpa<-apply(estrogen.a[,1:2],1,mean,na.rm=T)
estrogen.pc<-estrogen.rmp-estrogen.rmpp
estrogen.ac<-estrogen.rma-estrogen.rmpa
# Calculates change scores based on mean(pot)-mean(pre)
t.test(estrogen.pc, estrogen.ac)

# Analysis of covariance
group<-estrogen[,1]
covar<-c(estrogen.rmpp,estrogen.rmpa)
resp<-c(estrogen.rmp,estrogen.rma)
summary(aov(resp~group+covar))
```

$\Longrightarrow$ Table 6.4

6.6 Exercises

6.1 Repeat the summary measure analysis of the estrogen patch data using the mean but only using women with a complete set of post- treatment EPDS ratings. Do you think this type of analysis is advisable?

6.2 A well-known method of dealing with missing values in longitudinal data, particularly in the pharmaceutical industry, is the so called Last Observation Carried Forward (LOCF) method. Missing values for a subject are replaced by their last available value. Use this procedure in association with a summary measure analysis of the estrogen patch data using the mean, and compare the results with those in the text.

6.3 Comment on the LOCF approach.

6.4 Repeat all summary measure analyses of the estrogen patch data using a suitable nonparametric alternative to the t-test.

6.5 Repeat the summary measure analysis of the estrogen patch data using the slope of the regression of depression score on time for each individual.

6.6 Produce a graphical display of the estrogen patch data that includes the individual observations at each time point and a fitted linear regression of depression on time for each group.

6.7 Repeat the above exercise but use a locally weighted regression.

7

More Graphics

7.1 Introduction

The importance of displaying data graphically prior to more formal analyses has already been mentioned in Chapter 2. And in Chapter 4 the fundamental diagram for exploring relationships between pairs of variables, the scatterplot, was discussed. In this chapter, the use of a number of more ambitious graphical displays will be considered. Much of the material originates from the 'visualization' philosophy of William Cleveland as outlined in his two excellent books, *The Elements of Graphing Data* (Cleveland, 1985) and *Visualizing Data* (Cleveland, 1993). The approach can be summarized by the following two quotations from the most recent of these:

> Visualization is critical to data analysis. It provides a front line of attack, revealing intricate structure in data that cannot be absorbed in any other way. We discover unimagined effects, and we challenge imagined ones.

> There are two components to visualizing the structure of statistical data - graphing and fitting. Graphs are needed, of course, because visualization implies a process in which information is encoded in visual displays. Fitting mathematical functions to data is needed too. Just graphing raw data, without fitting them and without graphing the fits and residuals often leaves important aspects of data undiscovered.

7.2   The bubbleplot

The basic scatterplot described in Chapter 4 can only accommodate two variables. But there have been a number of suggestions as to how other variable values might be displayed on the diagram. In this section, we shall look at one of these, the *bubbleplot*. This is a technique for showing three-dimensional observations; two of the variables are chosen to form a scatterplot, and then the values of the third variable are represented by circles with radii proportional to these values centred on the appropriate point in the scatterplot. To illustrate this type of plot, we shall use the data obtained in a health survey of paint sprayers in a car assembly plant shown in Table 7.1. The variables are as follows:

HAEMO: haemoglobin concentration

PCV: packed cell volume

WBC: white blood cell count

LYMPHO: lymphocyte count

NEUTRO: neutrophil count

LEAD: serum lead concentration

A bubbleplot of the three variables, HAEMO, PCV and LEAD, is shown in Figure 7.1. The diagram illustrates the positive correlation among each pair of the three variables but also identifies one observation with an apparently abberant LEAD value, the other two variables being close to their means. (The observation is number 11 where the LEAD value is 62, perhaps a data entry error?)

TABLE 7.1. Health survey of paint sprayers in car assembly plant

	HAEMO	PCV	WBC	LYMPHO	NEUTRO	LEAD
1	13.4	39	4100	14	25	17
2	14.6	46	5000	15	30	20
3	13.5	42	4500	19	21	18
4	15.0	46	4600	23	16	18
5	14.6	44	5100	17	31	19
6	14.0	44	4900	20	24	19
7	16.4	49	4300	21	17	18
8	14.8	44	4400	16	26	29
9	15.2	46	4100	27	13	27
10	15.5	48	8400	34	42	36
11	15.2	47	5600	26	9	62
12	16.9	50	5100	28	17	23
13	14.8	44	4700	24	20	23
14	16.2	45	5600	26	25	19
15	14.7	43	4000	23	13	17
16	14.7	42	3400	9	22	13
17	16.5	45	5400	18	32	17
18	15.4	45	6900	28	36	24
19	15.1	45	4600	17	29	17
20	14.2	46	4200	14	25	28

TABLE 7.1: Health survey of paint sprayers in car assembly plant (continued)

	HAEMO	PCV	WBC	LYMPHO	NEUTRO	LEAD
21	15.9	46	5200	8	34	16
22	16.0	47	4700	25	14	18
23	17.4	50	8600	37	39	17
24	14.3	43	5500	20	31	19
25	14.8	44	4200	15	24	19
26	14.9	43	4300	9	32	17
27	15.5	45	5200	16	30	20
28	14.5	43	3900	18	18	25
29	14.4	45	6000	17	37	23
30	14.6	44	4700	23	21	27
31	15.3	45	7900	43	23	23
32	14.9	45	3400	17	15	24
33	15.8	47	6000	23	32	21
34	14.4	44	7700	31	39	23
35	14.7	46	3700	11	23	23
36	14.8	43	5200	25	19	22
37	15.4	45	6000	30	25	18
38	16.2	50	8100	32	38	18
39	15.0	45	4900	17	26	24
40	15.1	47	6000	22	33	16
41	16.0	46	4600	20	22	22
42	15.3	48	5500	20	23	23
43	14.5	41	6200	20	36	21
44	14.2	41	4900	26	20	20
45	15.0	45	7200	40	25	25
46	14.2	46	5800	22	31	22
47	14.9	45	8400	61	17	17
48	16.2	48	3100	12	15	18
49	14.5	45	4000	20	18	20
50	16.4	49	6900	35	22	24
51	14.7	44	7800	38	34	16
52	17.0	52	6300	19	21	16
53	15.4	47	3400	12	19	18
54	13.8	40	4500	19	23	21
55	16.1	47	4600	17	28	20
56	14.6	45	4700	23	22	27
57	15.0	44	5800	14	39	21
58	16.2	47	4100	16	24	18
59	17.0	51	5700	26	29	20
60	14.0	44	4100	16	24	18
61	15.4	46	6200	32	25	16
62	15.6	46	4700	28	16	16
63	15.8	48	4500	24	20	23
64	13.2	38	5300	16	26	20
65	14.9	47	5000	22	25	15
66	14.9	47	3900	15	19	16
67	14.0	45	5200	23	25	17
68	16.1	47	4300	19	22	22
69	14.7	46	6800	35	25	18
70	14.8	45	8900	47	36	17
71	17.0	51	6300	42	19	15
72	15.2	45	4600	21	22	18
73	15.2	43	5600	25	28	17
74	13.8	41	6300	25	27	15
75	14.8	43	6400	36	24	18
76	16.1	47	5200	18	28	25
77	15.0	43	6300	22	34	17
78	16.2	46	6000	25	25	24
79	14.8	44	3900	9	25	14
80	17.2	44	4100	12	27	18
81	17.2	48	5000	25	19	25
82	14.6	43	5500	22	31	19

TABLE 7.1: Health survey of paint sprayers in car assembly plant (continued)

	HAEMO	PCV	WBC	LYMPHO	NEUTRO	LEAD
83	14.4	44	4300	20	20	15
84	15.4	48	5700	29	26	24
85	16.0	52	4100	21	15	22
86	15.0	45	5000	27	18	20
87	14.8	44	5700	29	23	23
88	15.4	43	3300	10	20	19
89	16.0	47	6100	32	23	26
90	14.8	43	5100	18	31	19
91	13.8	41	8100	52	24	17
92	14.7	43	5200	24	24	17
93	14.6	44	9899	69	28	18
94	13.6	42	6100	24	30	15
95	14.5	44	4800	14	29	15
96	14.3	39	5000	25	20	19
97	15.3	45	4000	19	19	16
98	16.4	49	6000	34	22	17
99	14.8	44	4500	22	18	25
100	16.6	48	4700	17	27	20
101	16.0	49	7000	36	28	18
102	15.5	46	6600	30	33	13
103	14.3	46	5700	26	20	21

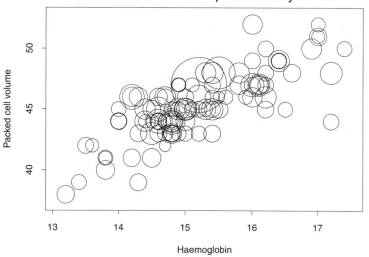

FIGURE 7.1. Bubbleplot for paint-sprayer data.

7.3   The scatterplot matrix

In the data from paint sprayers in a car assembly plant, the seven observed variables generate between them 21 possible scatterplots, and it is very important that the separate bivariate displays be presented in a way that aids in overall comprehension and understanding of the data. The *scatterplot matrix* is intended to accomplish exactly this objective.

A scatterplot matrix is defined as a square, symmetric grid of bivariate scatterplots. This grid has p rows and columns, each one corresponding to a different variable. Each of the grid's cells shows a scatterplot of two variables. Variable j is plotted against variable i in the ijth cell, and the same variables appear in cell ji with the x- and y-axes of the scatterplots interchanged. The reason for including both the upper and lower triangles of the grid, despite the seeming redundancy, is that it enables a row and a column to be visually scanned to see one variable against all others, with the scales for the one variable lined up along the horizontal or the vertical.

The scatterplot matrix of the data on paint sprayers is shown in Figure 7.2. One very noticeable feature of this plot is the clear indication of two outliers on the LEAD variable. Another is the very strong linear relationship between LYMPHO and WBC and between HAEMO and PCV. The plots involving the PCV cell suffer from the small number of discrete values observed for this variable. A possible solution is to produce a 'jittered' scatterplot matrix as shown in Figure 7.3.

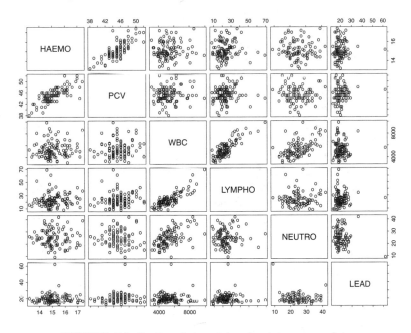

FIGURE 7.2. Scatterplot matrix of paint-sprayer data.

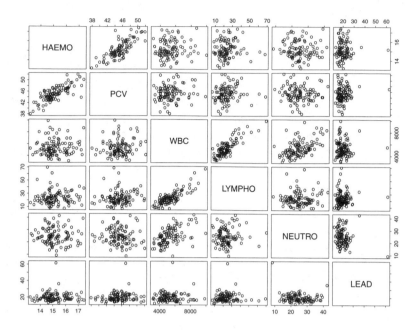

FIGURE 7.3. Jittered scatterplot matrix of paint-sprayer data.

Taking Cleveland's advice that simply plotting the raw data is not usually enough, Figure 7.4 shows the scatterplot matrix of the data on paint sprayers, with each cell in the grid displaying both the appropriate fitted linear and locally weighted regressions. This figure demonstrates again why it is essential to use to full, square scatterplot matrix, rather than a half-matrix, lower diagonal version; the dependence between pairs of variables is asymmetric. The smooth curve for a pair of variables will differ when one or another variable is placed on the vertical (or horizontal) axis. For example, consider the LEAD/NEUTRO and NEUTRO/LEAD cells of the grid. The overall message to be taken from Figure 7.4, however, is the remarkable similarity of the linear and locally weighted regression fits.

All methods discussed in Chapter 4 for enhancing scatterplots to make them more informative could be applied to each of the individual cells of a scatterplot matrix. Figure 7.5 shows an example of what can be done; here, a contour plot of the bivariate density estimate of each pair of variables is added to each panel. Implementing the many other possibilities is left as an exercise for the reader—see, for example, Exercise 7.1.

7.4   Conditioning plots

The *conditioning plot* or *coplot* is a particularly powerful visualization tool for studying how a response variable depends on two or more explanatory

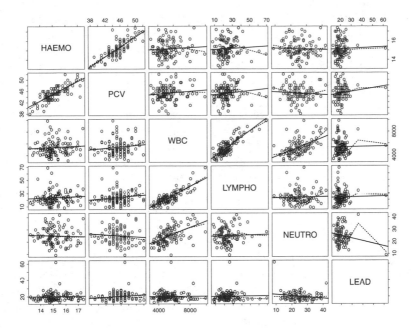

FIGURE 7.4. Scatterplot matrix with linear and locally weighted regression fits for paint-spayer data.

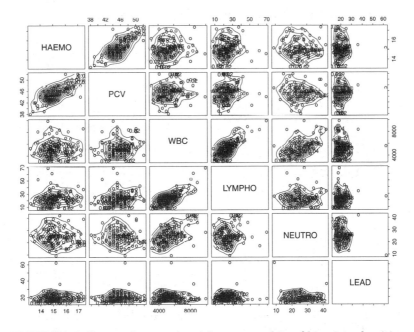

FIGURE 7.5. Scatterplot matrix with contour plots of bivariate densities.

variables. In essence, such a plot displays the bivariate relationship between two variables while holding constant (or 'conditioning upon') the values of one or more other variables. There are several varieties of conditioning plot, with the differences being largely a matter of presentation rather than real substance. The most useful way to describe this type of plot is by means of a number of examples.

The first data set we shall consider is shown in Table 7.2. This arises from a random sample of people responding to a newspaper advertisement for volunteers to participate in a medical research project and consists of a score on a test measuring level of knowledge of good health practices along with the recipient's age and area of residence.

Here, we shall examine conditioning plots of the relationship between age and the good health practices score, conditional on area of residence. So in this case, the conditioning plot is nothing more than three age/score scatterplots, one for each area of residence. These plots might be presented in a number of ways, two of which are shown in Figure 7.6. The only difference in the two plots is that the aspect ratio (see Chapter 4) of the scatterplots has been altered. Each scatterplot suggests that there is a negative relationship between age and health awareness score—older people do not appear to be as well informed about good health practices. This relationship appears to be somewhat stronger in area of residence B. We can add the fitted linear regression and locally weighted regression curves to each scatterplot to make the diagram more informative—see Figure 7.7. The relationship between age and the health awareness score appears predominately linear.

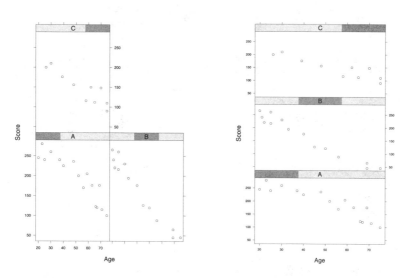

FIGURE 7.6. Conditioning plots: age against score for each area of residence using two different aspect ratios.

TABLE 7.2. Health survey volunteers in medical research project

Score	Age	Area
112	65	C
230	30	B
280	23	A
205	59	A
236	48	A
260	25	B
176	39	C
245	20	A
123	66	A
176	40	B
216	25	B
176	63	A
90	75	C
176	69	A
240	37	A
88	56	B
120	67	A
220	22	B
260	30	A
45	69	B
210	30	C
225	40	A
126	45	B
200	26	C
240	21	B
170	56	A
116	58	C
120	50	B
200	52	A
45	75	B
110	75	C
150	62	C
148	70	C
265	20	B
194	33	B
156	48	C
100	75	A
115	71	A
65	69	B
240	25	A

(a)   (b)

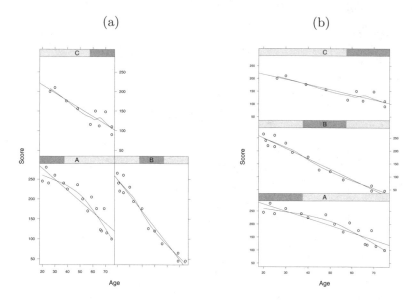

FIGURE 7.7. Conditioning plots with linear and locally weighted regression curves: age against score for each area of residence using two different aspect ratios.

Next, we shall construct conditioning plots for the data shown in Table 7.3 These relate to using a particular hypotensive drug to lower a patient's blood pressure during surgery. The sooner the blood pressure rises again to normal after the drug is discontinued, the better. The recovery time given is the time in minutes before the patient's systolic blood pressure returned to 100 mm of mercury. Also given are the logarithm (base 10) of the dose of the drug in milligrams and the average systolic blood pressure achieved while the drug was being administered. Primary interest is in how recovery time is related to the other two variables.

Here, we shall concentrate on the coplot of log(dose) on time given blood pressure. Because here the conditioning variable is continuous, it is divided into a number of (overlapping) intervals and scatterplots of log(dose) v. time plotted for each interval. The basic plot is shown in Figure 7.8. In this diagram, the panel at the top of the figure is known as the *given panel*; the panels below are *dependence panels*. Each rectangle in the given panel specifies a range of values of blood pressure. On a corresponding dependence panel, log(dose) is plotted against recovery time for those observations whose blood pressure values lie in the particular interval. To match blood pressure intervals to dependence panels, the latter are examined in order from left to right in the bottom row and then again from left to right in subsequent rows.

TABLE 7.3. Hypotensive drug to lower a patient's blood pressure during surgery

Logdose	BP	Time	Logdose	BP	Time
2.26	66	7	2.70	73	39
1.81	52	10	1.90	56	28
1.78	72	18	2.78	83	12
1.54	67	4	2.27	67	60
2.06	69	10	1.74	84	10
1.74	71	13	2.62	68	60
2.56	88	21	1.80	64	22
2.29	68	12	1.81	60	21
1.80	59	9	1.58	62	14
2.32	73	65	2.41	76	4
2.04	68	20	1.65	60	27
1.88	58	31	2.24	60	26
1.18	61	23	1.70	59	28
2.08	68	22	2.45	84	15
1.70	69	13	1.72	66	8
1.74	55	9	2.37	68	46
1.90	67	50	2.23	65	24
1.79	67	12	1.92	69	12
2.11	68	11	1.99	72	25
1.72	59	8	1.99	63	45
1.74	68	26	2.35	56	72
1.60	63	16	1.80	70	25
2.15	65	23	2.36	69	28
2.26	72	7	1.59	60	10
1.65	58	11	2.10	51	25
1.63	69	8	1.80	61	44
2.40	70	14			

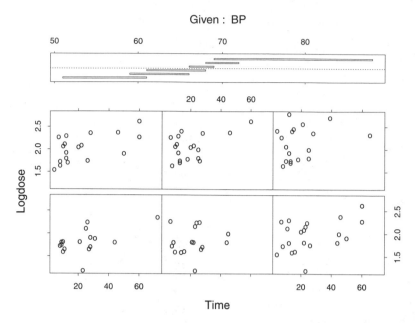

FIGURE 7.8. Conditioning plot for blood pressure data.

In Figure 7.9, least squares and locally weighted regressions are added to each panel. It appears that the basic relationship between log(dose) and time is very similar at all levels of blood pressure.

7.5   Trellis graphics

The conditional graphical displays illustrated above are simple examples of a more general scheme known as *trellis graphics* (Becker and Cleveland, 1994). This is an approach to examining high-dimensional structure in data by means of one-, two-, and three-dimensional graphs. The problem addressed is how observations of one or more variables depends on the observations of the other variables. The essential feature of this approach is the multipanel conditioning that allows some type of plot to be displayed for different values of a given variable (or variables). The aim is to help in understanding both the structure of the data and how well proposed models describe the structure.

In the coplot described previously, a simple scatterplot appears in each panel, but more complex graphics could be used. For example, Figure 7.10 shows scatterplot matrices for five of the variables in the paint sprayers data conditioning on WBC, and Figure 7.11 shows box plots of HAEMO for two groups of PCV (35 to 44 and 45 to 54) values conditioned on WBC.

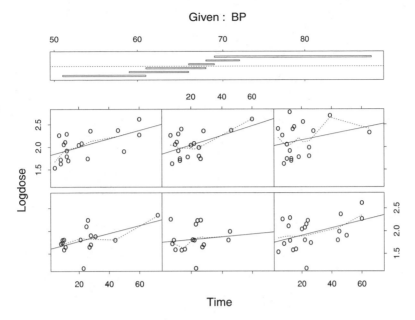

FIGURE 7.9. Conditioning plot for blood pressure data with linear and locally weighted regression curves.

Finally, Figure 7.12 shows a variety of graphical displays conditioned on various variables arranged on the same diagram.

A recent example of the use of trellis graphics in a longitudinal study is given in Verbyla *et al.*, 1999. Trellis graphics is a potentially very exciting and very powerful tool for the analysis of data from medical studies. But a word of caution is perhaps in order. With small or moderately sized data sets, the number of observations in each panel may be too few to make the panel graphic convincing.

7.6   Summary

There are now many exciting graphical displays for use with all types of data. Only a small subset of the possibilities have been investigated in this chapter, and readers are encouraged to explore the many other options available with S-PLUS.

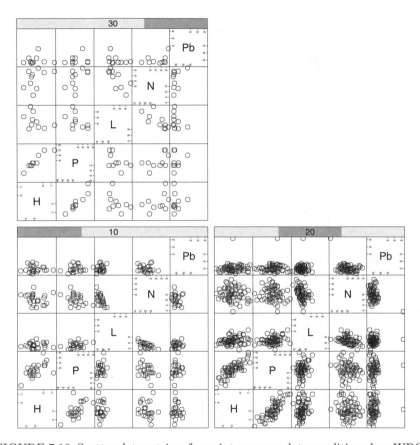

FIGURE 7.10. Scatterplot matrices for paint sprayers data conditioned on WBC.

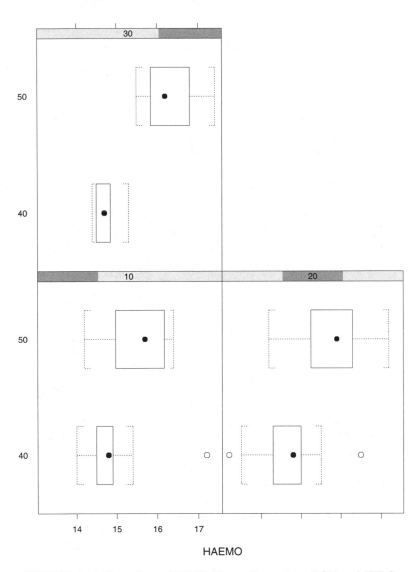

FIGURE 7.11. Box plots of HAEMO conditioned on PCV and WBC.

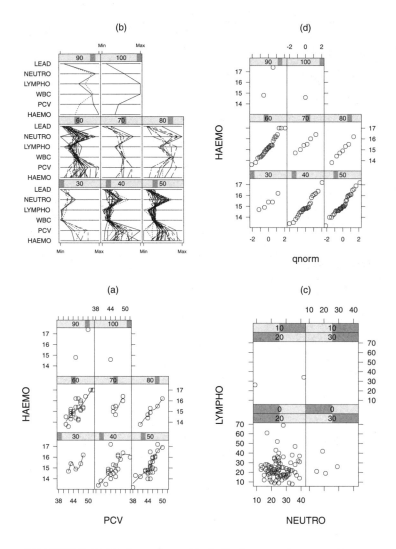

FIGURE 7.12. Variety of graphical displays on the same diagram.

7.7   Using S-PLUS

Section 7.2

A bubbleplot is constructed using the `symbols()` function. This function could also be used to construct displays that accommodate more than three variables. Readers are encouraged to explore these possibilities.

Script for Section 7.2

```
# Use data on paint sprayers
paint<-road.table("paint.dat",header=T)
attach(paint)

# Construct bubbleplot for HAEMO, PCV and LEAD
win.graph()
symbols(HAEMO,PCV,circles=LEAD,inches=0.5,xlab="Haemoglobin",
   ylab="Packed cell volume")
title("Scatterplot of haemoglobin concentration v packed
   cell volume with lead represented by circles")
```
$\Longrightarrow$ Figure 7.1

Section 7.3

Here, the `pairs()` function is used to produce scatterplot matrices. Each panel of such a display can be enhanced in many ways by using the argument `panel=function(x,y)`. A number of examples are given.

Script for Section 7.3

```
# Construct scatterplot matrix using the pairs function
paint1<-paint[,-1]
pairs(paint1)
```
$\Longrightarrow$ Figure 7.2

```
# Now jitter data before plotting
pairs(paint1,
   panel=function(x,y){
      x<-jitter(x)
      y<-jitter(y)
      points(x,y)
   }
)
```
$\Longrightarrow$ Figure 7.3

```
# Now add least-squares regression lines and locally weighted
# regressions to each panel
pairs(paint1,
```

```
      panel=function(x,y) {
          abline(lm(y~x),lwd=2)
          lines(lowess(x,y),lty=2,lwd=2)
          points(x,y)
      }
)
```

$\implies$ Figure 7.4

```
pairs(paint1,
    panel=function(x,y) {
        points(x,y)
        den<-tdden1(x,y)
        contour(den$seqx,den$seqy,
        den$den,add=T,nlevels=10,
        xlab="",ylab="")
    }
)
```

$\implies$ Figure 7.5

Section 7.4

In this section's codes, the trellis graphics function `xyplot()` is used to produce a coplot in addition to the `coplot()` function. Here, a model formula is used of the form y ~ x | z, where z is the conditioning variable. Use of the `panel=function(x,y)` argument for enhancing the plots is again demonstrated. The `par.strip.text`, `xlab` and `ylab` options are used to increase the size of the strip labels and axis labels and titles.

Script for Section 7.4

```
# Read health data
health<-read.table("health.dat",header=T)
attach(health)

# Open window for trellis graphics
trellis.device(win.graph)

# Conditioning plot
xyplot(Score~Age|Area,
    par.strip.text=list(cex=1.3),
    xlab=list(cex=1.3),ylab=list(cex=1.3)
)


# Changing the aspect ratio
xyplot(Score~Age|Area,aspect=1/2,
    par.strip.text=list(cex=1.3),
    xlab=list(cex=1.3),ylab=list(cex=1.3)
)
```

$\Longrightarrow$ Figure 7.6

```
# Conditioning plots with regression line and smooth
xyplot(Score~Age|Area,
    par.strip.text=list(cex=1.3),
    xlab=list(cex=1.3),ylab=list(cex=1.3),
    panel=function(x,y){
        panel.smooth(x,y,lty=1)
        abline(lm(y~x))
    }
)

# Changing the aspect ratio
xyplot(Score~Age|Area,aspect=1/2,
    par.strip.text=list(cex=1.3),
    xlab=list(cex=1.3),ylab=list(cex=1.3),
    panel=function(x,y){
        panel.smooth(x,y,lty=1)
        abline(lm(y~x))
    }
)
```

$\Longrightarrow$ Figure 7.7

```
# Read blood data
blood<-read.table("surgery.dat",header=T)
attach(blood)

# Conditioning on continuous variable: blood pressure
coplot(Logdose~Time|BP)
```

$\Longrightarrow$ Figure 7.8

```
# Adding regression line and smooth
coplot(Logdose~Time|BP,
    panel=function(x,y){
        lines(lowess(x,y),lty=2)
        abline(lsfit(x,y)$coef)
        points(x,y)
    }
)
```

$\Longrightarrow$ Figure 7.9

Section 7.5

The function splom() is used to create a scatterplot matrix conditioning on another variable. Several trellis graphs are displayed on a single display using the print() function with the split option.

Script for Section 7.5

```
# Calculate a series on intervals of WBC and store as a
# factor variable
WBC.int<-as.factor(10*round(WBC/3000))
trellis.device(win.graph)

# Construct a scatterplot matrix for each interval of WBC
splom(~paint[,-c(1,4)]|WBC.int,col=1,
    varnames=c("H","P","L","N","Pb"))
```
$\Longrightarrow$ Figure 7.10

```
# Construct a series of intervals for PCV
PCV.int<-as.factor(10*round(PCV/10))

# Produce box plots conditioned on WBC
trellis.device(win.graph)
bwplot(PCV.int~HAEMO|WBC.int,col=1)
```
$\Longrightarrow$ Figure 7.11

```
# Calculate new set of intervals for WBC and PCV and
# introduce intervals for LEAD
WBC.int<-as.factor(10*round(WBC/1000))
WBC.int1<-as.factor(10*round(WBC/5000))
PCV.int<-as.factor(10*round(PCV/20))
LEAD.int<-as.factor(10*round(LEAD/60))

# Arrange a number of trellis displays on the same page
# Graphs are first stored and then printed at the
# required postions using the split argument
trellis.device(win.graph)
gr1<-xyplot(HAEMO~PCV|WBC.int,main="(a)",
    panel=function(x,y) { if(length(y)>2) panel.loess(x,y,col=1)
                                          panel.xyplot(x,y,col=1)})
gr2<-parallel(~paint[,-1]|WBC.int,col=1,main="(b)")
gr3<-xyplot(LYMPHO~NEUTRO|PCV.int*LEAD.int,col=1,main="(c)")
gr4<-qqmath(~HAEMO|WBC.int,main="(d)")
print(gr1,split=c(1,1,2,2),more=T)
print(gr2,split=c(1,2,2,2),more=T)
print(gr3,split=c(2,1,2,2),more=T)
print(gr4,split=c(2,2,2,2),more=T)
```
$\Longrightarrow$ Figure 7.12

7.8   Exercises

7.1 The bubbleplot makes it possible to accommodate three variable values on a scatterplot. More than three values can be ac-
comodated by using what might be termed a *star plot* in which

the extra variable values are represented by the lengths of the sides of a star. Construct such a plot for the paint sprayer's data using the `symbols()` function.

7.2 Construct a scatterplot matrix of the data on paint sprayers, including in each panel information about the univariate marginal distribution of each variable.

7.3 Further investigate the use of the `coplot()` function of the paint sprayer's data set by selecting the ranges of the conditioning variable in various ways, including using the function `co.intervals()`.

7.4 Multivariate normality can be tested by a chi-square probability plot of ordered distances of observations from the sample mean, i.e.,

$$d_i = (\mathbf{x}_i - \bar{\mathbf{x}})'\mathbf{S}^{-1}(\mathbf{x}_i - \bar{\mathbf{x}})$$

where $\mathbf{S}$ is the sample covariance matrix. Write an S-PLUS function to produce such a plot for a set of multivariate data, and apply it to the data on paint sprayers.

8
Multiple Linear Regression

8.1 Introduction

Multiple linear regression represents a generalization to more than a single explanatory variable of the simple linear regression model introduced in Chapter 4. The aim of this type of regression is to model the relationship between a random response variable and a number of explanatory variables. Strictly speaking, the values of the explanatory variable are assumed to be known, or under the control of the investigator; in other words, they are not considered to be random variables. In most applications of multiple regression, however, the observed values of the explanatory variables will, like the response variable, be subject to random variation. Parameter estimation and inference is then considered conditional on the observed values of the explanatory variables.

8.2 The multiple linear regression model

The multiple linear regression model relates a response variable to a set of explanatory variables. The relationship assumed is linear (in terms of the parameters rather than in terms of the explanatory variables), and the parameters in the model (usually known as *regression coefficients*) are generally estimated by least squares. An inferential framework is added by making specific distributional assumptions about the error terms in the model. Details of the structure of the model are given in Display 8.1, and estimation and testing are described in Display 8.2.

8.2.1 Anesthesia example

As a first illustration of the application of the multiple regression model, it will be applied to the data shown in Table 8.1, which arise from a study reported in Cullen and van Belle (1975), dealing with the amount of anesthetic agent administered during an operation. The variables involved are as follows:

- Response variable y: percentage depression of lymphocyte transformation following anethesia.

- Explanatory variable x_1: duration of anesthesia (in hours).

- Explanatory variable x_2: trauma factor rated on a five-point scale.

The results of fitting the multiple regression model described in Display 8.1 to these data are shown in Table 8.2. Here, the F-test that the regression coefficients β_1 and β_2 are both zero has an associated p-value of 0.055, and the t-statistics given by the ratios of the estimated regression coefficients to their estimated standard errors have associated p-values of 0.76 and 0.17. It appears that neither duration of anesthesia nor degree of trauma are useful for predicting percentage of depression of lymphocyte transformation following anethesia. The R-squared value of just 0.17 underlines this finding. Only 17% of the variance in the response variable is accounted for by the two explanatory variables. The number of observations in this example is, however, rather small, and so inferences are not particularly powerful.

8.2.2 Cystic fibrosis example

Our second example uses data from a study of 25 patients with cystic fibrosis reported in O'Neill et al. (1983). The data are given in Altman (1991) and are shown here in Table 8.3. The dependent variable in this case, PEmax, is a measure of malnutrition in these patients; the explanatory variables relate largely to body size or lung function. In this example, the number of observations relative to the number of variables is clearly too low; so all results should be interpreted with caution.

Note that one of the explanatory variables in Table 8.3 is sex, a binary variable, coded as 0 for male subjects and 1 for female subjects. This causes no problem for the regression model because no distributional assumptions are made about the explanatory variables—indeed, as pointed out in the introduction, strictly speaking, they are not regarded as random variables at all. The regression coefficient for a binary variable will indicate the average

---

Display 8.1 The multiple regression model

- Assume y_i represents the value of the response variable on the ith individual, and that $x_{i1}, x_{i2}, \cdots, x_{in}$ respresent the individual's values on p explanatory variables, with $i = 1, 2 \cdots n$.

- The multiple linear regression model is given by

$$y_i = \beta_0 + \beta_1 x_{i1} + \cdots + \beta_p x_{ip} + \epsilon_i \qquad (1)$$

- The residual or error terms $\epsilon_i, i = 1, \cdots, n$ are assumed to be independent random variables having a normal distribution with mean zero and constant variance σ^2.

- Consequently, the distribution of the random response variable, y, is also normal with expected value.

$$E(y|x_1, x_2, \cdots, x_p) = \beta_0 + \beta_1 x_1 + \cdots + \beta_p x_p \qquad (2)$$

and variance σ^2.

- The parameters of the model $\beta_k, k = 1, 2, \cdots, p$ are known as *regression coefficients*. They represent the expected change in the response variable associated with a unit change in the corresponding explanatory variable, when the remaining explanatory variables are held constant.

- The 'linear' in multiple linear regression applies to the regression parameters, not to the response or explanatory variables. Consequently, models in which, for example, the logarithm of a response variable is modeled in terms of quadratic functions of some of the explanatory variables would still be included in this class of models.

- The multiple regression model can be written most conveniently for all n individuals by using matrices and vectors as

$$\mathbf{y} = \mathbf{X}\boldsymbol{\beta} + \boldsymbol{\epsilon} \qquad (3)$$

where $\mathbf{y}' = [y_1, y_2, \cdots, y_n]$, $\boldsymbol{\beta}' = [\beta_0, \beta_1, \cdots, \beta_p]$, $\boldsymbol{\epsilon}' = [\epsilon_1, \epsilon_2, \cdots, \epsilon_n]$ and

$$\mathbf{X} = \begin{bmatrix} 1 & x_{11} & x_{12} & \cdots & x_{1p} \\ 1 & x_{21} & x_{22} & \cdots & x_{2p} \\ \vdots & \vdots & \vdots & \vdots & \vdots \\ 1 & x_{n1} & x_{n2} & \cdots & x_{np} \end{bmatrix} \qquad (4)$$

- Each row in $\mathbf{X}$ (sometimes known as the *design matrix*) represents the values of the explanatory variables for one of the individuals in the sample, with the addition of unity to take account of the parameter β_0.

Display 8.2 Estimation and testing in multiple regression

- Assuming that $\mathbf{X'X}$ is nonsingular, (i.e., can be inverted), then the least-squares estimator of the parameter vector $\boldsymbol{\beta}$ is

$$\hat{\boldsymbol{\beta}} = (\mathbf{X'X})^{-1}\mathbf{X'y} \tag{1}$$

- This estimator $\hat{\boldsymbol{\beta}}$ has the following properties

$$
\begin{aligned}
E(\hat{\boldsymbol{\beta}}) &= \boldsymbol{\beta} & (2) \\
\text{cov}(\hat{\boldsymbol{\beta}}) &= \sigma^2(\mathbf{X'X})^{-1} & (3)
\end{aligned}
$$

- The diagonal elements of the matrix $\text{cov}(\hat{\boldsymbol{\beta}})$ give the variances of the $\hat{\beta}_j$, whereas the off diagonal elements give the covariances between pairs $\hat{\beta}_j, \hat{\beta}_k$. The square roots of the diagonal elements of the matrix are thus the standard errors of the $\hat{\beta}_j$.

- The regression analysis can be assessed using the following analysis of variance table.

Source of Variation	Sum of Squares	Degrees of Freedom	Mean Square
Regression	$\sum_{i=1}^{n}(\hat{y}_i - \bar{y})^2$	p	MSR=SS/df
Residual	$\sum_{i=1}^{n}(y_i - \hat{y}_i)^2$	$n-p-1$	MSE=SS/df
Total	$\sum_{i=1}^{n}(y_i - \bar{y})^2$	$n-1$	

where $\hat{y}_i$ is the predicted value of the response variable for the ith individual ($\hat{y}_i = \hat{\beta}_0 + \hat{\beta}_1 x_{ij} + \cdots + \hat{\beta}_p x_{ip}$) and $\bar{y}$ is the mean value of the response variable.

- The mean square ratio MSR/MSE provides an F-test of the general hypothesis

$$H_0 : \beta_1 = \beta_2 = \cdots = \beta_p = 0 \tag{4}$$

- An estimate of σ^2 is provided by s^2 given by

$$s^2 = \frac{1}{n-p-1}\sum_{i=1}^{n}(y_i - \hat{y}_1)^2 \tag{5}$$

- Under H_0, the mean square ratio has an F-distribution with $p, n-p-1$ degress of freedom.

- The correlation between the observed values y_i and the predicted values $\hat{y}_i$, R, is known as the multiple correlation coefficient. The value of R^2 gives the proportion of variance of the response variable accounted for by the explanatory variables.

- Individual regression coefficients can be assessed by using the ratio $\hat{\beta}_j/\text{SE}(\hat{\beta}_j)$, although these ratios should only be used as rough guides to the 'significance' or otherwise of the coefficients for reasons discussed in the text.

TABLE 8.1. Duration of anesthetic data

Duration	Trauma	Depression
4.0	3	36.7
6.0	3	51.3
1.5	2	40.8
4.0	2	58.3
2.5	2	42.2
3.0	2	34.6
3.0	2	77.8
2.5	2	17.2
3.0	3	−38.4
3.0	3	1.0
2.0	3	53.7
8.0	3	14.3
5.0	4	65.0
2.0	2	5.6
2.5	2	4.4
2.0	2	1.6
1.5	2	6.2
1.0	1	12.2
3.0	3	29.9
4.0	3	76.1
3.0	3	11.5
3.0	3	19.8
7.0	4	64.9
6.0	4	47.8
2.0	2	35.0
4.0	2	1.7
2.0	2	51.5
1.0	1	20.2
1.0	1	−9.3
2.0	1	13.9
1.0	1	−19.0
3.0	1	−2.3
4.0	3	41.6
8.0	4	18.4
2.0	2	9.9

TABLE 8.2. Results of applying the multiple linear regression model to the duration of anesthesia data

```
Call: lm(formula = Depress ~ Duration + Trauma)
Residuals:
   Min    1Q Median   3Q   Max
 -70.3 -17.4   2.22 17.2  56.3


Coefficients:
             Value Std. Error t value Pr(>|t|)
(Intercept) -2.555   12.395    -0.206   0.838
   Duration  1.105    3.620     0.305   0.762
     Trauma 10.376    7.460     1.391   0.174


Residual standard error: 25.7 on 32 degrees of freedom
Multiple R-Squared: 0.166
F-statistic: 3.18 on 2 and 32 degrees of freedom, the p-value is 0.0548


Correlation of Coefficients:
         (Intercept) Duration
Duration  0.148
   Trauma -0.712       -0.762
```

TABLE 8.3. **Cystic fibrosis data**

Sub	Age	Sex	Height	Weight	BMP	FEV	RV	FRC	TLC	PEmax
1	7	0	109	13.1	68	32	258	183	137	95
2	7	1	112	12.9	65	19	449	245	134	85
3	8	0	124	14.1	64	22	441	268	147	100
4	8	1	125	16.2	67	41	234	146	124	85
5	8	0	127	21.5	93	52	202	131	104	95
6	9	0	130	17.5	68	44	308	155	118	80
7	11	1	139	30.7	89	28	305	179	119	65
8	12	1	150	28.4	69	18	369	198	103	110
9	12	0	146	25.1	67	24	312	194	128	70
10	13	1	155	31.5	68	23	413	225	136	95
11	13	0	156	39.9	89	39	206	142	95	110
12	14	1	153	42.1	90	26	253	191	121	90
13	14	0	160	45.6	93	45	174	139	108	100
14	15	1	158	51.2	93	45	158	124	90	80
15	16	1	160	35.9	66	31	302	133	101	134
16	17	1	153	34.8	70	29	204	118	120	134
17	17	0	174	44.7	70	49	187	104	103	165
18	17	1	176	60.1	92	29	188	129	130	120
19	17	0	171	43.6	69	38	172	130	103	130
20	19	1	156	37.2	72	21	216	119	81	85
21	19	0	174	54.6	86	37	184	118	101	85
22	20	0	178	64.0	86	34	225	148	135	160
23	23	0	180	73.8	97	57	171	108	98	165
24	23	0	175	51.1	71	33	224	131	112	95
25	23	0	179	71.5	95	52	225	127	101	195

difference in the response variable between the groups defined by the binary variable, adjusted for any differences between the groups with respect to the other variables in the model. (A multiple regression model that includes both continuous and categorical explanatory variables is essentially equivalent to the analysis of covariance model introduced in Chapter 5.)

Before undertaking a multiple regression analysis, it is often useful to plot the data in some way. Here, we shall examine a number of scatterplot matrices, leaving out the binary variable sex.

Figure 8.1 shows a straightforward scatterplot matrix of the data. There are no obvious outliers, but the distribution of BMP values appears at first sight to be rather odd. A possible explanation is that the sample contains both men and women, whose body mass is likely to show a clear difference. We can examine this possibility by plotting the BMP variable against the binary variable used to code sex—see Figure 8.2. This graph suggests that the division of BMP values seen in Figure 8.1 does *not* relate directly to sex, but arises from a division in both males and females into individuals with large and individuals with small BMP values.

Figure 8.3 shows a scatterplot matrix of the data in which each panel is enhanced with both a linear regression and a locally weighted regression fit. There appears to be no strong evidence for using a nonlinear function for any explanatory variable in the regression model, although this possibility will be investigated in Chapter 14 using *generalized additive models*.

The results of fitting a multiple regression model to the cystic fibrosis data are shown in Table 8.4. Note that we are overfitting the data here by using nine explanatory variables when there are only 25 observations, but we will ignore this problem here. Here, the F-test that the regression coefficients of all the explanatory variables are zero has an associated p-value of 0.03, suggesting that at least some of the regression coefficients are not zero. The R-squared value of 0.64 shows that 64% of the variance of PE max is accountable for by the explanatory variables. The t-statistics associated with each regression coefficient are, however, all nonsignificant. It has to be remembered that both terms defining the t-statistic, namely, the estimated regression coefficient and its estimated standard error, are estimated *conditional* on the other variables in the model. If, for example, a variable is removed from consideration, then the regression coefficients of the remaining variables (and their standard errors) would need to be reestimated from a new analysis excluding the variable. Because the t-statistics can, for this reason, only give a rough guide to which explanatory variables are, and which are not, predictive of the response variable, other methods are generally used to try to identify informative subsets of the explanatory variables in multiple regression, as we shall see in the next section.

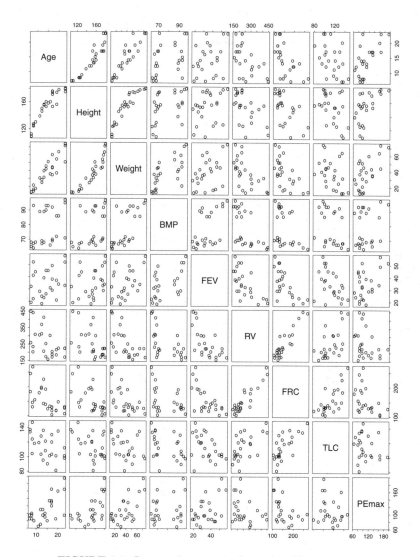

FIGURE 8.1. Scatterplot matrix for cystic fibrosis data.

TABLE 8.4. Multiple regression for cystic fibrosis data

```
Call: lm(formula = PEmax ~ Age + Sex + Height + Weight + BMP
+ FEV + RV + FRC + TLC)
Residuals:
  Min  1Q Median  3Q  Max
 -37.2 -12   1.41 13.6 33.3
```

Coefficients:

	Value	Std. Error	t value	Pr(>|t|)
(Intercept)	177.754	224.385	0.792	0.441
Age	-2.563	4.768	-0.538	0.599
Sex	-3.871	15.399	-0.251	0.805
Height	-0.478	0.908	-0.527	0.606
Weight	3.028	2.000	1.514	0.151
BMP	-1.718	1.130	-1.521	0.149
FEV	1.055	1.081	0.977	0.344
RV	0.208	0.196	1.060	0.306
FRC	-0.335	0.494	-0.679	0.508
TLC	0.207	0.496	0.418	0.682

```
Residual standard error: 25.4 on 15 degrees of freedom
Multiple R-Squared: 0.64
F-statistic: 2.97 on 9 and 15 degrees of freedom, the p-value is 0.0304
```

Correlation of Coefficients:

	(Intercept)	Age	Sex	Height	Weight	BMP	FEV	RV	FRC
Age	-0.624								
Sex	-0.422	0.369							
Height	-0.802	0.164	0.238						
Weight	0.888	-0.792	-0.326	-0.682					
BMP	-0.720	0.579	0.005	0.453	-0.776				
FEV	-0.593	0.498	0.706	0.356	-0.480	0.064			
RV	0.086	-0.265	-0.411	-0.083	0.170	0.235	-0.350		
FRC	-0.312	0.414	0.511	0.205	-0.301	-0.118	0.616	-0.852	
TLC	-0.529	0.323	0.160	0.278	-0.418	0.439	0.151	0.139	-0.250

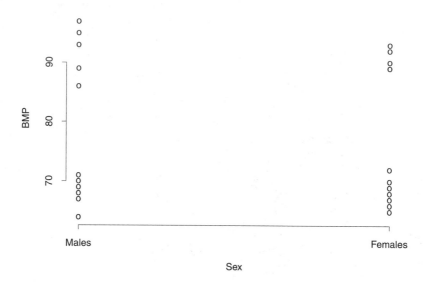

FIGURE 8.2. Scatterplot matrix of BMP against sex.

8.3   Identifying a good model

A multiple regression analysis begins with a set of observations on a response variable and a number of explanatory variables. After an initial analysis has established that some, at least, of the explanatory variables are predictive of the response, the question arises as to whether a subset of the explanatory variables might provide a simpler model that is essentially as useful as the full model in predicting, or explaining, the response. Because as pointed out at the end of the previous section, the t-statistics associated with each regression coefficient provide only a partial answer to this question, we need to consider other possible approaches. The best approach is to build a model based on theory, for example, by first considering the most important predictors and confounders and then sequentially considering inclusion of further variables believed to be associated with the response variable. Automatic approaches are available. These rely on testing many different combinations of variables and therefore suffer from all of the problems of multiple testing; spurious results (false-positives) are likely, and the analysis must be considered exploratory. Nevertheless, we shall briefly examine two automatic selection procedures.

8.3.1   All possible subsets regression

With p explanatory variables, there are a total of $2^p - 1$ possible regression models—each variable can be in or out of the model, and the model containing no explanatory variables is excluded. The advent of modern, high-

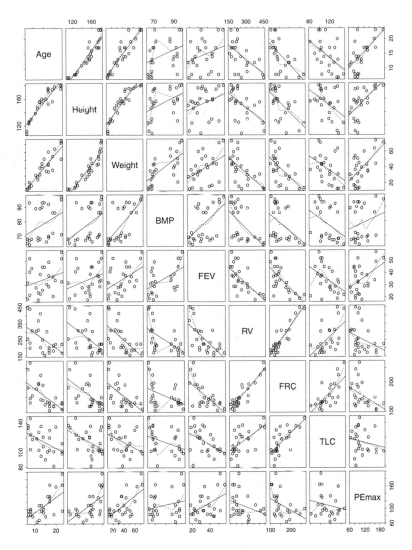

FIGURE 8.3. Scatterplot matrix for cystic fibrosis data with linear and locally weighted regression fits.

speed computing has made possible the development of *all possible subsets regression*. All possible models are estimated, and one or more criteria are computed that are useful in indicating the best models for consideration. The most commonly used among these criteria is *Mallows's C_k statistic*, which is described fully in Display 8.3.

Display 8.3 Mallows's C_k statistic

- Mallows C_k statistic is defined as

$$C_k = (\text{RSS}_k/s^2) - (n - 2k) \tag{1}$$

  where RSS_k is the residual sum of squares from a regression model with a particular set of $k - 1$ of the explanatory variables, plus an intercept, and s^2 is the estimate of σ^2 from the model, including all explanatory variables under consideration.

- C_k is an unbiased estimate of the mean square error, $E[\sum \hat{y}_i - E(y_i)]^2/n$, of the model's fitted values as estimates of the true expectations of the observations.

- If C_k is plotted against k, the subsets of variables worth considering in searching for a parsimonious model are those lying close to the line $C_k = k$.

- In this plot, the value of k is (roughly) the contribution to C_k from the variance of the estimated parameters, whereas the remaining $C_k - k$ is (roughly) the contribution from the bias of the model.

- This feature makes the plot a useful device for a broad assessment of the C_k values of a range of models.

- The criterion is described in detail in Mallows (1973, 1995) and Burman (1996).

Some of the models considered in the all subsets regression of the cystic fibrosis data are given in Table 8.5, together with their associated C_k values. But more useful is the plot of C_k against k, labelling the points by subset number from Table 8.5, particularly if we restrict plotting to subsets lying close to the line $C_k = k$. This is done in Figure 8.4. Some of the subsets suggested as promising in the figure are highlighted with an asterix in Table 8.5.

8.3.2 Stepwise methods

Perhaps the most common approach to selecting informative subsets of explanatory variables in a multiple regression is to use a method that relies on a significance test to select a particular explanatory variable for inclusion in, or deletion from, the current regression model. There are three main possibilities:

TABLE 8.5. Some of the models fitted in all subsets regression

Model	Size	Terms	C_k
7	2	Sex	17.24
14	3	Sex,Weight	4.63
21	4	Age,FEV,RV	2.62
28*	4	Age,BMP,FEV	4.5
35	5	Sex,Weight,BMP,FEV	2.95
42	6	Age,Weight,BMP,FEV,RV	2.8
49	6	Age,Sex,Height,FEV,TLC	6.99
56*	7	Age,Sex,Height,FEV,RV,TLC	7.06
63	8	Sex,Weight,BMP,FEV,RV,FRC,TLC	6.49
70	9	Age,Height,Weight,BMP,FEV,RV,FRC,TLC	8.06
77	9	Age,Sex,Height,BMP,FEV,RV,FRC,TLC	10.29

* models with $|C_k - k| \leq 0.5$

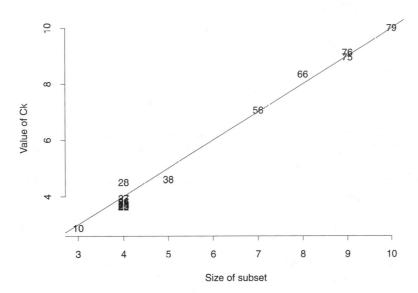

FIGURE 8.4. C_k versus k with for all subset regressions. The models close to the line $C_k = k$ are indicated by their labels.

- Forward selection

- Backward elimination

- Stepwise regression

The forward selection approach begins with an initial model that contains only a constant term and successively adds explanatory variables to the model from the pool of candidate variables until a stage is reached where none of the candidate variables, if added to the current model, would contribute information that is statistically important concerning the expected value of the response. This is generally decided by comparing a function of the decrease in the residual sum of squares with a threshold value set by the investigator; see Draper and Smith (1998) for details.

The backward elimination method begins with an initial model that contains all explanatory variables and then identifies the single variable that contributes the least information concerning the expected value of the response—again, this is decided by looking at changes in the residual sum of squares, in this case, of course, increases. (Again, details are given in Draper and Smith, 1998). If the increase in the residual sum of squares is deemed not to be significant, then the variable is eliminated from the current model. Successive iterations of the method result in a 'final' model from which no variables can be eliminated without adversely affecting, in a statistical sense, the predicted value of the expected response.

The stepwise regression method combines elements of both forward selection and backward elimination. The initial model for stepwise regression is one that contains only a constant term. Variables are then considered for inclusion as for forward selection, but in each step, variables included previously are also considered for possible elimination as in the backward method; this will occur if they no longer make any contribution to predicting the expected response.

The three procedures described depend crucially on the thresholds set by the investigator, an obvious danger when seeking a convincing simplified model. A separate factor that influences the results of all such automatic methods in an unpredictable fashion is the underlying correlation of the data. It is highly unlikely, for example, that any of the procedures would produce a final model that included both of two highly correlated explanatory variables. This is, of course, appropriate because including both variables might lead to *collinearity* problems. It does, however, mask the fact that the variable not selected might, if selected, lead to a somewhat different, but equally acceptable, final model. Caution is needed in using any automatic technique for variable selection.

Tables 8.6 and 8.7 show the complete results of forward selection and backward elimination on the cystic fibrosis data, respectively. To use these results to choose a particular model would require setting an appropriate value with which to compare the various $f.stat$ values. In the forward selection results, for example, setting a threshold value of 2.0 would result

TABLE 8.6. Results of forward selection

$rss:
[1] 15969 14078 11549 10336 10120 9964 9838 9691 9650

$size:
[1] 1 2 3 4 5 6 7 8 9

$which:

	Age	Sex	Height	Weight	BMP	FEV	RV	FRC	TLC
1(+4)	F	F	F	T	F	F	F	F	F
2(+5)	F	F	F	T	T	F	F	F	F
3(+6)	F	F	F	T	T	T	F	F	F
4(+7)	F	F	F	T	T	T	T	F	F
5(+9)	F	F	F	T	T	T	T	F	T
6(+8)	F	F	F	T	T	T	T	T	T
7(+3)	F	F	T	T	T	T	T	T	T
8(+1)	T	F	T	T	T	T	T	T	T
9(+2)	T	T	T	T	T	T	T	T	T

$f.stat:
[1] 15.6466 2.9558 4.5984 2.3477 0.4053 0.2821 0.2168 0.2432 0.0632

$method:
[1] "forward"

TABLE 8.7. Results of backward elimination

$rss:
[1] 9691 9829 9989 10129 10336 11549 14078 15969 26833

$size:
[1] 8 7 6 5 4 3 2 1 0

$which:

	Age	Sex	Height	Weight	BMP	FEV	RV	FRC	TLC
8(-2)	T	F	T	T	T	T	T	T	T
7(-9)	T	F	T	T	T	T	T	T	F
6(-8)	T	F	T	T	T	T	T	F	F
5(-1)	F	F	T	T	T	T	T	F	F
4(-3)	F	F	F	T	T	T	T	F	F
3(-7)	F	F	F	T	T	T	F	F	F
2(-6)	F	F	F	T	T	F	F	F	F
1(-5)	F	F	F	T	F	F	F	F	F
0(-4)	F	F	F	F	F	F	F	F	F

$f.stat:
[1] 0.0632 0.2290 0.2765 0.2510 0.3883 2.3477 4.5984 2.9558 15.6466

$method:
[1] "backward"

in choosing a model with the four variables Weight, BMP, FEV and RV. In the backward elimination results, choosing a threshold of 3.0 leads to selection of the same model.

8.4   Checking model assumptions: residuals and other regression diagnostics

A regression analysis should not end without an attempt to check assumptions such as those of constant variance and normality of the error terms. Violation of these assumptions may invalidate conclusions based on the regression analysis. The estimated residuals $r_i = y_i - \hat{y}_i$ play an essential role in diagnosing a fitted model, although because these do not have the same variance (the precision of $\hat{y}_i$ depends on x_i), they are sometimes standardized before use; see Cook and Weisberg (1982) for details. The following diagnostic plots are generally useful when assessing model assumptions:

- Residuals versus fitted values; if the fitted model is appropriate, the plotted points should lie in an approximately horizontal band across the plot. Departures from this appearance may indicate that the functional form of the assumed model is incorrect, or alternatively, that there is nonconstant variance.

- Residuals versus explanatory variables; systematic patterns in these plots can indicate violations of the constant variance assumption or an inappropriate model form.

- Normal probability plot of the residuals; the plot checks the normal distribution assumptions on which all statistical inferences procedures are based.

A further diagnostic that is often very useful is an index plot of the *Cook's distances* for each observation. This statistic is defined as follows:

$$D_k = \frac{1}{(p+1)s^2} \sum_{i=1}^{n} [\hat{y}_{i(k)} - \hat{y}_i]^2 \tag{8.1}$$

where $\hat{y}_{i(k)}$ is the fitted value of the ith observation when the kth observation is omitted from the model. The values of D_k assess the impact of the kth observation on the estimated regression coefficients. Values of D_k greater than one are suggestive that the corresponding observation has undue influence on the estimated regression coefficients (see Cook and Weisberg, 1982).

A number of diagnostic plots for the model chosen by forward selection and backward elimination are shown in Figures 8.5 to 8.7. None of them give cause for concern as to violations of model assumptions. The details of

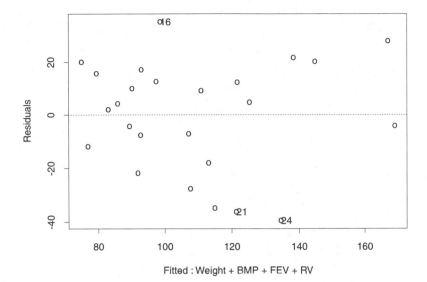

FIGURE 8.5. Residuals versus fitted values for cystic fibrosis data.

TABLE 8.8. Regression coefficients for cystic fibrosis data

	Value	Std. Error	t value	Pr(>|t|)
(Intercept)	62.445	53.243	1.173	0.255
Weight	1.748	0.380	4.603	0.000
BMP	-1.364	0.563	-2.422	0.025
FEV	1.548	0.577	2.682	0.014
RV	0.127	0.083	1.532	0.141

the estimated model are shown in Table 8.8. Note that now the t- statistics corresponding to Weight, BMP and FEV are statistically significant.

8.5 The linear model

We have so far discussed ANOVA, ANCOVA and linear regression as though they were separate models. In fact, all of these models are equivalent and can be viewed as special cases of a *general linear model* in which the residuals have a normal distribution with constant variance σ^2. The only difference between ANOVA, ANCOVA and linear regression models as described in this and previous chapters is that ANOVA uses categorical explanatory variables, linear regression uses continuous (or binary) explanatory variables and ANCOVA uses a mixture of the two.

But such apparent differences can easily be accommodated by a general formulation in which a continuous response variable is modeled as a linear function of explanatory variables.

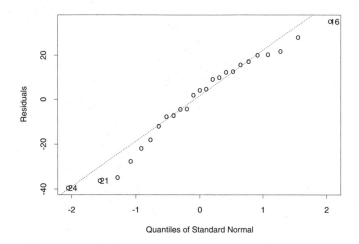

FIGURE 8.6. Normal Q-Q plot of residuals for cystic fibrosis data.

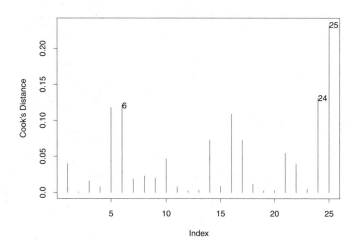

FIGURE 8.7. Cook's distance for cystic fibrosis data.

TABLE 8.9. One way ANOVA via linear regression

```
Coefficients:
              Value Std. Error  t value Pr(>|t|)
(Intercept) 316.625   16.164     19.588   0.000
     group2 -60.181   22.216     -2.709   0.014
     group3 -38.625   26.064     -1.482   0.155

Residual standard error: 45.7 on 19 degrees of freedom
Multiple R-Squared: 0.281
F-statistic: 3.71 on 2 and 19 degrees of freedom, the p-value is 0.0436
```

We have already seen one example in which what is essentially an AN-
COVA model was estimated by linear regression. In the analysis of the cystic fibrosis data in Section 8.2.2, the explanatory variable sex was coded 0
for men and 1 for women. As mentioned previously, the corresponding regression coefficient represents the mean difference between women and men
when all other variables are held constant; i.e., it represents the *adjusted
mean difference*. If the variable was coded the opposite way, 1 for men and 0
for women, then the sign of the regression coefficient would change because
we would now be estimating the difference between men and women. The
variable sex is an example of a *dummy* or *indicator variable*. If we had a
factor with three levels, this could be represented by two dummy variables.
For example, in the bypass surgery example in Chapter 5, three different
ventilation groups were compared. We will now fit this model using linear
regression by defining two dummy variables *group2*, equal to 1 for subjects
in Group II and 0 otherwise and *group3*, equal to 1 for subjects in Group
III and 0 otherwise. The output is shown in Table 8.9.

The ANOVA test is the same as before; i.e., the effect of group is significant ($F_{2,19} = 3.71, p = 0.044$). The regression coefficients represent the
differences groups II - group I and group III - group I. The group not represented by a dummy variable is always the *reference group*. (See Display 8.4
to see the equivalence of regression with dummy variables and one-way
ANOVA.) In Chapter 5, we tested the Helmert contrasts with coefficients
(-1,1,0) and (-1,-1,2). We can obtain the same results using linear regression
by defining two variables, x1, and x2, where x1 takes on the values -1,1 and
0 for groups I, II and III and variable x2 takes on the values -1,-1 and 2 for
groups I, II and III. The result in Table 8.10 shows that the p-values are
the same as those for the two contrasts obtained using one-way ANOVA.

Interactions between two factors can be modeled in linear regression by
using as explanatory variables the dummy variables for both factors as
well as the products of each of the dummy variables of factor 1 with all
of the dummy variables of factor 2. For the biofeed example in Chapter 5,
we can represent all three factors by dummy variables. We therefore have
two dummy variables, drugY and drugZ, for the three drugs (drug X is
the reference category), one dummy variable for biofeedback present and

TABLE 8.10. Helmert contrasts linear regression

Coefficients:

	Value	Std. Error	t value	Pr(>|t|)
(Intercept)	283.690	10.064	28.188	0.000
x1	-30.090	11.108	-2.709	0.014
x2	-2.845	7.756	-0.367	0.718

Residual standard error: 45.7 on 19 degrees of freedom
Multiple R-Squared: 0.281
F-statistic: 3.71 on 2 and 19 degrees of freedom, the p-value is 0.0436

TABLE 8.11. Three way ANOVA via linear regression

Coefficients:

	Value	Std. Error	t value	Pr(>|t|)
(Intercept)	188.000	5.110	36.791	0.000
drugY	12.000	7.226	1.661	0.102
drugZ	21.000	7.226	2.906	0.005
bio	-20.000	7.226	-2.768	0.007
diet	-15.000	7.226	-2.076	0.042
drugYbio	24.000	10.220	2.348	0.022
drugZbio	0.000	10.220	0.000	1.000
drugYdiet	2.000	10.220	0.196	0.846
drugZdiet	-12.000	10.220	-1.174	0.245
bio:diet	16.000	10.220	1.566	0.123
drugYbiodiet	-35.000	14.453	-2.422	0.018
drugZbiodiet	-5.000	14.453	-0.346	0.731

Residual standard error: 12.5 on 60 degrees of freedom
Multiple R-Squared: 0.584
F-statistic: 7.66 on 11 and 60 degrees of freedom, the p-value is 4.64e-008

one variable for diet present (absent is the reference category for both variables). The result is shown in Tabe 8.11.

Interpretation of the terms is relatively involved. The three-way interaction terms drugYbiodiet and drugZbiodiet represent the differences between the means in those two subgroups and the means that would be predicted if there was no three-way interaction. The term drugY represents the difference between drug Y and drug X when biofeedback and diet are absent. The term bio represents the difference between biofeedback present and absent when drug X is used and diet is absent. The term drugYbio represents the difference among the mean in the drug Y, biofeedback no diet group and the sum of the constant and the two effects drugY and bio (the expected mean if there were no interaction). We can test the significance of the three-way interaction by omitting the two terms drugYbiodeit and drugZbiodiet from the model and comparing the two models using ANOVA.

Display 8.4 Fitting one-way ANOVA via regression with dummy variables

- Let y_{ij} be the value of the dependent variable for group i, person j (i=1,2). A linear regression model with a single explanatory variable, for group,

$$z_{ij} = \begin{cases} 0 & \text{if } i = 1 \\ 1 & \text{if } i = 2 \end{cases}$$

can be written as

$$
\begin{aligned}
y_{ij} &= \beta_0 + \beta_1 z_{ij} + \epsilon_{ij} & (1) \\
&= (\mu + \alpha_1) + (\alpha_2 - \alpha_1) z_{ij} + \epsilon_{ij} & (2) \\
&= \mu + \alpha_i + \epsilon_{ij} & (3)
\end{aligned}
$$

showing that it is equivalent to a one-way ANOVA. The intercept β_0 represents the mean for group 1, and the coefficient β_1 represents the difference in means between groups 2 and 1. Unlike the ANOVA formulation, the linear regression model does not require a constraint for the parameters because only two (not three) prameters are estimated to fit two means.

- Note that the test-statistic for the regression coefficient β_1, $\hat{\beta}_1/\text{SE}(\hat{\beta}_1)$, is equal to the t-statistic of an independent samples t-test.

- A variable like z_{ij} that is equal to 1 when the observation belongs to a given group is called an *indicator variable* for that group or a *dummy variable*.

8.6 Summary

Multiple regression is one of the most used (one is tempted to say over used) statistical techniques. It can be helpful for assessing the relationship between a response variable and a number of explanatory variables, but researchers using the technique should take care to check assumptions using a variety of regression diagnostics, and they should not accept blindly the results of the automatic techniques for selecting subsets of explanatory variables. The multiple regression model and the ANOVA and ANCOVA models described in previous chapters are all essentially the same model, one that can be further subsumed into an even more general setting of generalized linear models, as we shall see in the next chapter.

8.7   Using S-PLUS

Section 8.2

This section uses the `lm()` function to fit multiple regression models. Scatterplot matrices are plotted using the `pairs()` function, and the panels are enhanced with linear and locally weighted regressions.

Script for Section 8.2

```
# Read in anesthesia data
anesth<-read.table("anesth.dat",header=T)
attach(anesth)

# Use the lm() function to regress the response variable on
# the two explanatory variables-Table 6.2
summary(lm(Depress~Duration+Trauma))
```
$\implies$ Table 8.2

```
# Data for 25 patients with cystic fibrosis
# PEmax is a measure of the malnutrition of the patients
cystic<-read.table("cystic.dat",header=T)
attach(cystic)

# Use the pairs function to produce a variety of scatterplot
# matrices
win.graph()
pairs(cystic[,-c(1,3)])
```
$\implies$ Figure 8.1

```
# Produce a scatterplot to check the relationship between
# Sex and BMP
win.graph()
plot(Sex,BMP,axes=F)
axis(1,at=c(0,1),labels=c("Males","Females"))
axis(2)
```
$\implies$ Figure 8.2

```
# Enhanced scatterplot matrix
win.graph()
pairs(cystic[,-c(1,3)],
   panel=function(x,y) {
      points(x,y)
      abline(lm(y~x))
      lines(lowess(x,y),lty=2)
   {
)
```
$\implies$ Figure 8.3

```
# Now regress PEmax on all the explanatory variables using the
# lm() function
cystic.lm<-lm(PEmax~Age+Sex+Height+Weight+BMP+FEV+RV+FRC+TLC)
summary(cystic.lm)
```
$\implies$ Table 8.4

Section 8.3

Here, the `leaps()` function is used to apply all subset regressions and a plot of C_k values lying close to the line $c_k = k$ is made. The `stepwise()` function is used for forward and backward selections of subsets of explanatory variables.

Script for Section 8.3

```
# Read in cystic fibrosis data again
cystic<-read.table("cystic.dat",header=T)
attach(cystic)

# Now use leaps to identify possible good models
cystic.leaps<-leaps(cystic[,-c(1,11)],cystic[,11])

# Identify models with Cp close to size
index<-seq(1,79)[abs(cystic.leaps$size-cystic.leaps$Cp)<=0.5]

# Plot Ck against k
win.graph()
plot(cystic.leaps$size[index],cystic.leaps$Cp[index],
    xlab="Size of subset",
    ylab="Value of Ck",type="n",axes=F)
axis(1,at=2:10,labels=2:10)
axis(2)
text(cystic.leaps$size[index],cystic.leaps$Cp[index],
    labels=index)
abline(a=0,b=1)
```
$\longrightarrow$ Figure 8.4

```
# Print details for every 7th model
cbind(7*(1:11),cystic.leaps$size[7*(1:11)],
    cystic.leaps$label[7*(1:11)],
    round(cystic.leaps$Cp[7*(1:11)],digits=2))
```
$\implies$ Table 8.5

```
# Examples of forward selection and backward elimination
stepwise(cystic[,2:10],cystic[,11],method="forward")
```
$\implies$ Table 8.6

```
stepwise(cystic[,2:10],cystic[,11],method="backward")
```

$\Longrightarrow$ Table 8.7

Section 8.4

Section 8.4 uses `plot()` with the option `ask=T` to request a number of useful diagnostic plots.

Script for Section 8.4

```
# Fit model chosen by forward and backward methods
# and check assumptions by examining some diagnostics
cystic.lm1<-lm(PEmax~Weight+BMP+FEV+RV)
win.graph()
par(mfrow=c(1,3))

# Use plot() with ask=T and select number of plot required
# (here 2,5,6) type 0 to finish
plot(cystic.lm1,ask=T)
```
$\Longrightarrow$ Figures 8.5 to 8.7

```
# Regression results
summary(cystic.lm1)
```
$\Longrightarrow$ Table 8.8

Section 8.5

Section 8.5 uses the `contrast` option in `lm()` to specify contrasts for categorical predictors. An alternative way of specifying contrasts for a factor, via the `contrasts()` function, is also illustrated.

Script for Section 8.5

```
# Read in data on patients undergoing cardiac bypass surgery
redcell<-read.table("redf.dat",header=T)
attach(redcell)

# Create dummy variables
group2 <- rep(0,length(Group))
group3<-group2
group2[Group=="g2"]<-1
group3[Group=="g3"]<-1
summary(lm(Folate~group2+group3))
```
$\Longrightarrow$ Table 8.9

```
# Get same result using contrasts option
summary(lm(Folate~Group,
   contrasts=list(Group=contr.treatment)))
```

```
# Alternatively, set the contrast for group before
# running lm()
contrasts(Group)<-contr.treatment(3)
summary(lm(Folate~Group))

# Helmert contrasts
x1<-rep(0,length(Group))
x1[Group=="g1"] <- -1
x1[Group=="g2"] <-  1
x2<-x1
x2[Group=="g1"] <- -1
x2[Group=="g2"] <- -1
x2[Group=="g3"] <-  2
summary(lm(Folate~x1+x2))
```
$\implies$ Table 8.10

```
# Using contrasts option
summary(lm(Folate~Group, contrasts=list(Group=contr.helmert)))

# Read in Biofeed data
bp<-scan("biofeed.dat")
bio<-factor(rep(c("P","A"),c(36,36)))
drug<-factor(rep(rep(c("X","Y","Z"),c(12,12,12)),2))
diet<-factor(rep(rep(c("A","P"),c(6,6)),6))
biofeed<-data.frame(bio,drug,diet,bp)
attach(biofeed)
biofeed.lm<-lm(bp~drug*bio*diet,
    contrasts=list(drug=contr.treatment,bio=contr.treatment,
    diet=contr.treatment))
summary(biofeed.lm)
```
$\implies$ Table 8.11

```
# Fit model without three way interaction
biofeed.lm2<-lm(bp~(drug+bio+diet)^2,
    contrasts=list(drug=contr.treatment,bio=contr.treatment,
    diet=contr.treatment))
anova(biofeed.lm,biofeed.lm2)
```

8.8 Exercises

8.1 Produce an index plot of Cook's distances for the duration of
anesthesia data. Does the plot give any evidence of outliers?

8.2 Construct a scatterplot matrix for the duration of anethesia
data. On each panel, plot the linear regression of the two variables.

8.3 For the cystic fibrosis data, produce plots of residuals against explanatory variables for each of the models suggested by the all subsets regression procedure.

8.4 Investigate the use of alternative criteria to Mallows's C_k for assesing models for the cystic fibrosis data.

8.5 Investigate the use of the `step()` function as an alternative to using the `stepwise()` function for identifying informative subsets of explanatory variables.

9
Generalized Linear Models I: Logistic Regression

9.1   Introduction

All of the models discussed so far assume that the dependent variable is continuous and normally distributed. In this chapter, we introduce *generalized linear models*, which include the regression and ANOVA models of previous chapters, but can also be used for modeling non-normally distributed response variables, in particular categorical variables.

As the term implies, generalized linear models generalize the linear model. Both linear models and generalized linear models model the mean of the response variable as a function of the explanatory variables. The generalization consists of allowing the following three assumption of linear models to be modified:

1. The response variable is normally distributed with a mean determined by the model.

2. The mean can be modeled as a linear function of (possibly nonlinear transformations of) the covariates; i.e., the effects of the covariates on the mean are additive.

3. The variance of the response variable, given the (predicted) mean, is constant.

None of these assumptions are, for example, satisfied in the case of a dichotmous response variable. Here, we require a model for the mean (or expectation) of the dichotomous variable, namely, a probability. It is clear that the first assumption of normality cannot be satisfied here because the variable is not continuous. The second assumption that the probability depends linearly on the variables is problematic because it could yield predicted values outside of the required range of 0 and 1. Finally, the third assumption of a constant variance does not apply because the variance of a dichotomous variable depends on its mean, i.e., the probability. For example, if for a given set of values of the explanatory variables, the predicted probability is 0.5, we expect about half the observations to be 1, giving an expected variance of $0.5(1 - 0.5)^2 + 0.5(0 - 0.5)^2 = 0.25$. For a probability of 0.9, about 90% of the observations are 1, giving a much smaller expected variance of $0.9(1 - 0.9)^2 + 0.1(0 - 0.9)^2 = 0.09$. In general, the variance of the responses for a given probability p is $p(1 - p)$. Therefore, unlike the linear model, the variance is not constant and is completely determined by the mean (the probabability).

Display 9.1 summarizes the main features of generalized linear models. For a more thorough introduction to such models, see McCullagh and Nelder (1989). In the rest of the chapter, we consider a particularly useful generalized linear model capable of modeling a binary response, namely, *logistic regression*. We shall consider the method in two situations, first where the data are grouped and second where they are not.

9.2   Logistic regression for grouped data

As an example of logistic regression for grouped data, we will analyze the data shown in Table 9.1. Here, a sample of male residents of Framingham, Massachusetts, aged 40-59, are classified according to blood pressure category and serum cholesterol category. The cells in Table 9.1 give the number of men in each combination of blood pressure and cholesterol category who had heart disease divided by the total number of men. The data appear in Agresti (1990).

The outcome here is the proportion of men with heart disease derived from an individual level binary response indicating whether a man had heart disease. For both binary variables and proportions, linear models are not sensible for the reasons given in the previous section, namely, because they can lead to fitted values outside of their range and the normality and constant variance assumptions are clearly violated. The specific type of generalized linear model most commonly used for binary variables or proportions is a logistic regression model, as described in Display 9.2. (See Collett, 1991, Clayton and Hills, 1993, and Agresti, 1990, 1996 for more information on logistic regression.)

Initially, we will just consider the effect of one predictor, blood pressure, on heart disease. The proportions of men with heart disease for each blood pressure category are given in Table 9.2. If we treat the blood pressure category as a factor, a separate parameter is estimated for each of the

---

Display 9.1 Generalized linear models

- Generalized linear models are a general class of models that include linear models as a special case.

- Generalized linear models model the mean μ of the response variable as a function of the explanatory variables.

- The explanatory variables are combined to form a *linear predictor* of the form

$$
\begin{aligned}
\eta &= \beta_0 + \beta x_1 + \beta x_2 + \cdots + \beta x_p \\
&= \beta' \mathbf{x}
\end{aligned} \tag{1}
$$

- The linear predictor is not directly equated with the mean of the response variable but with a monotonic function of μ, called the *link function*, $g(\mu)$,

$$
\eta = g(\mu) \tag{2}
$$

In linear regression, the link function is the identity. Other link functions include the log, logit, probit, inverse and power transformations.

- The distribution of the response variable given its mean μ is a distribution from the exponential family of the form

$$
f(y; \theta, \phi) = \exp\{(y\theta - b(\theta))/a(\phi) + c(y, \phi)\}. \tag{3}
$$

In linear regression, a normal ditribution is assumed with mean μ and constant variance σ^2

$$
\begin{aligned}
f(y; \theta, \phi) &= \frac{1}{\sqrt{(2\pi\sigma^2)}} \exp\{-(y - \mu)^2/2\sigma^2\} \\
&= \exp\{(y\mu - \mu^2/2)/\sigma^2 - \frac{1}{2}(y^2/\sigma^2 + \log(2\pi\sigma^2))\} \tag{4}
\end{aligned}
$$

so that $\theta = \mu$, $b(\theta) = \theta^2/2$, $\phi = \sigma^2$ and $a(\phi) = \phi$. Other distributions in the exponential family include the binomial, Poisson, gamma, inverse Gaussian and exponential distributions.

- The choice of probability distribution determines the relationship between the variance of the response variable (conditional on the explanatory variables) and its mean. This relationship is known as the *variance function*, denoted $V(\mu)$. For the Gaussian distribution, $V(\mu) = \sigma^2$, so that the variance does not vary with the mean and is estimated freely. For the Poisson distribution, the variance equals the mean, $V(\mu) = \mu$, so that the variance is not constant and cannot be estimated freely.

- The models are estimated by maximizing the joint likelihood of the observed responses given the parameters of the model and the explanatory variables. This generally requires iterative algorithms.

TABLE 9.1. Proportions of men with heart disease by blood pressure and serum cholesterol cross-classification

Blood Pressure	Serum Cholesterol (mg/100ml)						
	<200	200-209	210-219	220-244	245-259	260-284	>284
<117	2/53	0/21	0/15	0/20	0/14	1/22	0/11
117-126	0/66	2/27	1/25	8/69	0/24	5/22	1/19
127-136	2/59	0/34	2/21	2/83	0/33	2/26	4/28
137-146	1/65	0/19	0/26	6/81	3/23	2/34	4/23
147-156	2/37	0/16	0/6	3/29	2/19	4/16	1/16
157-166	1/13	0/10	0/11	1/15	0/11	2/13	4/12
167-186	3/21	0/5	0/11	2/27	2/5	6/16	3/14
>186	1/5	0/1	3/6	1/10	1/7	1/7	1/7

eight blood pressure categories and the model yields fitted proportions equal to the observed proportions regardless of the link used. This *full model* or *saturated model* is completely uninformative. Further, it does not take into account the fact that the blood pressure categories are ordered and, if assigned values equal to the midpoints of the ranges 111.5 121.5 131.5 141.5 151.5 161.5 176.5 191.5 even fall on an interval scale. The risk of heart disease is likely to monotonically increase (or decrease) with blood pressure, making it reasonable to assume that a monotonic transformation $g(\mu)$ of the mean depends linearly on blood pressure; i.e.,

$$g(\mu) = \beta_0 + \beta_1 x$$

where x are the midpoints of the blood pressure ranges. Now, the choice of link makes a difference to the fitted proportions because it determines the shape of the relationship between the predicted proportion μ and the blood pressure x. As discussed in Display 9.2, the most common link for binary data or proportions in medical statistics is the *logit* link

$$g(\mu) = \log(\frac{\mu}{1 - \mu})$$

The logit link has been applied to the proportions in Table 9.2. Overall, there is a steady increase in the logits with blood pressure category and it seems reasonable to assume that this increase is linear by fitting a logistic regression model. The model yields predicted logits shown in the third column of the table. There appears to be reasonable agreement between the observed and the predicted logits.

The regression coefficients and their standard errors are given in Table 9.3. The coefficient of blood pressure, 0.0243, represents the expected change in the logit when blood pressure increases by one unit. This is not easy to interpret. However, as shown in Display 9.2, the exponential of a difference in logits is an *odds ratio* (see also Chapter 3). Here, the odds ratio is 1.025. This corresponds to a 2.5% increase in the odds of heart

---

Display 9.2 Logistic regression

- Response variables are frequently dichotomous; i.e., they represent a 'yes'/'no' answer to a question such as 'is the disease present?', 'has the woman had a child?', and so on. By convention, the responses are coded as 1 for 'yes' (or present) and 0 for 'no' (or absent). Logistic regression is a specific generalized linear model that is almost always used in medical statistics when the response variable is dichotomous.

- Because of the way the response variable is coded, its mean represents the proportion of subjects with the characteristic or event, and its expectation represents the corresponding probability. The expectation must therefore lie in the range $0 \leq \mu \leq 1$. To ensure this, the *logit link* may be used given by

$$\text{logit}(\mu) = \log(\mu/(1-\mu)) = \beta' \mathbf{x}_i \qquad (1)$$

  Note that this is the log of the *odds*. The predicted probability as a function of the linear predictor is

$$\begin{aligned} \pi(\beta' \mathbf{x}_i) &= \frac{\exp(\beta' \mathbf{x}_i)}{1 + \exp(\beta' \mathbf{x}_i)} \\ &= \frac{1}{1 + \exp(-\beta' \mathbf{x}_i)} \end{aligned} \qquad (2)$$

- The Bernouilli distribution (binomial distribution with a denominator of 1) is the only reasonable distribution to select; i.e., the probability of a positive response is μ, and the probability of a negative response is $1 - \mu$.

- The variance function is given by $V(\mu) = \mu(1 - \mu)$.

- Logistic regression can also be used when the response variable is a proportion, e.g., the proportion of headache-free days on a number of subjects. The appropriate distribution is then the binomial distribution with the correct denominator, e.g., the number of days over which headache status has been recorded.

- Although other link functions such as the probit and complimentary log-log can be used to ensure that the expectation μ lies in the premitted range, the logit is the most popular choice in medical statistics for the following reasons:

  - Because the logit link can be interpreted as representing the log-odds, the exponentiated coefficients of the linear predictor represent adjusted odds ratios.

  - Unlike the relative risk, the odds ratio is a measure of association between risk factors and disease status that can be estimated from retrospective, case-control studies.

TABLE 9.2. Proportion of men with heart disease by blood pressure category together with observed and fitted logits using a logistic regression model

Blood pressure	Proportion	Observed logit	Fitted logit
<117	0.0192	-3.93	-3.37
117-126	0.0675	-2.63	-3.12
127-136	0.0423	-3.12	-2.88
137-146	0.0590	-2.77	-2.64
147-156	0.0863	-2.36	-2.39
157-166	0.0941	-2.26	-2.15
167-186	0.1616	-1.65	-1.79
>186	0.1860	-1.48	-1.42

TABLE 9.3. Coefficients of logistic regression model for heart disease data

```
Coefficients:
              Value Std. Error t value
(Intercept) -6.08203   0.724091  -8.400
         bp  0.02434   0.004842   5.026
```

disease when blood pressure increases by a unit. When blood pressure increases by 10 units (from one category in the table to the next), the odds ratio is $\exp(10 \times 0.0243) = 1.025^{10} = 1.28$; i.e., the odds of heart disease increases approximately by 28%. Note that it is the *odds* of heart disease that depends multiplicatively on blood pressure, not the *risk*. The odds are defined as $\mu/(1-\mu)$, where μ is the predicted probability or risk. For small values of μ, the denominator is approximately equal to 1, so that the odds is aproximately equal to the probability or risk and the odds ratio is approximately equal to the probability ratio or *relative risk*. In Table 9.2, the proportions are mostly low enough for this approximation to be reasonable, e.g., 0.02/(1-0.02)=0.020,0.06/(1-0.06)=0.064 and 0.2/(1-0.2)=0.25. We can therefore say that the relative risk of heart disease associated with an increase in blood pressure by 10 units is approximately 1.28.

The predicted probabilities (risks) can be found from the predicted logits $\hat{\eta}$ by applying the inverse link function,

$$\mu = \frac{1}{1 - \exp(-\hat{\eta})}$$

A graph of the predicted probability versus blood pressure is given in Figure 9.1, together with the observed proportions.

Display 9.3 discusses goodness of fit and model comparisons for generalized linear models. We can test the significance of the association between blood pressure and heart disease using the Wald test-statistic given under "t-value" in Table 9.3. This is clearly significant ($p = 5 \times 10^{-7}$). A more accurate test is a likelihood ratio test, based on the difference in deviance

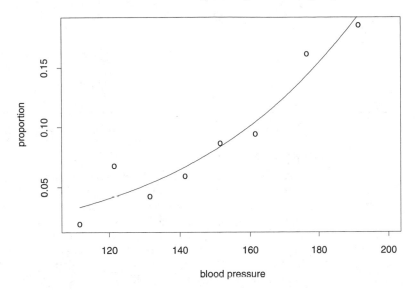

FIGURE 9.1. Predicted probabilities and observed proportions versus blood pressure for heart disease data.

between the model including just the intercept β_0 (the *null deviance*) and the model including blood pressure (the *model deviance* or *residual deviance*) given by $30.02 - 5.91 = 24.11$. This likelihood ratio statistic has a χ^2 distribution with 1 degree of freedom. The p-value is 9×10^{-7}.

For the model treating blood pressure category as an unordered factor, the difference in deviance between the null model and the model including blood pressure is $(30.02 - 0)$ with 6 degrees of freedom, giving a larger p-value of $4 \ 10^{-5}$. Testing the null hypothesis of independence is more powerful against the narrow alternative of a monotonic increase in probability with increasing blood pressure than against the very general alternative of any association between blood pressure and heart disease (see, for example, Agresti, 1996).

We can also test whether the residual deviance of the model treating blood pressure as continuous is significant. Here, the null hypothesis is that the model fits (i.e., that the model generated the data). The residual deviance is 5.91 with 6 degrees of freedom (8 proportions - 2 parameters) and $p = 0.43$. The observed proportions are therefore consistent with the model.

This does not imply that other variables are not important predictors of heart disease. If we fit the same models to the 56 proportions in Table 9.1, we get the same parameter estimates as previously but now the model treating blood pressure as categorical no longer fits the proportions perfectly and the residual deviance now is 77.60 with 48 degrees of freedom, giving $p = 0.004$, so that the model ignoring cholesterol is rejected.

Display 9.3 Goodness of fit and model comparison

- There are two commonly used methods of assessing goodness of fit of generalized linear models, the *deviance* and the generalized *Pearson X^2* statistic.

- Consider a *full model* or *saturated model* having as many parameters (n) as there are observations. The full model fits the data perfectly, and the maximized likelihood of the full model therefore represents the maximum achievable likelihood. A useful way of assessing goodness of fit of a given model with $p < n$ parameters is to compare the maximized likelihood of that model with the maximized likelihood of the full model. This is the rationale behind the deviance defined as twice the difference in log-likelihoods between the model under investigation and the full model.

- For a linear model, the deviance is the residual sum of squares.

- Let $\hat{\mu}_i$ be the predicted mean of a given model for subject i. The generalized Pearson X^2 is defined as the weighted sum of squared deviations between the observed value y_i and the predicted mean $\hat{\mu}_i$ with weight given by the reciprocal of the predicted variance of y_i; i.e.,

$$X^2 = \sum (y_i - \hat{\mu}_i)^2 / V(\hat{\mu})$$

- The Pearson X^2 test introduced in Chapter 3 for cross-tabulations is just the generalized Pearson X^2 for a generalized linear model with a log link and a Poisson distribution (see Chapter 11).

- Both the deviance and the generalized Pearson X^2 have asymptotic χ^2 distributions with p degrees of freedom.

- The difference in deviance between a model with p_1 parameters and a nested model with a subset $p_2 < p_1$ parameters, where the $p_1 - p_2$ terms have been omitted, has an asymptotic χ^2 with $p_1 - p_2$ degrees of freedom under the null hypothesis that the $p_1 - p_2$ parameters are zero. This *likelihood ratio test* can be used to assess the joint significance of the omitted terms.

- The Wald test is based on the estimated parameters and their covariance matrix. This test provides an approximation to the likelihood ratio test.

TABLE 9.4. Logistic regression model with blood pressure and cholesterol level as main effects

Coefficients:			
	Value	Std. Error	t value
(Intercept)	-8.78924	1.013122	-8.675
bp	0.01941	0.004865	3.988
ch	0.01384	0.003174	4.361

A very parsimonious model would be a model including only the main effects of blood pressure and cholesterol, treating both as continuous. Here, we use the values 195.5, 204.5, 214.5, 232, 252, 272 and 297 for the cholesterol categories. The estimated coefficients are shown in in Table 9.4.

Both main effects are significant using the Wald test since the ratios of the parameter estimates divided by their standard errors (listed under t-value) are much greater than 2. The residual deviance is 63.9 with 53 degrees of freedom, which is not significant ($p = 0.15$). Therefore, it seems reasonable to assume a linear relationship between the logits and both explanatory variables and to omit the interaction. Comparing the deviance of the main effects model with that of the model including an interaction gives a p-value of 0.54.

9.3   Logistic regression for individual level data

The outcome in the previous example was a proportion because large numbers of men shared the same values of the explanatory variables. We will now analyze a much smaller data set that is not aggregated into a table of proportions. Here, the outcome is a binary variable, whether or not patients with leukemia lived for at least 24 weeks after diagnosis. Possible explanatory variables are the white blood cell count and presence or absence of a morphological characteristic of the white blood cells (AG). The data are taken from Venables and Ripley (1994) and are given in Table 9.5.

We will fit a model including both explanatory variables and their interaction. The variable ag has been coded as a dummy variable (1 = present, 0 = absent). Because the white blood cell counts are very large, we divide this variable by 1,000 to avoid obtaining regression coefficients very close to 0 (and odds ratios very close to 1). The estimated log-odds ratios with their standard errors are given in Table 9.6. The odds ratios are obtained by exponentiating the coefficients, and the 95% confidence interval of the odds ratios are obtained by exponentiating the upper and lower confidence limits of the log odds (based on log odds ± 2 standard errors).

The interaction is significant at the 5% level. When AG is present, the white blood cell count has a smaller effect on the chances of survival than

TABLE 9.5. Survival of leukemia patients in weeks

wbc	ag	surv	wbc	ag	surv
2300	present	65	4400	absent	56
750	present	156	3000	absent	65
4300	present	100	4000	absent	17
2600	present	134	1500	absent	7
6000	present	16	9000	absent	16
10500	present	108	5300	absent	22
10000	present	121	10000	absent	3
17000	present	4	19000	absent	4
5400	present	39	27000	absent	2
7000	present	143	28000	absent	3
9400	present	56	31000	absent	8
32000	present	26	26000	absent	4
35000	present	22	21000	absent	3
100000	present	1	79000	absent	30
100000	present	1	100000	absent	4
52000	present	5	100000	absent	43
100000	present	65			

TABLE 9.6. Coefficients and odds ratios for leukemia data

	Value	Std. Error	odds ratio	95% CI
Intercept	−1.77	0.89		
ag	3.28	1.16	26.67	2.77,256.69
wbc/1000	0.020	0.017	1.02	0.99,1.05
ag:I(wbc/1000)	−0.049	0.024	0.95	0.91,1.00

when AG is absent. The best way of understanding the model is to plot
the predicted values as shown in Figure 9.2.

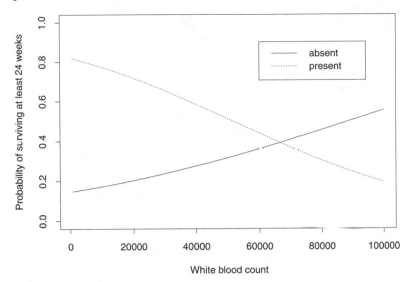

FIGURE 9.2. Predicted probabilities as a function of white blood cell count for
ag absent and present.

We can again use the difference in deviance as an alternative to the
Wald test. However, in small data sets as the one here, we cannot test the
residual deviance because the χ^2 distribution only applies asymptotically.
Including observed values on the graph is also not very informative because
we only have one or very few observations for most white blood cell counts.
Other diagnostics for generalized linear models will be discussed in the next
chapter.

9.4   Case-control studies

Table 9.7 summarizes data from a study investigating whether BCG vaccination in early childhood, whose purpose it is to protect against tuber-
culosis, is also protective of leprosy, which is caused by a closely related
bacillus. New cases of leprosy during a given period were examined for the
presence or absence of the characteristric scar left by a BCG vaccination.
During approximately the same period, a 100% survey of the population in
the same area had also been carried out. The subjects of this survey provide the controls to compare with the cases. The data are given in Clayton
and Hills (1993).

The main question is whether presence of a BCG scar is associated with
a lower incidence of leprosy. However, because the data are not from a

TABLE 9.7. BCG scar status in new leprosy cases and in a healthy population survey

Cases	Total	Scar	Age
1	7594	0	0–4
1	11720	1	0–4
11	7154	0	5–9
14	10198	1	5–9
28	5639	0	10–14
22	7583	1	10–14
16	2224	0	15–19
28	8145	1	15–19
20	2458	0	20–24
19	5607	1	20–24
36	4392	0	25–29
11	1636	1	25–29
47	5292	0	30–34
6	1240	1	30–34

single cohort, there is no information in the proportion of cases in this sample and the incidence or risk of leprosy cannot be estimated. This is an example of a case-control study (although the large number of controls is unusual). An alternative to the relative risk that can be estimated from a case-control study is the odds ratio. Because age is an important predictor of almost any disease, we need to adjust the odds ratio for age to eliminate any possible confounding effects. One way of doing this would be to use the Mantel-Haenszel test discussed in Chapter 3. Another alternative is to estimate a logistic regression model. Because we merely want to control for age and are not particulary interested in the relationship between age and leprosy, we will include age as a categorical variable. The estimated odds ratio of being a case if vaccinated compared with not being vaccinated (adjusted for age) is 0.58, with a 95% confidence interval from 0.44 to 0.76. The vaccination therefore appears to protect against leprosy.

9.5 Summary

In this chapter, generalized linear models were introduced. These models can be used to model the mean of a response variable as a function of explanatory variables without assuming that the response variable has a normal distribution. The explanatory variables are combined linearly to form a linear predictor. The link function specifies the relationship between the mean of the response and the linear predictor. A distribution from the exponential family is then selected as the assumed distribution of the response given its mean. For binary responses or proportions, particularly from case-control studies, by far, the most common generalized linear model used for medical data is the logistic regression model with a logit link and a binomial (or Bernoulli) distribution. The model provides estimates of odds ratios and their confidence intervals for both prospective and retrospective studies.

9.6 Using S-PLUS

Section 9.2

The glm() function is used to fit generalized linear models. For porportions, the dependent variables is a matrix with two columns, giving the number of 'successes' and the number of 'failures'. The aggregate.data.frame() function is used to collapse a table. The predict() function is used to plot the predicted probabilities. The expand.grid() function is used to generate all combinations of values of two vectors. The functions pnorm() and pchisq() are used to calculate p-values.

Script for Section 9.2

```
# Read heart data
heart<-read.table("hdis.dat", header=T)

# Define factors
heart$bpress<-factor(heart$bpress,
    labels=c("<117","117-126","127-136","137-146","147-156",
    "157-166","167-186",">186"))
heart$chol<-factor(heart$chol,
    labels=c("<200","200-209","210-219","220-244","245-259",
    "260-284",">284"))

# Collapse table over cholesterol levels
short<-aggregate.data.frame(heart[,c("hdis","total")],
    data.frame(bpress=heart[,"bpress"]),FUN=sum)
# the first argment gives the variables to be aggregated
# and the second gives the grouping variables

short<-data.frame(short,obs=short$hdis/short$total)

# Fit full model for blood pressure
heart.glm<-glm(cbind(hdis, total-hdis)~bpress,family=binomial,
    data=short)
cbind(short$obs,predict(heart.glm,type="response"))
summary(heart.glm)
heart.glm

# Treat blood pressure factor as continuous
bp<-seq(111.5,191.5,by=10)
bp<-c(bp[1:6],(bp[7]+bp[8])/2,bp[9])
# bp are the mid-points of the intervals of the categories
# of blood pressure

# Add bp to data-frame
short<-data.frame(short,bp=bp)
```

```
heart.glm2<-glm(cbind(hdis, total-hdis)~bp,family=binomial,
    data=short)
summary(heart.glm2)
```
⟹ Table 9.3

```
# Table of proportions, observed logits and predicted logits
cbind(short$obs,log(short$obs/(1-short$obs)),
    predict(heart.glm2,type="link"))
```
⟹ Table 9.2

```
# Graph of observed and predicted proportions
win.graph()
plot(short$bp,short$obs,xlab="blood pressure",
    ylab="proportion",xlim=c(110,200))
bp<-seq(111.5,191.5,length=200)
lines(bp,predict(heart.glm2,data.frame(bp=bp),type="response"))
```
⟹ Figure 9.1

```
# Test effect of blood pressure as continuous variable
# Wald test:
2*(1-pnorm(summary(heart.glm2)$coefficients[2,3]))

# Likelihood ratio test:
1-pchisq(heart.glm2$null.deviance-heart.glm2$deviance,1)

# Test effect of blood pressure as categorical variable
1-pchisq(heart.glm$null.deviance-heart.glm$deviance,6)

# Test of model fit with blood pressure continuous
1- pchisq(heart.glm2$deviance,heart.glm2$df)

# Consider both blood pressure and cholesterol level
heart.glm<-glm(cbind(hdis, total)~bpress,family=binomial,
    data=heart)
# This model ignores cholesterol level

summary(heart.glm)
heart.glm$deviance
1- pchisq(heart.glm$deviance,heart.glm$df)
# This is the p-balue of the residual deviance of the model
# that ignores cholesterol level

# Fit model with blood pressure and cholesterol continuous
bp<-seq(111.5,191.5,by=10)
bp<-c(bp[1:6],(bp[7]+bp[8])/2,bp[9])
ch<-c(195.5,204.5,214.5,232,252,272,297)
```

```
# Check the order in which the levels of blood pressure
# and cholesterol appear in the data
cbind(heart$bpress, heart$chol)

# Use expand.grid() to create all combinations of the
# ch and bp values with ch varying first
junk<-expand.grid(ch,bp)

# Include expanded ch and bp in dataframe
heart<-data.frame(heart,ch=junk[,1],bp=junk[,2])

# Check that it is correct
cbind(heart$bpress,heart$bp,heart$chol,heart$ch)

# Fit logistic regression model with main effects only
heart.glm2<-glm(cbind(hdis, total)~bp+ch,family=binomial,
   data=heart)
summary(heart.glm2)
```

$\implies$ ⬛ Table 9.4

```
# Check goodness of fit
1- pchisq(heart.glm2$deviance,heart.glm2$df)

# Include interaction
heart.glm3<-glm(cbind(hdis, total)~bp*ch,family=binomial,
   data=heart)

# Test significance of interaction
anova(heart.glm2,heart.glm3)
1-pchisq(0.3682483,1)
```

Section 9.3

The contrasts() function is used to set the coding of a binary variable to 0,1 (a treatment contrast). (The default coding is -1,1. If this is used, the regression coefficient represents *half* the required log odds ratio.) The model formula includes a logical expression for the dependent variable. The I() notation is used to transform an explanatory variable within the formula. The predict() function is used to plot the predicted probabilities as a function of a continuous variable and a categorical variable.

Script for Section 9.3

```
# Read Leukemia data
leuk<-matrix(scan("leuk.dat"),ncol=3,byrow=T)
leuk<-data.frame(wbc=leuk[,1],ag=leuk[,2],surv=leuk[,3])
leuk$ag<-factor(leuk$ag,level=c(1,2),
```

```
          label=c("absent", "present"))

# Check contrasts for ag
contrasts(leuk$ag)
# default is Helmert

# Change contrast so that absent=0 and present=1
contrasts(leuk$ag)<-contr.treatment(levels(leuk$ag),2)

# Logistic regression with main effects and interactions
nleuk.lr<-glm(surv>=24~ag*wbc, family=binomial,data=leuk)
# default link is logit

# Use white blood cell count in thousands
nleuk.lr<-glm(surv>=24~ag*I(wbc/1000), family=binomial,
    data=leuk)
# The I() notation allows functions of variables to be
# specified as explanatory variables
summary(nleuk.lr)

# Display odds ratios and confidence intervals
lor<-summary(nleuk.lr)$coefficients[,1]
se<-summary(nleuk.lr)$coefficients[,2]
or1<-exp(lor-1.96*se)
or2<-exp(lor+1.96*se)
or<-exp(lor)
cbind(or,or1,or2)

# Get column labels as well:
cbind(OR=or,lower=or1,upper=or2)
```
$\Longrightarrow$ Table 9.6

```
# Graph of predicted probabilities
attach(leuk)
nleuk.lr<-glm(surv>=24~ag*wbc, family=binomial,data=leuk)
w<-seq(min(wbc),max(wbc),length=100)

# Generate values of wbc to be plotted
plot(c(w[1],w[100]),c(0,1),type="n",xlab="White blood count",
    ylab="Probability of surviving at least 24 weeks")
pframe1<-data.frame(wbc=w,ag=rep(0,100))

# Dataframe for predictions for ag=absent
lines(w, predict(nleuk.lr,pframe1,type="response"))
pframe2<-data.frame(wbc=w,ag=rep(1,100))

# Dataframe for predictions for ag=present
lines(w, predict(nleuk.lr,pframe2,type="response"),lty=2)
legend(70000,.9,c("absent","present"),lty=1:2)
```
$\Longrightarrow$ Figure 9.2

Section 9.4

Section 9.4 uses the same functions used in the previous sections.

Script for Section 9.4

```
# Read leprosy data
leprosy<-read.table("leprosy.dat",header=T)

# Define age to be a factor
leprosy$age<-factor(leprosy$age,
    labels=c("0-4","5-9","10-14","15-19","20-24",
    "25-29","30-34"))

# Set contrasts
contrasts(leprosy$age)<-contr.treatment(
    levels(leprosy$age),7)

# Fit logistic regression model
leprosy.glm<-glm(cbind(cases,total-cases)~scar+age,
    family=binomial(link=logit),data=leprosy)

# Compute odds ratio and 95% CI
coeffs<-summary(leprosy.glm)$coefficients
c(exp(coeffs[2,1]), exp(coeffs[2,1]-1.96*coeffs[2,2]),
    exp(coeffs[2,1]+1.96*coeffs[2,2]))
```

9.7   Exercises

9.1 Model the probability of lung disease by fitting a logistic regression model to the data described in Chapter 2 Section 2.3. Use a matrix with the number of cases in column 1 and the number of noncases in column 2 as the dependent variable and include dust, smoking and emp as independent variables (where dust and emp are treated as continuous).

9.2 Use polynomial contrasts for emp and dust. Is the quadratic effect significant?

9.3 Use the step() function to consider adding race and sex as main effects.

9.4 Consider adding interactions among selected variables.

10

Generalised linear models II: Poisson regression

10.1 Introduction

In the previous chapter, we used logistic regression to model binary variables and proportions. In this chapter, we will use another type of generalized linear model, *Poisson regression*, to model counts. Many medical and epidemiological investigations are concerned with the incidence of diseases in populations. Here, a number of people are followed up and the onset of a disease recorded for each person. The data can then be summarized by counting the total number of occurrences of the disease in different subgroups of subjects sharing the same values of the important explanatory variables. The dependent variable is therefore a count.

The *incidence rate* in each subgroup can be estimated by dividing the number of occurrences of the disease by the total observation time, the sum of the observation times of all subjects in the subgroup, usually measured in *person years*. If the incidence rate is constant within a subgroup, and if the individuals in the group are independent (we assume that the disease can occur only once per person), then the observed count follows a Poisson distribution with expected count given by the product of the incidence rate and the total person-years of observation. A Poisson model is a special case of a generalized linear model with a log link and a Poisson distribution; see Display 10.1 for details. The book *Statistical Models in Epidemiology* by Clayton and Hills (1993) is a very good reference on Poisson modeling in epidemiology.

Display 10.1 Poisson regression

- If events occur independently of one another and have a constant probability of occurring at any point in continuous time (or space), then the number of events observed over a time interval (or region) has a Poisson distribution given by

$$f(y; \mu) = \mu^y e^{-\mu}/y!, \quad y = 0, 1, 2, \cdots \tag{1}$$

where μ is the expected count. Many epidemiological studies have response variables that are counts, such as the number of cases of cancer observed in different regions within a given period of observation.

- The variance function is $V(\mu) = \mu$.

- Because counts must be positive, the log link is frequently used

$$\ln(\mu) = \eta \tag{2}$$

This yields a multiplicative model whose regression coefficients may be interpreted as the logarithms of ratios between expected counts.

- However, it is not useful to compare expected *numbers* of events, μ, between groups of subjects (e.g., men and women) when the number of subjects or length of follow-up in each group may differ. Therefore, Poisson models often include an *offset* equal to the log of the demoninator d of a 'rate' μ/d that can be compared between groups. The model is

$$\ln(\mu) = \eta + \ln(d) \tag{3}$$

so that the log rate is modeled as a linear combination of the covariates,

$$\ln(\mu/d) = \eta \tag{4}$$

and the regression coefficients represent log *rate ratios*. The most common 'denominator' used in epidemiology is the person-years of observation, the sum of all the subjects' periods of observation.

TABLE 10.1. Subset of lung cancer data

Age	Smoker	Cigscat	Death	Follow	Freq
61	1	2	1	1	13
70	1	1	1	3	12
36	1	1	1	3	1
60	1	2	2	5	7
60	1	2	0	6	2010
51	1	2	1	4	17
59	0	0	1	5	53
80	1	1	1	1	3
73	0	0	1	3	78
57	1	2	1	5	16
53	1	1	2	1	1
49	1	2	0	5	1
69	0	0	0	5	1
62	1	2	1	4	22
72	1	2	2	1	1
69	1	1	1	3	10
60	0	0	1	1	37
40	1	1	1	2	1
66	0	0	1	2	53
61	1	2	2	1	3

10.2 Poisson regression examples

The first example is from a large prospective cohort study carried out by the American Cancer Society. In 1982, over 1 million volunteers were enrolled in the United States and followed up every two years until 1988. During the six-year follow-up period, 98.2% of subjects were traced (dead or alive). For every reported death, the cause of death was determined from death certificates where available. The study is described by Stellman *et al.* (1988) and a subset of the data is available on a disk accompanying the book *Case Studies in Biometry* edited by Lange *et al.* (1994).

We consider here only women smokers and nonsmokers (not including exsmokers) and three explanatory variables: age, smoking status and number of cigarettes smoked per day, categorized as less than 20 or at least 20. The data are in the form of a table. For every year of follow-up (`follow`), the variable `freq` gives the number of subjects followed up for that length of time and the variable `death` gives the number of subjects who died of lung cancer in that year for each combination of the explanatory variables. The data set is too large to present here, but Table 10.1 gives a small subset of the data.

The people included in this data set varied in age between 35 and 80 in 1982. Obviously, subjects got older during follow-up so that it would not

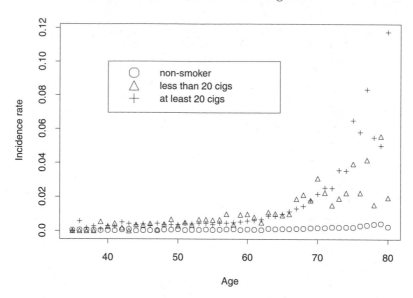

FIGURE 10.1. Incidence rate versus age for different cigarette categories.

make sense to analyze the entire follow-up period using age in 1982 as a constant covariate. Another problem with analyzing the entire follow-up period is that some individuals were lost to follow-up. A person who died of a different cause or emigrated after a year can no longer be observed as dying of lung cancer. This is reflected in the variable `freq` decreasing appropriately between successive follow-up periods.

To begin, we will therefore consider only the first year of follow-up. To achieve this, everyone followed up for more than a year is simply coded as not dying in year 1. Figure 10.1 shows a graph of the 'raw' estimated incidence rate (number of deaths divided by number of people followed up in each `age` and `cigscat` group) as a function of `age` and `cigscat`.

There is an obvious increase in incidence rate with age and a consistently larger incidence rate among smokers than among nonsmokers. The distinction between those smoking less than 20 or at least 20 cigarettes is less marked. We can fit a Poisson regression model using the number of deaths as the dependent variable and the log of freq as an offset. As explained in Display 10.1, this implies that we are modeling the *log incidence rate* as a linear function in the predictors. Using age and smoking status as main effects results in the estimates shown in Table 10.2.

Both `smoker` and `age` have significant effects (*t*-values much greater than 2). Confidence intervals (CI) can be obtained by using the estimate ± 1.96 times the standard error. Exponentiating the regression coefficients and 95% confidence limits yields an estimated incidence rate ratio for smokers compared with nonsmokers of 8.6 (95% CI from 7.5 to 8.9). To assess the effect of an increase in age by five years, we multiply the coefficient and

TABLE 10.2. Poisson regression for year 1 follow-up data

```
Coefficients:
                Value Std. Error t value
(Intercept) -11.24380   0.221380  -50.79
    smoker     2.15160   0.067283   31.98
       age     0.07214   0.003326   21.69

(Dispersion Parameter for Poisson family taken to be 1 )

Null Deviance: 12157 on 1382 degrees of freedom

Residual Deviance: 10822 on 1380 degrees of freedom
```

standard error for age by five first giving an incidence rate ratio estimate of 1.43 (95% CI from 1.39 to 1.48). To assess goodness of fit, we can add the predicted incidence rates to Figure 10.1, giving the curves in Figure 10.2.

Note that the estimated (absolute) effect of age increases with age because the model is linear on the log scale and the *relative* increase is constant. However, the fitted curve does not appear to increase sharply enough to fit the data for smokers. We therefore add a quadratic effect of age. The new model and analysis of deviance table comparing the new model with the previous one are given in Table 10.3. The quadratic effect is highly significant ($\chi^2(1) = 23.4$, $p < 0.001$). Adding the new predicted curves to Figure 10.2 gives Figure 10.3.

The new model fits the data more closely.

We have been wasteful by only using the first year of follow-up data. The reasons for this were that the important predictor, age, increases over the follow-up period and that the number of subjects followed up decreases over time. We can determine how many subjects were followed up during the second year (their follow-up will be greater than 1) and how many of them died of lung cancer during that year. Adding one year to these people's ages gives data for the second year of follow-up. These data can be combined with the year 1 follow-up data. Repeating this for follow-ups 3 to 6 gives a larger data set that can be analyzed as before. Note that the same subject now contributes to the data of several follow-up years. The parameter estimates for the model including smoker, age and age squared are given in Table 10.4 using just the one-year follow-up period and using all six years.

The parameter estimates have not changed substantially, and the standard errors have approximately halved. A graph of the observed and predicted incidence rates is given in Figure 10.4. The fit does not appear to be adequate. Note, however, that the data for ages over 80 are much less precise than are the remaining data because only subjects who were 80 at recruitment and subsequently did not die of other causes contributed to these estimates. These observations could be excluded from the analysis. Further analyses of the data set are suggested in the exercises.

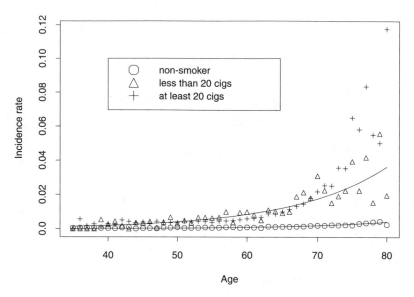

FIGURE 10.2. Observed and fitted incidence rates for lung cancer data

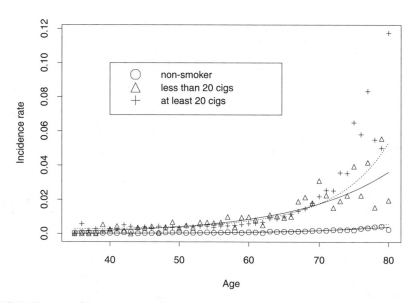

FIGURE 10.3. Observed and fitted incidence rates for lung cancer data (solid curve: log rate linear in age; dotted curve: log rate quadratic in age).

TABLE 10.3. Poisson regression including quadratic effect of age and analysis of deviance to asses significance of quadratic effect

```
Coefficients:
                Value Std. Error t value
(Intercept) -6.617308  0.9366805  -7.065
     smoker  2.189847  0.0681444  32.135
        age -0.086352  0.0316335  -2.730
   I(age^2)  0.001313  0.0002616   5.020

(Dispersion Parameter for Poisson family taken to be 1 )

    Null Deviance: 12157 on 1382 degrees of freedom

Residual Deviance: 10799 on 1379 degrees of freedom
```

Analysis of deviance table

```
Analysis of Deviance Table

Response: death

                                     Terms Resid. Df Resid. Dev
1            smoker + age + offset(log(freq))      1380       10822
2 smoker + age + I(age^2) + offset(log(freq))      1379       10799
      Test Df Deviance
1
2 +I(age^2)  1     23.39
```

TABLE 10.4. Poisson models using year 1 data and all data

Year 1 data			
	Value	Std. Error	t value
(Intercept)	-6.617308	0.9366805	-7.065
smoker	2.189847	0.0681444	32.135
age	-0.086352	0.0316335	-2.730
I(age^2)	0.001313	0.0002616	5.020

All data			
	Value	Std. Error	t value
(Intercept)	-5.484609	0.4628297	-11.850
smoker1	2.131828	0.0342329	62.274
age1	-0.124756	0.0151458	-8.237
I(age1^2)	0.001494	0.0001214	12.309

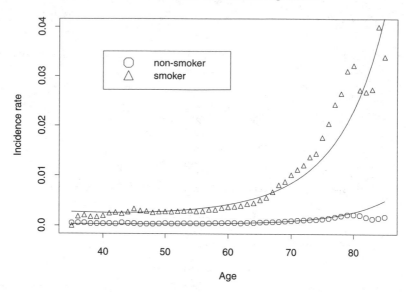

FIGURE 10.4. Observed and fitted incidence rates for lung cancer data for entire follow-up period.

10.3 Overdispersion

Overdispersion is the phenomenon when observed counts or proportions are more variable than predicted by the model. Both the Poisson and binomial distributions have variance functions that are completely determined by the expectation μ. There is no free parameter for the variance. The models are appropriate if all variability between observations with the same predicted value of μ is due to Poisson variability and binomial variability, respectively. For example, if the response variable is the number of GP visits in one year observed on each subject and the only explanatory variable used is sex, then the variability in the number of visits in a year between *different* women is assumed to be the same as the variability between the number of visits per year of the *same* woman in different years. This is clearly not a reasonable assumption because some women will be more prone to visit their GP than will others, and these differences in proneness are likely to persist over time. Therefore, observing the same woman over several years should give a smaller variance than observing different women for one year each. Some of this extra variability in the counts for different women may be due to omitted covariates, for example, age. Overdispersion should always be suspected when counts are observed on subjects (rather than subjects being counted) because in most situations we cannot hope to account for all sources of heterogeneity. The same phenomenon is likely if the counts are observed on 'higher level' units such as GP practices or regions. Note that in the lung cancer example, we had at most one occurrence of lung cancer per subject so that overdispersion due to subjects was not possible. If we had had separate counts for different states, there may have been overdispersion due to states. However, by using aggregate counts, we cannot detect this possible source of heterogeneity.

As an example of counts on units of observation, we will analyze counts of lip cancer in 56 Scottish counties. The data have previously been analyzed by Clayton and Kaldor (1987). The observed number of cases and a potential predictor affpct, the percentage of the employed population working in agriculture, fishing and farming, are available for each county. Other important predictors, age and sex, have been used to compute the 'expected' number of lip cancer cases. This was done by multiplying age and sex-specific expected rates by the number of individuals within the corresponding age and sex group within each county. The data are tabulated in Table 10.5.

In order for the exponentiated coefficients of the model to be interpretable as rate ratios, we need to use an appropriate variable as an offset. An interpretable rate in this case is the number of observed cases divided by the number of expected cases—this can be interpreted as an age- and sex-adjusted rate. We will therefore include the log of the expected number of cases as an offset.

The output is shown in Table 10.6. The coefficient of affpct is 0.073 with a standard error of 0.006. The effect is highly significant. The rate ratio per percentage increase in population working in agriculture, fisheries and foods is given by the exponential of this coefficient, 1.077.

However, the model assumes that all variability in the counties' true rates has been explained by this covariate together with the age and sex distribution and that all variance of the counts given the predicted mean is due to Poisson variablity only. This assumption appears to be unrealistic because there are likely to be other important differences between regions. In Display 10.2, the estimated dispersion parameter is suggested as a diagnostic for detecting overdispersion. The dispersion parameter can be estimated by dividing the residual deviance by the residual degrees of freedom, giving $238.6/54 = 4.4$. This is much greater than one suggesting that there is overdispersion and that the standard error of the regression coefficient has been underestimated.

As discussed in Display 10.2, we can scale the t-statistics using the square root of the estimated dispersion parameter or use a method analogous to analysis of variance to test the effect of the covariate, as shown in Table 10.7. Here, the dispersion parameter is based on the Pearson X^2 statistic. The effect of affpct is still highly significant. Equivalently, we can use *quasi-likelihood* to estimate the overdispersed Poisson model given in Table 10.8.

TABLE 10.5. Lip cancer data: observed and expected numbers of cases and percentage of population working in agriculture, fishing and forestry for 56 counties

County	Obs	Exp	Affpct	County	Obs	Exp	Affpct
1	9	1.4	16	29	9	1.4	16
2	39	8.7	16	30	39	8.7	16
3	11	3.0	10	31	11	3.0	10
4	9	2.5	24	32	9	2.5	24
5	15	4.3	10	33	15	4.3	10
6	8	2.4	24	34	8	2.4	24
7	26	8.1	10	35	26	8.1	10
8	7	2.3	7	36	7	2.3	7
9	6	2.0	7	37	6	2.0	7
10	20	6.6	16	38	20	6.6	16
11	13	4.4	7	39	13	4.4	7
12	5	1.8	16	40	5	1.8	16
13	3	1.1	10	41	3	1.1	10
14	8	3.3	24	42	8	3.3	24
15	17	7.8	7	43	17	7.8	7
16	9	4.6	16	44	9	4.6	16
17	2	1.1	10	45	2	1.1	10
18	7	4.2	7	46	7	4.2	7
19	9	5.5	7	47	9	5.5	7
20	7	4.4	10	48	7	4.4	10
21	16	10.5	7	49	16	10.5	7
22	31	22.7	16	50	31	22.7	16
23	11	8.8	10	51	11	8.8	10
24	7	5.6	7	52	7	5.6	7
25	19	15.5	1	53	19	15.5	1
26	15	12.5	1	54	15	12.5	1
27	7	6.0	7	55	7	6.0	7
28	10	9.0	7	56	10	9.0	7

TABLE 10.6. Poisson model for lip cancer data

```
Coefficients:
              Value Std. Error t value
(Intercept) -0.54227   0.069520   -7.80
     affpct  0.07373   0.005955   12.38

(Dispersion Parameter for Poisson family taken to be 1 )

Null Deviance: 380.7 on 55 degrees of freedom

Residual Deviance: 238.6 on 54 degrees of freedom
```

Display 10.2 Diagnostics for generalized linear models

- The *deviance residuals* are defined as

$$r_i^D = \text{sign}(y_i - \hat{\mu}_i)\sqrt{d_i} \qquad (1)$$

  where d_i is the contribution of the ith subject to the deviance, with total deviance given by $D = \sum_i (r_i^D)^2$.

- The *Pearson residuals* are defined as the contribution of the ith subject to the Pearson X^2 statistic,

$$r_i^P = \frac{(y_i - \hat{\mu}_i)}{\sqrt{V(\hat{\mu}_i)}} \qquad (2)$$

  so that the $X^2 = \sum (r_y^P)^2$

- Both the the Pearson and deviance statistics can be used for detecting observations not well fitted by the model. The deviance residuals are more commonly used because their distribution tends to be closer to normal than that of the Pearson residuals.

- The *dispersion* parameter is estimated as X^2/ν or D/ν, where ν are the degrees of freedom of the model. For normally distributed responses, these two estimates are identical and are estimates of the residual variance.

- For the Poisson and binomial distributions, the dispersion parameter is assumed to be 1. The estimated dispersion parameter can be used to assess *overdispersion* or *underdispersion*.

- If overdispersion or underdispersion exists, the assumption that $\phi = 1$ can be relaxed. In the Poisson case, the variance is assumed to be

$$V(\mu) = \phi\mu \qquad (3)$$

  and in the binomial case,

$$V(\mu) = \phi\mu(1 - \mu) \qquad (4)$$

  Although there are no likelihoods with these variance functions, the parameters can be estimated because the algorithm only requires the mean and variance functions. The method is known as *quasi-likelihood*. Analysis of variance must now be used instead of analysis of deviance to compare models.

- Instead of reestimating the model by quasi-likelihood, we can simply scale the t-statistics for the regression coefficients using the square root of the estimated dispersion parameter and use analysis of variance instead of comparing deviances.

TABLE 10.7. Analysis of variance for Poisson model

	Df	Sum of Sq	Mean Sq	F Value	Pr(F)
affpct	1	153.3	153.3	31.19	7.836e-007
Residuals	54	265.5	4.9		

TABLE 10.8. Quasi-likelihood for lip cancer data

```
Coefficients:
            Value Std. Error t value
(Intercept) -0.54227    0.1541  -3.518
    affpct   0.07373    0.0132   5.584
```

(Dispersion Parameter for Quasi-likelihood family taken to be 4.916)

Null Deviance: 380.7 on 55 degrees of freedom

Residual Deviance: 238.6 on 54 degrees of freedom

10.4 Diagnostics

Display 10.2 describes various possible diagnostics for generalized linear models. We can assess the fit of the lip cancer model using deviance residuals that should be approximately normally distributed if the model is appropriate. In the presence of overdispersion, we can standardize the residuals by dividing by the square root of the estimated dispersion parameter. A normal quantile plot of these scaled deviance residuals is shown in Figure 10.5.

The distribution appears to be close to normal. Plotting the same residuals against the predicted counts using county codes as labels gives the graph in Figure 10.6. Note that the offset was included in determining the predicted counts so that the counties to the right are likely to be large counties.

A graph of the deviance residuals against age for the lung cancer data over the entire follow-up period is shown in Figure 10.7 with different symbols for smokers and nonsmokers. Lowess curves are superimposed. The fact that the deviance residuals vary systematically with age suggests that the age dependence is not adequately modeled, as was previously suggested by Figure 10.4. In addition, the difference between the lowess curves for smokers and nonsmokers suggests that an interaction between smoking status and age may be needed.

10.5 Summary

Poisson regression can be used to model the effect of risk factors and confounders on diseases from cohort data. Here, the count is the dependent

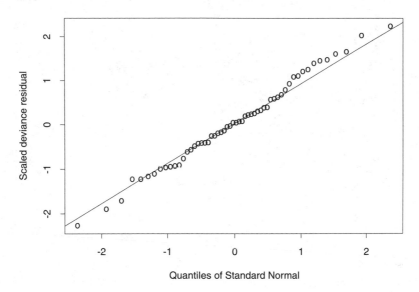

FIGURE 10.5. Normal quantile plot of standardized deviance residuals for lip cancer data.

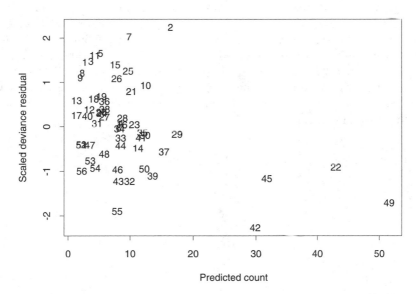

FIGURE 10.6. Standardized deviance residuals versus predicted counts for lip cancer data with county codes used as labels.

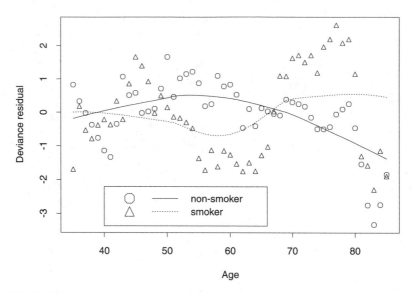

FIGURE 10.7. Deviance residuals versus age for smokers and nonsmokers with lowess curves.

variable, and an offset is used to ensure that the exponentiated regression coefficients can be interpreted as rate ratios. Overdispersion is a frequent problem when applying Poisson regression to medical data. There are many other aplications of Poisson models. For example, we could model the number of epileptic fits or the number of visits to GPs. In the first example discussed in this chapter, we assumed that the incidence rate increases with age but is piecewise constant during each year of follow-up. If the exact dates of death are recorded, the incidence rate could be modeled as varying continuously with time. Such models, known as survival models, will be discussed in Chapters 16 and 17.

10.6   Using S-PLUS

Section 10.2

Some data manipulation is used to prepare the data, making use of the
tapply() function. Poisson models are fitted using glm() with the option
family=poisson (the log link is the default) and with an offset, specified via
the offset() function in the model formula. The control option is used
to increase the maximum number of iterations used by glm(). predict()
is used to compute and plot predicted counts. The anova() function is used
to compare two nested generalized linear models using analysis of deviance.
The marks option is used in the legend() function to provide a legend for
symbols used to represent points on a scatterplot.

Script for Section 10.2

```
# Read lung cancer data
lung<-read.table("lungcanc.dat", header=T)

# Analyze year 1 data
lung1<-lung

# Deaths that occurred after 1 year are not counted
death1<-lung$death
death1[death1==1&lung$follow>1]<-0

# Replace death by death1
lung1$death<-death1

# Plot incidence against age for smokers and nonsmokers
win.graph()
attach(lung1)

# Compute incidence for each combination of age and cigscat
den<-tapply(freq,list(age=age,cigscat=cigscat),FUN=sum)
num<-tapply(death,list(age=age,cigscat=cigscat),FUN=sum)
inc<-num/den

# Work out corresponding values of age and cigscat
age1<-tapply(age,list(age=age,cigscat=cigscat),FUN=mean)
cigs1<-tapply(cigscat,list(age=age,cigscat=cigscat),FUN=mean)

plot(age1,inc,type="n",ylab="Incidence rate",xlab="Age")
points(age1[cigs1==0],inc[cigs1==0],pch=1)
points(age1[cigs1==1],inc[cigs1==1],pch=2)
points(age1[cigs1==2],inc[cigs1==2],pch=3)
legend(40,.1,legend=
    c("nonsmoker","less than 20 cigs","at least 20 cigs"),
```

```
    marks=c(1,2,3))                                    ⟹  Figure 10.1


# Fit Poisson model
lung.glm<-glm(death~smoker+age+offset(log(freq)),
    family=poisson,data=lung1)
# did not converge after 10 iterations

# Fit Poisson model using up to 15 iterations
lung.glm<-glm(death~smoker+age+offset(log(freq)),
    family=poisson,data=lung1,
    control = glm.control(maxit = 15))
summary(lung.glm)
                                                       ⟹  Table 10.2


# Compute incidence rate ratios and 95% CI
exp( 2.15160)
exp( 2.15160 - 1.96* 0.067283)
exp( 2.15160 + 1.96* 0.067283)


exp(5*0.07214)
exp(5*0.07214- 1.96*5* 0.003326)
exp(5*0.07214+ 1.96*5* 0.003326)


# Add fitted curves to figure
new<-data.frame(age=rep(35:80,2),smoker<-rep(0:1,each=46),
    freq=rep(20,92))
# use follow-up period of 20, then divide predicted count by 20

pred<-predict(lung.glm,newdata=new,type="response")/20
lines(35:80,pred[1:46])
lines(35:80,pred[47:92])
                                                       ⟹  Figure 10.2


# Use second-order polynomial for age
lung.glm2<-glm(death~smoker+age+I(age^2)+offset(log(freq)),
    family=poisson,data=lung1,
    control = glm.control(maxit = 15))
summary(lung.glm2)
# Likelihood ratio test
anova(lung.glm,lung.glm2)
                                                       ⟹  Table 10.3

1-pchisq(23.29,1)
# This gives the p-value


# Add new fitted curves
pred<-predict(lung.glm2,newdata=new,type="response")/20
lines(35:80,pred[1:46],lty=2)
lines(35:80,pred[47:92],lty=2)
                                                       ⟹  Figure 10.3
```

```
# Use all data up to follow-up 6
attach(lung)
# lung1 is as before

# lung2: everyone followed for at least two years
lung2<-lung[follow>=2,]
# Those who die later survived up to end of follow-up 2
death1<-death[follow>=2]
death1[death1==1&lung2$follow>2]<-0
lung2$death<-death1
# Age has increased by one year
lung2$age<-lung2$age+1

# Repeat for other follow-up periods
lung3<-lung[follow>=3,]
death1<-death[follow>=3]
death1[death1==1&lung3$follow>3]<-0
lung3$death<-death1
lung3$age<-lung3$age+2

lung4<-lung[follow>=4,]
death1<-death[follow>=4]
death1[death1==1&lung4$follow>4]<-0
lung4$death<-death1
lung4$age<-lung4$age+3

lung5<-lung[follow>=5,]
death1<-death[follow>=5]
death1[death1==1&lung5$follow>5]<-0
lung5$death<-death1
lung5$age<-lung5$age+4

lung6<-lung[follow>=6,]
death1<-death[follow>=6]
death1[death1==1&lung6$follow>6]<-0
lung6$death<-death1
lung6$age<-lung6$age+5

# Fit glm to all data
Lung<-rbind(lung1,lung2,lung3,lung4,lung5,lung6)
lung.glm3<-glm(death~smoker+age+I(age^2)+offset(log(freq)),
   family=poisson,data=Lung,
   control = glm.control(maxit = 15))
summary(lung.glm3)$coefficients
summary(lung.glm2)$coefficients                    ⟹ Table 10.4

# Plot data and fitted curves
```

```
# First, collapse data to one observation for each combination
# of age and smoker
attach(Lung)
age1<-as.vector(tapply(age,list(age=age,smoker=smoker),
    FUN=mean))
# tapply() returns a matrix and as.vector() stacks
# this in a vector
smoker1<-as.vector(tapply(smoker,list(age=age,smoker=smoker),
    FUN=mean))
death1<-as.vector(tapply(death,list(age=age,smoker=smoker),
    FUN=sum))
freq1<-as.vector(tapply(freq,list(age=age,smoker=smoker),
    FUN=sum))
lung.glm4<-glm(death1~smoker1+age1+I(age1^2)+offset(log(freq1)),
    family=poisson)

# Check that we made no mistake and model is the same as before
summary(lung.glm3)$coefficients
summary(lung.glm4)$coefficients

inc<-death1/freq1
plot(age1, inc, type="n",ylab="Incidence rate",xlab="Age")
points(age1[smoker1==0],inc[smoker1==0],pch=1)
points(age1[smoker1==1],inc[smoker1==1],pch=2)
new<-data.frame(age1=rep(35:85,2),smoker1<-rep(0:1,each=51),
    freq1=rep(20,102))
# use arbitrary offset of log(20), then divide
# predicted count by 20

pred<-predict(lung.glm4,newdata=new,type="response")/20
lines(35:85,pred[1:51])
lines(35:85,pred[52:102])
legend(40,.035,legend=c("non-smoker","smoker"),
    marks=c(1,2))
```
$\implies$ Figure 10.4

Section 10.3

In this section, the summary.aov() function is used to obtain tests for the regression coefficients that are correct if there is overdispersion. The family=quasi() option of glm() is illustrated to fit an overdispersed Poisson model.

Script for Section 10.3

```
# Read lip cancer data
Lip<-matrix(scan("lips.dat"),ncol=3,byrow=T)
```

```
Lip<-as.data.frame(list(obs=Lip[,1],exp=Lip[,2],
   affpct=Lip[,3]))
attach(Lip)

lip.pr<-glm(obs~affpct+offset(log(exp)),family=poisson,
   data=Lip)
summary(lip.pr)

# assumes no overdispersion, phi=1

summary.aov(lip.pr)
# allows for overdispersion by assuming that
# phi would be estimated

# Quasilikelihood
lip.q<-glm(obs~affpct+offset(log(exp)),
   family=quasi(link=log, variance=mu),
   data=Lip)
# assumes overdispersion
summary(lip.q)
```

$\Longrightarrow$ Table 10.6

$\Longrightarrow$ Table 10.7

$\Longrightarrow$ Table 10.8

Section 10.4

In this section, the residuals() function is used with the type="deviance" option to compute deviance residuals. Fitted values are obtained from the object returned by glm(). The qqnorm() and qqline() functions are used to plot a normal quantile plot.

Script for Section 10.4

```
# Compute deviance residuals
resids<-residuals(lip.pr,type="deviance")
resids<-resids*sqrt(54/238.6)
# divide by dispersion parameter

# Q-Q plot of scaled deviance residuals
qqnorm(resids,ylab="Scaled deviance residual")
qqline(resids)

# Deviance residuals versus predicted
fit<-lip.pr$fitted
plot(fit,resids,xlab="Predicted count",
   ylab="Scaled deviance residual",type="n")
text(fit,resids,labels=as.character(row.names(Lip)))
```

$\Longrightarrow$ Figure 10.5

$\Longrightarrow$ Figure 10.6

```
# Deviance residuals versus age for lung cancer data
# (use age1, etc. from before)
resids<-residuals(lung.glm4,type="deviance")
plot(age1,resids,type="n",ylab="Deviance residual",xlab="Age")
points(age1[smoker1==0],resids[smoker1==0],pch=1)
points(age1[smoker1==1],resids[smoker1==1],pch=2)
lines(lowess(age1[smoker1==0],resids[smoker1==0]),lty=1)
lines(lowess(age1[smoker1==1],resids[smoker1==1]),lty=2)
legend(40,-2.5,legend=c("nonsmoker","smoker"),
    marks=c(1,2),lty=1:2)
```

$\implies$ Figure 10.7

10.7 Exercises

10.1 Analyze the lung cancer data from the whole six-year follow-up period using `cigscat` instead of `smoker` as the explanatory variable. Exclude observations with `age` > 80. Include `age` and `age`^{2}, and use treatment contrasts for `cigscat`.

10.2 What contrasts will give you a test of smokers versus nonsmokers and a test of frequent smokers versus infrequent smokers (consider recoding the variable)? Refit the model using this contrast, and compute the incidence rate ratios and their confidence intervals.

10.3 Plot the raw incidence estimates and the fitted curves for this model.

10.4 Plot the deviance residuals against age. Does this plot indicate that third- and higher order polynomial terms of age may be required?

10.5 Consider including further terms in the model, for example, an interaction between smoking frequency and age or higher order polynomial terms for age.

11
Linear Mixed Models I

11.1 Introduction

Observations often fall into groups or clusters. For example, longitudinal data consist of repeated observations on the same subjects. Hierarchical data sets typically consist of subjects nested in higher level units, such as families or GP practices. In both types of data, we cannot assume that observations on the same subject (or cluster) are independent. Standard methods of analysis such as ANOVA or multiple regression, which assume that observations are independent, are therefore not valid for clustered data. Fortunately, these methods can be extended by explicitly modeling the covariances among observations within a cluster. In this chapter, we discuss how this can be done using *linear mixed models*.

11.2 Variance components

An example of clustered data is given by the repeated measurements of peak expiratory flow rate (PEFR) on 17 subjects presented in Bland and Altman (1986). Two measurements were taken with each of two instruments, the Wright peak flow meter and the mini Wright meter, in random order. The data are given in Table 11.1.

The first and second recordings on the mini Wright meter are plotted against the subject idenitfier in Figure 11.1(a). The horizontal line represents the overall mean measurement.

(a) First and second measurements

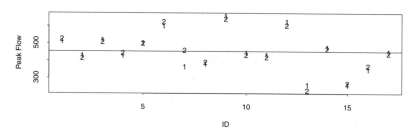

(b) First measurement and second measurements+100

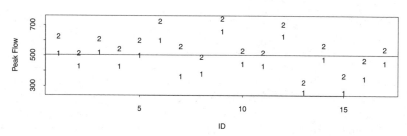

FIGURE 11.1. (a) First and second recordings of peak expiratory flow using mini Wright meter versus subject number. (b) 100 added to second recording. The horizontal lines represent the overall means.

TABLE 11.1. Peak expiratory flow rate measured twice using both the Wright peak flow meter and the mini Wright meter

Subject	Wright peak flow meter		Mini Wright meter	
	First	Second	First	Second
1	494	490	512	525
2	395	397	430	415
3	516	512	520	508
4	434	401	428	444
5	476	470	500	500
6	557	611	600	625
7	413	415	364	460
8	442	431	380	390
9	650	638	658	642
10	433	429	445	432
11	417	420	432	420
12	656	633	626	605
13	267	275	260	227
14	478	492	477	467
15	178	165	259	268
16	423	372	350	370
17	427	421	451	443

It is clear from the figure that the repeated measurements on the same subject tend to be closer to each other than to the measurements on a different subject. In fact, if this was not the case, the mini Wright meter would be useless as a tool for discriminating between the individuals in this particular sample. We can model the measurements y_{ij} of subject i on occasion j as

$$y_{ij} = \mu + u_i + \epsilon_{ij}, \quad \epsilon_{ij} \sim N(0, \sigma^2) \tag{11.1}$$

where u_i is the difference between the overall mean and subject i's mean measurement and ϵ_{ij} is the measurement error for subject i on occasion j. This looks like a one-way ANOVA model with subjects as a factor. However, instead of fitting an ANOVA model by estimating the u_i as *fixed effects*, we shall assume that the u_i are *random effects* that are independently normally distributed, $u_i \sim N(0, \tau^2)$, and independent of the ϵ_{ij}. Each measurement therefore differs from the overall mean μ by the sum of two error terms, u_i, which is shared between measurements on the same subjects, and ϵ_{ij}, which is not. Because the error terms are independent, the total variance is the sum of the *variance components*, $\tau^2 + \sigma^2$, and the proportion of the total variance that is due to subjects is

$$\rho = \frac{\tau^2}{\tau^2 + \sigma^2} \tag{11.2}$$

TABLE 11.2. Estimates of mean and standard deviations

```
Approximate 95% confidence intervals

Fixed effects:
              lower   est. upper
(Intercept)   397 453.9 510.9

Random Effects:
  Level: id
                 lower   est. upper
sd((Intercept)) 67.09 110.4 181.7

Within-group standard error:
lower   est. upper
12.38 19.91 32.03
```

This coefficient, known as the *intraclass correlation*, directly measures the 'closeness' of observations on the same subject relative to the closeness of observations on different subjects. In the measurement context, τ^2 is the variance between subjects' 'true' scores (defined as the long-term average measurement), σ^2 is the measurement error variance and the intraclass correlation is a *reliability* index (see, for example, Streiner and Norman, 1989).

The model in (11.1) is an example of a *random effects model* or *random intercept model* as described in Display 11.1. Using the multilevel terminology of Goldstein (1995) and Bryk and Raudenbush (1992), we will refer to the levels of the grouping variable, in this case, subjects, as level 2 units and to the individual observations, in this case, repeated measurements, as level 1 units. There are several ways of estimating the variance components. Using REML, for example (see Display 11.1), gives the estimates and 95% confidence intervals of τ and σ shown in Table 11.2.

The overall mean is estimated as 453.9. The standard deviation of the effect of subjects, τ, is estimated as 110.4, and the within-subject standard deviation, σ, is estimated as 19.91. The intraclass correlation is therefore estimated as $110.4^2/(19.91^2 + 110.4^2) = 0.97$. This is very close to one, indicating that the instrument is very reliable. (Note, however, that the reliability depends on the variability between subjects, τ^2, and that this can differ between populations.)

Figure 11.1(b) shows the result of shifting the second measurements up by 100 units (this could be interpreted as a practice effect). As the graph suggests, such a shift reduces the reliability, with an intraclass correlation of 0.63. Note that the Pearson correlation is 0.97 for both cases (a) and (b) because it is based on deviations of the first and second measurements from their *respective* means. The Pearson correlation is therefore not a suitable measure of reliability. Unlike the Pearson correlation, the intraclass

---

Display 11.1 Random intercept models

- When the observations (level 1 units) are clustered within level 2 units, e.g., subjects in families, we cannot use ordinary linear models because the observations are not independent. A random intercept model is a linear model that includes random effects for the level 2 units. Writing i for the level 2 units and j for the level 1 units, the model with a single random factor can be written as

$$y_{ij} = \boldsymbol{\beta}' \mathbf{x}_{ij} + u_i + \epsilon_{ij} \tag{1}$$

where $u_i \sim N(0, \tau^2)$ and $\epsilon_{ij} \sim N(0, \sigma^2)$ are independent. Instead of estimating the values u_i, as in a *fixed effects* model, the variance of the distribution of u_i, τ^2, is estimated. The model can also be described as a linear regression model with a *random intercept* for the level 2 units.

- The total (predicted) variance of a level 1 unit conditional on the covariates is

$$\text{var}(y_{ij}|\mathbf{x}_{ij}) = \tau^2 + \sigma^2 \tag{2}$$

The two variances τ^2 and σ^2 that make up the total variance are therefore also known as *variance components*.

- The covariance between two level 1 units j and l is

$$\text{cov}(y_{ij}, y_{kl}|\mathbf{x}_{il}, \mathbf{x}_{kl}) = \begin{cases} \tau^2 & \text{if } i = k \\ 0 & \text{otherwise} \end{cases} \tag{3}$$

so that the correlation is $\tau^2/(\tau^2 + \sigma^2)$ for any pair of units within the same level 2 unit and zero otherwise. This correlation structure (constant variance and constant within-cluster covariance) is known as an *exchangeable* correlation structure or as *compound symmetry*. The within-cluster correlation is known as the *intraclass correlation*.

- Conditionally on the random and fixed effects, any pair of level 1 units within the same level 2 unit is assumed to be independent. This is the *conditional independence assumption*. The marginal correlations (conditional on fixed effect but not on random effects) are correlations are due to the tendency of the units within the same level 2 unit to lie on the same side of the overall mean.

- The model can be estimated by maximum likelihood. However, this method tends to underestimate the variance components. A modified version of maximum likelihood, known as *restricted maximum likelihood* (REML), provides consistent estimates of the variance components. See Diggle *et al.* (1994) or Longford (1993) for more details.

- Different models can be compared using a likelihood ratio test. If the models have been estimated by REML, this is essentially based on transforming the dependent variable to error contrasts. Because the transformation and therefore the "data" used in the estimation depend on the fixed effects, the likelihood ratio test can only be used if both models have the same set of fixed effects (see Longford, 1993).

---

correlation is defined both for more than two observations per subject and for unequal numbers of observations per subject.

11.3   Mixed effects ANOVA model

Another example of clustered data are longitudinal data arising, for example, in clinical trials. Here, we wish to estimate the effect of factors such as treatments while taking into account that observations on the same subject are correlated. Table 11.3 gives the results of a small two-period, two-treatment cross-over trial reported in Maqs *et al.* (1987) and analyzed in Gelfand *et al.* (1990). Here, subjects were randomized to receive either a new chewable tablet formulation of carbamezepine (treatment A) or standard carbamezepine tablets (treatment B). After a four-week washout period, subjects crossed over to the other treatment. Blood samples were collected over 48 hours following a 200 mg dose to derive concentration time curves for each subject and each formulation. The logarithms of the maxima of these curves are given in Table 11.3.

Treating subject as a random factor, we can model the response y_{ijk} for subject i in period j receiving treatment k as

$$y_{ijk} = \mu + \alpha_j + \beta_k + u_i + \epsilon_{ij} \tag{11.3}$$

with $u_i \sim N(0, \tau^2)$ and $\epsilon_{ij} \sim N(0, \sigma^2)$. The model assumes that the residuals $u_i + \epsilon_{ij}$ are correlated within subjects with a correlation equal to the intraclass correlation in (11.2) and uncorrelated between subjects. The parameter estimates are shown in Table 11.4.

The treatment effect is very close to zero with 95% CI from -0.09 to 0.10. There is a significant period effect. The intraclass correlation of the residuals is 0.69. We now consider including a treatment by period interaction. In order to compare the models using a likelihood ratio test, both models must be estimated by maximum likelihood because REML can only be used to compare models with the same fixed effects (see Display 11.1). The likelihood ratio test, shown in Table 11.5, is not significant, implying that the treatment by period interaction is not present.

The observed and fitted values of the model with main effects only are plotted in Figure 11.2. Here, the values of the random effects have been 'predicted' using BLUP estimates; see Display 11.2. Because the effect of treatment is negligible, the 'slopes', representing the differences between periods, appear constant. It is clear that some subjects have consistently higher outcomes than have others. This is captured by including the random intercepts u_i in the model.

A great advantage of this type of model is that subjects with missing values on some of the occasions can contribute to the analysis. If the data are *missing at random*, i.e., the probability that y_{ijk} is missing is independent of the value of y_{ijk} given the explanatory variables included in the model,

TABLE 11.3. Cross-over trial results (logarithm of maxima of concentration-time curves

Sequence	Sequ. code	Period 1	Period 2
AB	1	1.40	1.65
AB	1	1.64	1.57
BA	−1	1.44	1.58
BA	−1	1.36	1.68
BA	−1	1.65	1.69
AB	1	1.08	1.31
AB	1	1.09	1.43
AB	1	1.25	1.44
BA	−1	1.25	1.39
BA	−1	1.30	1.52

TABLE 11.4. Parameter estimates for cross-over trial

```
Linear mixed-effects model fit by REML
 Data: equiv2
       AIC   BIC logLik
 -0.8715 3.295  5.436

Random effects:
 Formula:  ~ 1 | id
         (Intercept) Residual
StdDev:      0.1399  0.09319

Fixed effects: y ~ period + treat
             Value Std.Error DF t-value p-value
(Intercept) 1.154    0.1010  9   11.42  <.0001
    period 0.180    0.0417  8    4.32  0.0025
     treat 0.008    0.0417  8    0.19  0.8526
 Correlation:
         (Intr) period
period -0.619
 treat -0.619  0.000

Standardized Within-Group Residuals:
    Min     Q1     Med    Q3   Max
 -1.158 -0.3306 -0.1629 0.355 1.713

Number of Observations: 20
Number of Groups: 10
```

TABLE 11.5. Likelihood ratio test for period by treatment interaction

Model	df	AIC	BIC	logLik	Test	L.Ratio	p-value
1	5	-14.39	-9.411	12.19			
2	6	-13.62	-7.650	12.81	1 vs 2	1.235	0.2665

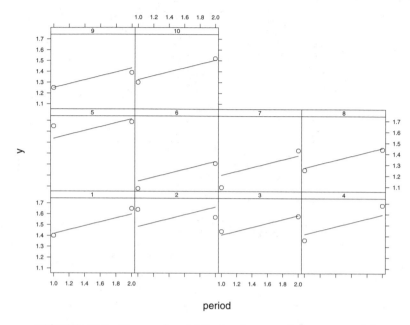

FIGURE 11.2. Observed and fitted outcomes of cross-over trial.

Display 11.2 Prediction of random effects

- The random effects are not estimated as part of the model. However, having estimated the model, we can *predict* the values of the random effects.

- According to Bayes Theorem, the *posterior probability* of the random effects is given by

$$\Pr(\mathbf{u}|\mathbf{y}, \mathbf{x}) = f(\mathbf{y}|\mathbf{u}, \mathbf{x})g(\mathbf{u}) \qquad (1)$$

where $f(\mathbf{y}|\mathbf{u}, \mathbf{x})$ is the conditional density of the responses given the random effects and covariates (a product of normal densities) and $g(\mathbf{u})$ is the *prior* density of the random effects (multivariate normal). The means of this posterior distribution can be used as estimates of the random effects and are known as *empirical Bayes* estimates.

- The empirical Bayes estimator is also known as a shrinkage estimator because the predicted random effects are smaller in absolute value than their fixed effect counterparts.

- *Best linear unbiased predictions* (BLUP) are linear combinations of the responses that are unbiased estimators of the random effects and minimize the mean square error.

TABLE 11.6. Result of fitting mixed effects model to cross-over trial data with three missing values

```
Linear mixed-effects model fit by REML
  Data: equiv3
      AIC   BIC logLik
    4.942 8.137  2.529

Random effects:
 Formula:  ~ 1 | id
           (Intercept) Residual
 StdDev:       0.1299   0.1157

Fixed effects: y ~ period + treat
               Value Std.Error DF t-value p-value
 (Intercept) 1.130     0.1416  9   7.978  <.0001
      period 0.189     0.0595  5   3.172  0.0247
       treat 0.018     0.0595  5   0.306  0.7722
 Correlation:
            (Intr) period
 period -0.677
  treat -0.709  0.099

Standardized Within-Group Residuals:
    Min      Q1     Med      Q3     Max
 -1.017 -0.4267 -0.1602 0.3264 1.602

Number of Observations: 17
Number of Groups: 10
```

then maximum likelihood (or REML) yields consistent parameter estimates (see Diggle et al., 1994, or Everitt and Pickles, 2000). To illustrate this, we drop the three responses y_{111}, y_{321} and y_{622} and repeat the analysis. The results shown in Table 11.6 agree very closely with those in Table 11.4 for the full data set. The standard errors of the fixed effects reflect the loss of observations.

11.4   Linear regression with a random intercept

In order to demonstrate that neonates have a deflation reflex that causes them to inhale when the lungs are deflated, Hannam et al. (2001) carried out the following experiment. The strength of inspiration (inhaling) following a gentle compression of the chest was repeatedly measured for 27 babies while altering the timing, magnitude and rate of the applied pressure. Table 11.7 gives the logarithm linsp of the measurements of the strength of inspiration (rise in oesophagael pressure on squeezing), applied pressure, maxp, and 'squeeze number', squeezen, for five of the babies. Here, squeeze number is just the sequence number of the experiment. The logarithm of the strength of inspiratory response will be analyzed because this is less skewed than are the original measurements.

The aim of the analysis is to demonstrate a dose-response relationship between the rise in oesophagael pressure and the srength of inspiration. In Chapter 6, the nonindependence of repeated measures on the same person was taken into account by analyzing summary measures. The main variable of interest was the treatment group, which differed *between* subjects. However, here, it would not be efficient to regress the average inspiratory response on the average applied pressure (between baby analysis) because the variables of interest vary mostly *within* babies. We can see this by looking at some summary statistics for each baby as shown in Table 11.8. A better approach would be to investigate the relationship between the two variables *within* babies, with the additional advantage that any between-baby differences are then controlled for.

This could be done by computing the linear regression coefficient for each baby and deriving a pooled estimate, or by including a dummy variable for each baby in a single linear regression model as follows:

$$y_{ij} = \beta_0 + \beta_1 x_{ij} + \beta_2 z_{ij} + \epsilon_{ij} \qquad (11.4)$$

where i and j are the baby and observation indices, respectively, and z_{ij} is an indicator variable for the ith baby. (Because of the constant β_0, one baby's dummy variable must be omitted.) This *fixed effects* model allows babies to have different intercepts but assumes that the slopes and residual error variances are the same for all babies.

Obviously, this approach ignores overall differences in the explanatory variable *between* babies. For example, if baby 6 had a lower average respiratory response than did baby 4, this would provide some evidence for a dose-response relationship because baby 6 has a lower average rate of applied pressure. But this information does not contribute to the estimate of the slope β_1.

One advantage of using random effects models is that they combine both within-cluster and between-cluster information. The random intercept model is

$$y_{ij} = \beta_0 + \beta_1 x_{ij} + u_i + \epsilon_{ij} \qquad (11.5)$$

Fitting the between-baby, fixed effects (within-baby) and random effects models yields the following estimates for the effect of the rate of applied pressure on log inspiratory response:

Method	Estimate	Standard error	p-value
between-baby	0.009	0.012	0.48
fixed effects	0.047	0.003	<0.001
random effects	0.045	0.003	<0.001

TABLE 11.7. Sample of inspiration data. For five babies, a label is tabulated, followed by the variable's squeeze number (sqeezen), applied pressure (maxp), and the logarithm of the strength of the inspiratory response (linsp)

1

sqeezen	2	3	4	5	7	8	9	10	11	12	16	18	19	21	22	23
maxp	7.7	13.9	16.2	11.6	21.6	11.6	16.9	13.1	10.8	22.3	14.6	17.7	13.9	21.6	17.7	18.5
linsp	5.7	3.5	5.1	5.5	3.7	4.7	4.6	5.7	4.2	4.4	3.9	5.6	4.5	4.2	5.8	3.8

2

sqeezen	2	4	6	7	8	9	10	11	12	13	14
maxp	15.4	19	17.7	21	19.3	13.9	22.3	19.3	10	9.2	5.8
linsp	13.4	11.5	12	8.9	9.2	15	13.3	15	8.9	4.9	4.4

3

sqeezen	1	2	3	4	6	8	9	10	11	12	13	14	15	16	17	19	20	21
maxp	8.8	8.8	10.4	12	13.6	11.2	12	13.6	14.4	14.4	16	13.6	16.3	5.6	14.4	16	13.6	
linsp	3.9	2.9	5.2	1.8	5.4	9.5	4.2	5.5	5.6	2.9	4.9	3.3	4.6	4.6	8.9	7.1	4.7	

4

sqeezen	5	6	7	9	11	12	13	14	15	16
maxp	22.2	16.7	26.6	16.3	15.4	15.4	19.4	19.2	19.2	22.9
linsp	3.5	3.7	2.3	4.4	7.9	5.1	3.3	5.9	1.8	4.8

5

sqeezen	1	2	3	4	5	6	7	9	10	11	12	13	16	18	19	21	23	24
maxp	9.2	13.9	12.3	10	8.5	7.7	8.5	6.2	6.9	6.9	13.1	9.2	6.9	8.5	9.2	10	10	10
linsp	0.8	2.7	2.8	5.3	4.4	5.5	7.4	5.6	5.6	4.8	4.3	7.1	4.7	4.2	4.6	2.4	6.3	7.1

TABLE 11.8. Summary measures of applied pressure for each baby

Baby	Min.	1st Qu.	Median	Mean	3rd Qu.	Max.
1	7.7	12.73	15.4	15.61	17.9	22.3
2	5.8	11.95	17.7	15.72	19.3	22.3
3	5.6	9	12	11.69	14.2	16.8
4	15.4	16.4	19.2	19.33	21.5	26.6
5	6.2	7.8	9.2	9.327	10	13.9
6	3.1	8.1	11.6	13.91	19.65	33.9
7	5.2	8.1	11.45	11.24	14.23	19.3
8	2.3	6.275	9.6	10.17	12.6	22.3
9	2.8	7.55	8.4	8.267	9.8	11.6
10	7.7	11.4	14.25	14.86	18.7	23.1
11	6.9	10	11.6	13.45	15.4	24.6
12	3.7	7.775	11.1	11.77	16.03	19.2
13	3.3	6.8	11.7	11.69	15	25
14	8	12	14.4	13.81	16	19.2
15	2.5	5.85	6.6	6.593	7.6	8.8
16	3	5.85	8.7	9.394	11.7	21.6
17	2.8	7.3	9.75	10.36	14.08	17.9
18	2.5	5.5	7.5	7.272	9.25	11
19	5.8	6.4	8.25	9.786	11.92	17.5
20	5.6	7.7	9.65	9.536	11.02	13.3
21	7.4	11.63	16.3	16.98	22.77	27
22	5.5	8.7	21.65	20.38	28.33	36.3
23	6.1	17.52	18.9	18.65	22.9	30.1
24	8	11	15	15.62	21	23
25	7	10	19	15.68	20.88	22
26	8	15.25	18.2	23.46	32.6	47
27	5.9	10.4	14.3	13.08	16.12	19.5

TABLE 11.9. Random effects model for effect of pressure on the logarithm of the strength of inspiration

```
Linear mixed-effects model fit by REML
 Data: new
     AIC   BIC logLik
   659.9 677.2   -326

Random effects:
 Formula:   ~ 1 | baby
         (Intercept) Residual
StdDev:       0.277    0.4092

Fixed effects: linsp ~ maxp
               Value Std.Error  DF t-value p-value
(Intercept) 0.9339    0.07083 523   13.19  <.0001
       maxp 0.0447    0.00324 523   13.79  <.0001
 Correlation:
      (Intr)
maxp -0.603

Standardized Within-Group Residuals:
    Min      Q1     Med     Q3    Max
 -4.097 -0.6469 0.05924 0.6495 2.753

Number of Observations: 551
Number of Groups: 27
```

The similarity in the estimates from the random effects and fixed effects models indicates that most of the information contributing to the estimates of the random effects model is due to within-baby variability. This is also reflected in the low estimate of the regression coefficient and large standard error for the between-baby analysis. The output from the random effects model is given in Display 11.9 (page 255).

The standard deviation of the random intercept is estimated as 0.28, and the standard deviation of the within-baby residual error is estimated as 0.41. The latter is identical to the fixed-effects estimate of the residual standard deviation (not shown).

So far, we have assumed that there is a linear relationship between applied pressure and the logarithm of the strength of the inspiratory response. To see whether this is a reasonable assumption, we can create a scatterplot in which the profiles for some babies are connected. Such a graph is shown in Figure 11.3 (page 256). There appears to be a flattening of the curves for larger values of applied pressure.

We will thus investigate whether quadratic and cubic polynomial terms significantly improve the model fit. Another variable that may be a predictor of response is the squeeze number. Table 11.10 (page 256) shows the like-

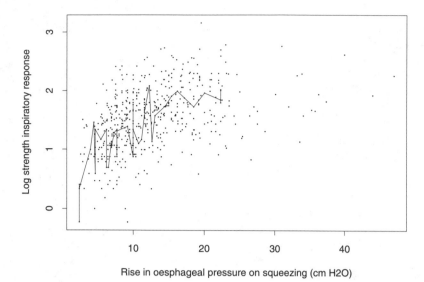

FIGURE 11.3. Scatterplot of the log strength of the inspiratory response against rise in oesophagael pressure for 27 babies. The trajectory of baby 14 has been connected.

TABLE 11.10. Likelihood ratios of sequentially adding squeeze number, quadratic and cubic terms of pressure

	Model	df	AIC	BIC	logLik	Test	L.Ratio	p-value
maxp.lme0	1	4	646.4	663.6	-319.2			
maxp.lme1	2	5	639.9	661.5	-315.0	1 vs 2	8.45	0.0036
maxp.lme2	3	6	599.3	625.2	-293.7	2 vs 3	42.62	<.0001
maxp.lme3	4	7	586.8	616.9	-286.4	3 vs 4	14.54	0.0001

lihood ratios for sequentially adding first the squeeze number (maxp.lme1) and then a quadratic (maxp.lme2) and cubic term (maxp.lme3).

The best-fitting random intercept model is therefore the full model, including a cubic polynomial in applied pressure and a linear effect of squeeze number (see Table 11.11, page 257).

11.5   Random coefficient models

The models considered so far for the inspiratory response data assume that the effect of changing applied pressure is the same for all babies. An alternative model would be to assume that, in addition to having different intercepts, the babies also have different slopes. The model becomes

$$y_{ij} = \beta_0 + u_{0i} + (\beta_1 + u_{1i})x_1 + \beta_2 x_1^2 + \beta_3 x_1^3 + \beta_4 x_2 \qquad (11.6)$$

TABLE 11.11. Random intercept model including third-order polynomial of applied pressure and squeeze number

```
Linear mixed-effects model fit by maximum likelihood
 Data: new
    AIC   BIC  logLik
  586.8 616.9 -286.4

Random effects:
 Formula:  ~ 1 | baby
         (Intercept) Residual
StdDev:       0.2709   0.3842

Fixed effects: linsp ~ poly(maxp, 3) + squeezen
                 Value Std.Error  DF t-value p-value
    (Intercept)  1.568    0.0611 520   25.65  <.0001
  poly(maxp, 3)1 6.877    0.4787 520   14.37  <.0001
  poly(maxp, 3)2 -2.897   0.4291 520   -6.75  <.0001
  poly(maxp, 3)3 1.564    0.4092 520    3.82  0.0001
        squeezen -0.005   0.0016 520   -2.80  0.0054
  Correlation:
                 (Intr) p(,3)1 p(,3)2 p(,3)3
  poly(maxp, 3)1 -0.062
  poly(maxp, 3)2  0.054 -0.017
  poly(maxp, 3)3  0.049 -0.023 -0.007
        squeezen -0.427  0.085 -0.095 -0.104

Standardized Within-Group Residuals:
    Min     Q1     Med     Q3    Max
 -4.557 -0.628 0.03407 0.6418 2.571

Number of Observations: 551
Number of Groups: 27
```

where x_1 is the applied pressure, x_2 is the squeeze number and there are now two random effects, a random intercept u_{0i} and a *random slope* (or *random coefficient*) u_{1i}. The random effects are assumed to have a bivariate normal distribution. (See Display 11.3, page 258 for the general form of a random coefficient model.)

Display 11.3 Random coefficient models

- A random intercept model assumes that the relationship between explanatory and response variables has the same slope within all level 2 units. However, in may cases, the effect of a variable can differ hugely between level 2 units. For example, if the data are pre-treatment and post-treatment data on a number of subjects taking part in a clinical trial, the treatment effect may differ between subjects.

- A random coefficient model can be written as

$$y_{ij} = \beta' \mathbf{x}_{ij} + \mathbf{u}_i' \mathbf{z}_{ij} + \epsilon_{ij} \qquad (1)$$

  where $\mathbf{z}_{ij}$ are covariates whose effect is assumed to vary between level 2 units and $\mathbf{u}$ are *random coefficients* assumed to have a multivariate normal distribution with mean zero and covariance matrix $\mathbf{\Sigma}_u$. The $\mathbf{u}_i$ and ϵ_{ij} are mutually independent. One of the elements of $\mathbf{z}_{ij}$ is normally equal to one so that one of the elements of $\mathbf{u}$ is a random intercept. Typically, the variables $\mathbf{z}_{ij}$ will be a subset of the variable $\mathbf{x}_{ij}$. (The $\mathbf{z}_{ij}$ must vary within level 2 units, but the $\mathbf{x}_{ij}$ can also be cluster-specific.)

- In matrix notation, the model can be written as

$$\mathbf{y} = \mathbf{X}\beta + \mathbf{Z}\mathbf{u} + \epsilon \qquad (2)$$

  where $\mathbf{y}$ and ϵ are vectors of the y_{ij} and ϵ_{ij}, $\mathbf{X}$ is the design matrix with rows equal to $\mathbf{x}_{ij}'$ and similarly for $\mathbf{Z}$.

- The variance of y_{ij} given $\mathbf{x}_{ij}$ and $\mathbf{z}_{ij}$ is

$$\mathrm{var}(y_{ij}|\mathbf{X}, \mathbf{Z}) = \mathbf{z}_{ij}\mathbf{\Sigma}_u \mathbf{z}_{ij}' + \sigma^2 \qquad (3)$$

  and the covariance between two level 1 units, j and l in the same level 2 units is

$$\mathrm{cov}(y_{ij}, y_{il}|\mathbf{X}, \mathbf{Z}) = \mathbf{z}_{ij}\mathbf{\Sigma}_u \mathbf{z}_{il}' \qquad (4)$$

  whereas level 1 units belonging to different level 2 units are uncorrelated. Therefore, the random coefficient model allows the (marginal) variances and covariances to depend on covariates.

This model fits significantly better than does the model without a random slope (likelihood ratio = 8.7, d.f. = 2 p = 0.01).

The results of fitting the model including a random slope are given in Table 11.12. Note that the covariance matrix of the random intercept and slope is difficult to interpret because it will change when a constant is added to the explanatory variable.

TABLE 11.12. Model including random slope

```
Linear mixed-effects model fit by maximum likelihood
Data: new
    AIC   BIC logLik
  582.1 620.9   -282

Random effects:
 Formula:  ~ maxp | baby
 Structure: General positive-definite
             StdDev   Corr
(Intercept) 0.13175 (Inter
       maxp 0.01136 1
   Residual 0.38016

Fixed effects: linsp ~ poly(maxp, 3) + squeezen
               Value Std.Error  DF t-value p-value
   (Intercept)  1.590    0.0618 520   25.70  <.0001
poly(maxp, 3)1  7.250    0.6338 520   11.44  <.0001
poly(maxp, 3)2 -2.556    0.4711 520   -5.43  <.0001
poly(maxp, 3)3  1.238    0.4157 520    2.98  0.0030
      squeezen -0.005    0.0016 520   -2.85  0.0045
 Correlation:
                (Intr) p(,3)1 p(,3)2 p(,3)3
poly(maxp, 3)1  0.433
poly(maxp, 3)2  0.048  0.155
poly(maxp, 3)3  0.029 -0.040  0.045
      squeezen -0.421  0.109 -0.077 -0.056

Standardized Within-Group Residuals:
    Min      Q1      Med     Q3    Max
 -4.539 -0.6305 0.004411 0.6467 2.664

Number of Observations: 551
Number of Groups: 27
```

A graph representing the fitted model and raw data for each baby is shown in Figure 11.4. Here, BLUP estimates of the random intercept and slope for each baby have been used to plot the individual curves. In order to obtain smooth curves, the effect of squeeze number has been removed from both the 'raw' data and the fitted curves. A logarithmic scale (base 2) is used for the y-axis so that the effect of pressure on strength of inspiratory response can be assessed (as opposed to the effect on the log inspiratory strength).

11.6 Summary

Linear mixed models can be used for hierarchical data when observations may be correlated within clusters. A random intercept simultaneously models the heterogeneity between clusters and the correlation between observations within clusters. Random coefficients can be used to represent heterogeneity between clusters in the effects of particular covariates. The models allow investigation of the effects of covariates that vary within clusters, between clusters, or both, and they can be used to model unbalanced longitudinal data, for example when data are missing 'at random'.

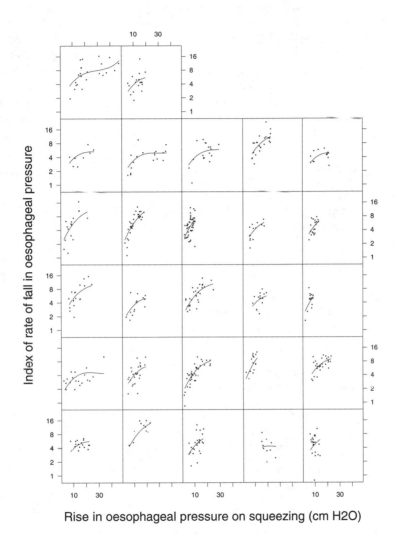

FIGURE 11.4. Scatterplots of inspiratory strength against applied pressure with fitted curves for 27 babies.

11.7   Using S-PLUS

Section 11.2

The data in *pefr.dat* contain one row per subject and a column for each measurement. To prepare the data for analysis using the S-PLUS function for linear mixed models, lme(), we first need to stack the responses into one long vector and replicate the explanatory variables appropriately. The lme() function is then used to fit a random intercept model. Here, two options are specified, **fixed** gives the model formula for the fixed part (including the dependent variable) and **random** gives the model formula for the random coefficients (without dependent variable). If the random effects consist of an intercept and coefficients of z1 and z2, the syntax is random = ~ z1+z2|clus, where clus is the clustering variable. The intervals() function is used to display 95% confidence intervals of the parameter estimates.

Script for Section 11.2

```
# Read Peak flow data
pefr<-read.table("pefr.dat",header=T)

# Construct a single response vector
y<-as.vector(as.matrix(pefr[,2:5]))
# stacks columns of matrix into supervector

# Define factors: method and id
meth<-c(rep(1,34),rep(2,34))
occ<-rep(c(rep(1,17),rep(2,17)),2)
id<-rep(pefr[,1],4)
pefr2<-data.frame(id=id,y=y,meth=meth,odd=occ)

# Plot mini Wright meter values
win.graph()
par(mfrow=c(2,1))
plot(id[meth==1],y[meth==2],type="n",xlab="ID",
    ylab="Peak Flow")
text(id[meth==2],y[meth==2],labels=occ[meth==2])
title("(a) First and second measurements")

# Draw line for mean peak flow measurement
mn<-mean(y[meth==2])
abline(mn,0)

# Add 100 to second mini Wright meter measurement
y1<-y[meth==2]+(occ[meth==2]-1)*100
plot(id[meth==2],y1,type="n",xlab="ID",ylab="Peak Flow")
```

```
text(id[meth==2],y1,labels=occ[meth==2])
title("(b) First measurement and second measurements+100")


# Draw line for mean peak flow measurement
mn<-mean(y1)
abline(mn,0)
```
                                              $\Longrightarrow$ Figure 11.1

```
# Pearson correlation between two mini Wright measurements
cor(pefr[,4:5])


# Fit random intercept model to mini Wright meter data
pefr.lme<-lme(fixed=y~1,random=~1|id,subset=meth==2,data=pefr2)
intervals(pefr.lme)
```
                                              $\Longrightarrow$ Table 11.2

```
# Compute intraclass correlation
110.4^2/(19.91^2+110.4^2)
y2<-y


# Repeat when second measurement increased by 100 units
y2[meth==2]<-y1
pefr2<-data.frame(pefr2,y2=y2)
pefr.lme<-lme(fixed=y2~1,random=~1|id,subset=meth==2,
   data=pefr2)
intervals(pefr.lme)
97.69^2/(75.4^2+97.69^2)
```

Section 11.3

Here, the update() function is used to add terms to the model and anova()
is used to compare nested linear mixed models using a likelihood ratio
test. The augPred() function is used to create an object containing both
predicted and observed values. When passed as an argument to the plot()
function, a trellis graph of observed and predicted values is plotted with a
separate panel for each cluster.

Script for Section 11.3

```
# Read equiv.dat
equiv<-matrix(scan("equiv.dat"),byrow=T,nrow=10)
attach(equiv)

# Stack responses into one vector
y<-as.vector(equiv[,2:3])

# Define factors
period<-c(rep(1,10),rep(2,10))
seq<-rep(equiv[,1],2)
treat<-rep(1,20)
treat[seq==1&period==2]<-2
```

```
treat[seq==-1&period==1]<-2
id<-rep(1:10,2)
equiv2<-data.frame(id=id,period=period,treat=treat,seq=seq,y=y)


# Fit mixed model
equiv.lme<-lme(fixed=y~period+treat,random=~1|id,data=equiv2)
summary(equiv.lme)
```
$\implies$ | Table 11.4 |
```
0.1399^2/(0.1399^2+ 0.09319^2)
intervals(equiv.lme)


equiv.lme<-update(equiv.lme,method="ML")
# fit same model by maximum likelihood
equiv.lme2<-update(equiv.lme,fixed=y~period*treat)
anova(equiv.lme,equiv.lme2)
```
$\implies$ | Table 11.5 |
```
# Plot observed and predicted values
win.graph()
plot(augPred(equiv.lme))
```
$\implies$ | Figure 11.2 |
```
# set y11 y32 y62 to missing
equiv3<-equiv2
equiv3$y[id==1&period==1]<-NA
equiv3$y[id==3&period==2]<-NA
equiv3$y[id==6&period==2]<-NA
equiv3$y
equiv.lme3<-lme(fixed=y~period+treat,random=~1|id,data=equiv3,
    na.action=na.omit)
summary(equiv.lme3)
```
$\implies$ | Table 11.6 |

Section 11.4

Various models are fitted using lme(). The poly(var,order) function is used to add polynomial terms (orthogonal polynomials) of a variable up to a given order to the model formula. A function is written to produce a scatterplot for longitudinal data with the data for a subset of cases connected.

Script for Section 11.4

```
# Read Stata file babies.dta using file -> import data

# List summaries of maxp (pressure) for each baby
for (i in unique(babies$baby)){
```

```
    print(i)
    print(summary(babies$maxp[babies$baby==i]))
}                                                   ⟹  Table 11.8


# Add log-transformed strength of inspiration to data frame
babies<-data.frame(babies,linsp=log(babies$inspirat))

# Exclude observations with missing values of maxp
new<-babies[!is.na(babies$maxp),]

# Create summary measures for each baby
smaxp<-tapply(new$maxp,new$baby,mean,simplify=T)
slinsp<-tapply(new$linsp,new$baby,mean,simplify=T)

# Between-baby estimate of effect of maxp on linsp
summary(lm(slinsp~smaxp))

# Within-baby analysis
new$baby<-factor(new$baby)
summary(lm(linsp~maxp+baby,data=new))

# Random effects analysis
summary(lme(linsp~maxp,random=~1|baby,data=new))    ⟹  Table 11.9


# Define function to plot scatterplot of y v x,
# with data for a subset of clusters connected
plotlong<-
function(x, y, cluster,subset=NULL,...)
{
    plot(x, y, type = "n",...)
    ord <- order(cluster,x)
    x1 <- x[ord]
    y1 <- y[ord]
    for(i in unique(cluster)) {
        points(x1[cluster == i], y1[cluster == i], pch = ".")
    }
    for (i in subset){
        lines(x1[cluster == i], y1[cluster == i], lty = 1)
    }
}


# Plot graph using plotlong
attach(new)
win.graph()
par(mfrow=c(1,1))
plotlong(maxp,linsp,baby,subset=c(8),
    xlab="Rise in oesphageal pressure on squeezing (cm H20)",
    ylab="Log strength inspiratory response")
```

$\Longrightarrow$ Figure 11.3

```
# Fit random effects model by ML
maxp.lme0<-lme(fixed=linsp~maxp,random=~1|baby,method="ML",
   data=new)

# Include squeeze number
maxp.lme1<-update(maxp.lme0,fixed=linsp~maxp+squeezen)

# Include quadratic
maxp.lme2<-update(maxp.lme1,fixed=linsp~poly(maxp,2)+squeezen)

# Include cubic
maxp.lme3<-update(maxp.lme2,fixed=linsp~poly(maxp,3)+squeezen)
anova(maxp.lme0,maxp.lme1,maxp.lme2,maxp.lme3)
```
$\Longrightarrow$ Table 11.10

```
summary(maxp.lme3)
```
$\Longrightarrow$ Table 11.11

Section 11.5

The lme() function is used to fit random coefficient models. The observed and fitted data are plotted by extracting the fixed and random coefficients from the lme object and using the trellis graphics function xyplot() with a logarithmic y-axis and various other options.

Script for Section 11.5

```
# Include a random slope for maxp
maxp.lme4<-update(maxp.lme3,random=~maxp|baby)
anova(maxp.lme3,maxp.lme4)
summary(maxp.lme4)
```
$\Longrightarrow$ Table 11.12

```
# Plot data and predicted curves
new<-data.frame(new,maxp2=new$maxp^2)
new<-data.frame(new,maxp3=new$maxp^3)
maxp.lme<-lme(fixed=linsp~maxp+maxp2+maxp3+squeezen,
   random=~maxp|baby,data=new)

# Extract random coefficients
coeffr<-maxp.lme$coefficients$random$baby

# Extract fixed coefficients
coeff<-maxp.lme$coefficients$fixed
# first column is intercepts, second is slopes
```

```
# Create ncoeff with one row per baby and four columns for
# all the coefficients except the coefficient of squeezen
ncoeff<-coeffr
ncoeff[,1]<-ncoeff[,1]+coeff[1]
ncoeff[,2]<-ncoeff[,2]+coeff[2]
# First two columns are total intercept and slope
# (fixed + random)

# Add coeffs of maxp2 and maxp3
ncoeff<-cbind(ncoeff,rep(coeff[3],nrow(coeffr)))
ncoeff<-cbind(ncoeff,rep(coeff[4],nrow(coeffr)))

# Subtract effect of squeeze number from linsp and
# exponentiate
linsp1 <- exp(new$linsp - coeff[5]*new$squeezen)
# this is so that we can plot on the log-scale

new<-data.frame(new,linsp1)

trellis.device(win.graph)
par(cex=1.5)
xyplot(linsp1~maxp|baby1,data=new,subscripts=T,
    # subscripts=T allows panel function to access observation
    # number used in each panel
    xlab=list("Rise in oesophageal pressure on squeezing (cm H20)",
        cex=1.3),
    ylab=list("Index of rate of fall in oesophageal pressure",
        cex=1.3),
    scales=list(draw=T,cex=0.7,y=list(log=2)),
    # uses logarithmic axis for y
    strip=F,
    # strip = F suppresses labels above panels
        panel=function(x,y,subscripts,degree=1,span=1){
            ind<-new$baby[subscripts]
            ind<-ind[1]
            # ind is the baby whose data is being plotted in
            # current panel
            s<-paste(ind)
            x1<-seq(min(x),max(x),length=100)
            y1<-(ncoeff[s,1]+ncoeff[s,2]*x1+ncoeff[s,3]*x1^2
                +ncoeff[s,4]*x1^3)/log(2)
            # predicted curve on log base 2 scale
            lines(x1,y1)
            points(jitter(x),jitter(y),pch=".")
    }
)
```

$\Longrightarrow$ Figure 11.4

11.8   Exercises

11.1 Fit a variance components model to the measurement of peak expiratory flow using the Wright Peak Flow meter, and estimate the reliability coefficient. Which instrument appears to be more reliable? Are the variance component estimates for the two instruments very different?

11.2 Assuming that the true residual variance and random effects variance are the same for both methods, fit a linear mixed model to test for a bias (change in mean) between the first and second applications of the Wright Peak Flow meter.

11.3 Analyze the postnatal depression data of Chapter 6 by treating the baseline measures and the visit 1 to visit 6 measures of depression as level 1 units, time (assesment numbers 1 to 8) as a fixed covariate and subjects as level 2 units. Include a main effect of group and a group by time interaction. Is a quadratic effect of time required?

11.4 Add a random slope for time to the model in 11.3.

11.5 Repeat the analysis, treating the mean of the two baseline measures as a further covariate and visits 1 to 6 as level 1 units. How does inclusion of the baseline measures as a covariate affect the estimated variance of the random intercepts?

12

Linear Mixed Models II

12.1   Introduction

In this chapter, we extend the methods of the previous chapter in several ways. First, we will relax the assumption of conditional independence of the responses given the random effects by introducing serial autocorrelations for longitudinal data. Then, we will discuss relaxing the assumption of constant variances of the random error terms. Finally, we consider models for *multilevel* data in which there are several levels of clustering. Examples are repeated measures on subjects in hospitals, patients in wards in hospitals, or patients of GPs in cities.

12.2   Autocorrelated residuals

Random intercept models for longitudinal data induce equal residual correlations between all pairs of observations belonging to the same subject (compound symmetry). However, in longitudinal data, it is often the case that observations separated by a smaller time interval are more highly correlated than are observations further apart in time.

This can be modeled by using a *first-order autoregressive* (AR(1)) model for the level 1 residuals ϵ_{ij}, as described in Display 12.1. Here, we are relaxing the conditional independence assumption that given the covariates and random effects, the observations are mutually independent.

For the babies data, the 'time scale', t_j, that determines the distance between observations is the sequence number of the experiment (squeeze number). We can assume that conditional on the covariates and random effects, the correlations between pairs of observations on the same baby decrease when the difference in squeeze number increases; i.e.,

$$\text{cor}(\epsilon_{t_j}, \epsilon_{t'_j}) = \phi^{t_j - t_{j'}} \tag{12.1}$$

where $\phi < 1$.

Adding this correlation structure for the level 1 residuals to the model selected in the previous chapter significantly improves model fit with a likelihood ratio of 6.9, giving a p-value of 0.009. The results of fitting this model are given in Table 12.1. The correlation between adjacent experiments, ϕ, is estimated as 0.15. The fixed parameter estimates have not changed substantially.

Display 12.1 Serial autocorrelation

- In the random effects models considered so far, the correlations between residuals induced by the random effects are constant for all pairs of units belonging to the same level 2 unit. Conditionally on the random effects and covariates, the observations are independent.

- For longitudinal data, it may not be reasonable to assume that residuals at adjacent time points are no more correlated with each other than residuals further apart. Unobserved influences varying smoothly over time could induce *serial* dependence between nearby observations so that conditional independence no longer holds.

- Random effects models can be extended to allow the 'level 1' errors ϵ_{ij} to be correlated.

- If the level 1 units correspond to equally spaced time points t, the error at time t can be modeled using a first-order *autoregressive* (AR(1)) model

$$\epsilon_{it} = \phi \epsilon_{t-1} + a_t \tag{1}$$

This generates correlations equal to

$$\text{cor}(\epsilon_t, \epsilon_{t+k}) = \phi^k \tag{2}$$

If the level 1 units do not correspond to equally spaced time points, the correlation structure can be generalized to continuous time using

$$\text{cor}(\epsilon_{t_j}, \epsilon_{t_{j'}}) = \phi^{t_j - t_{j'}} \tag{3}$$

where t_j is the time associated with the jth level 1 unit.

TABLE 12.1. Model including AR(1) structure for within-baby error term

```
Linear mixed-effects model fit by REML
 Data: new
  AIC BIC logLik
  636 679   -308

Random effects:
 Formula:  ~ maxp | test
 Structure: General positive-definite
            StdDev    Corr
(Intercept) 0.1441 (Inter
       maxp 0.0108 0.922
   Residual 0.3845

Correlation Structure: ARMA(1,0)
 Parameter estimate(s):
  Phi1
 0.1466
Fixed effects: linsp ~ maxp + maxp2 + maxp3 + squeezen
             Value Std.Error  DF t-value p-value
(Intercept)  0.4362    0.1209 520   3.609  0.0003
       maxp  0.1488    0.0221 520   6.749  <.0001
      maxp2 -0.0046    0.0012 520  -3.751  0.0002
      maxp3  0.0001    0.0000 520   2.640  0.0085
   squeezen -0.0048    0.0018 520  -2.687  0.0074
 Correlation:
          (Intr)   maxp  maxp2  maxp3
    maxp -0.859
   maxp2  0.788 -0.966
   maxp3 -0.702  0.903 -0.976
squeezen -0.284  0.003  0.035 -0.052

Standardized Within-Group Residuals:
    Min     Q1      Med     Q3    Max
 -4.493 -0.613 0.0005388 0.6303 2.609

Number of Observations: 551
Number of Groups: 27
```

TABLE 12.2. Simple linear mixed model for peak expiratory flow measurements

```
Linear mixed-effects model fit by REML
 Data: pefr2
    AIC   BIC logLik
  692.9 701.7 -342.5

Random effects:
 Formula:  ~ 1 | id
           (Intercept) Residual
 StdDev:       112.6    23.82

Fixed effects: y ~ meth
              Value Std.Error DF t-value p-value
(Intercept) 441.9     28.79 50   15.35  <.0001
       meth   6.0      5.78 50    1.04  0.3016
 Correlation:
    (Intr)
meth -0.301

Standardized Within-Group Residuals:
    Min      Q1    Med      Q3    Max
 -2.202 -0.3637 0.0322 0.4487  1.951

Number of Observations: 68
Number of Groups: 17
```

12.3   Heteroscedasticity

We now return to the peak expiratory flow measurements in Table 11.1. We have so far analyzed the measurements on a single instrument. However, because both instruments are measuring peak expiratory flow, it may be reasonable to assume that

$$y_{ijk} = \mu + \alpha_j + u_i + \epsilon_{ijk}, \quad u_i \sim N(0, \tau^2), \quad \epsilon_{ijk} \sim N(0, \sigma^2) \quad (12.2)$$

where y_{ijk} is the kth measurement of the peak expiratory flow of the ith subject using instrument j. This model allows for constant bias α_j between the two methods and assumes that both instruments have the same measurement error variance. The results of fitting this model are given in Table 12.2. There is no significant bias between the methods, the mean difference being estimated as 6, $t = 1.04$, $p = 0.32$.

We can relax the assumption of equal error variances by specifying that

$$\epsilon_{ijk} \sim N(0, \sigma_j^2) \quad (12.3)$$

giving the output in Table 12.3. The model is parameterized as $\sigma_j = \sigma \delta_j$ with $\delta_1 = 1$. Therefore, the measurement errors of the Wright peak flow meter (meth = 1) have an estimated standard deviation of 17.35, compared with 17.35×1.731 for the mini Wright meter. According to a likelihood ratio test, this difference is not significant ($p = 0.23$).

TABLE 12.3. Measurement error model with different error variances for the instruments

```
Linear mixed-effects model fit by REML
 Data: pefr2
    AIC   BIC logLik
  693.5 704.5 -341.8

Random effects:
 Formula:  ~ 1 | id
         (Intercept) Residual
StdDev:       114.6    17.35

Variance function:
 Structure: Different standard deviations per stratum
 Formula:  ~ 1 | meth
 Parameter estimates:
 1     2
 1 1.731
Fixed effects: y ~ meth
            Value Std.Error DF t-value p-value
(Intercept) 441.9     28.88 50   15.30  <.0001
       meth   6.0      5.95 50    1.01  0.3158
 Correlation:
     (Intr)
meth -0.258

Standardized Within-Group Residuals:
   Min      Q1     Med      Q3     Max
 -1.81 -0.3783 0.02032 0.5078 2.223

Number of Observations: 68
Number of Groups: 17
```

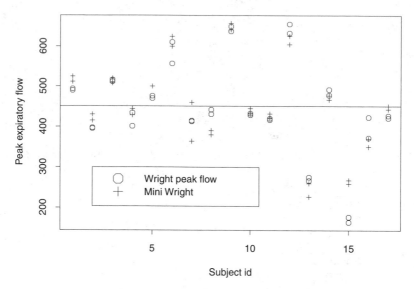

FIGURE 12.1. Scatterplot of peak expiratory flow measured by two instruments versus subject id.

12.4 Multilevel models

The models used for the peak flow measurements so far assume that the four measurements using the two instruments are all mutually independent if we condition on the random effect. To see if this appears reasonable, we can plot all four measurements against subject id, as shown in Figure 12.1.

The figure suggests that for a given individual, the measurements using the same instrument tend to resemble each other more than do measurements on different instruments. We can model this by including another random effect that takes on a different value for each combination of method and subject. The model is

$$y_{ijk} = \mu + \alpha_j + u_i^{(3)} + u_{ij}^{(2)} + \epsilon_{ijk} \tag{12.4}$$

where

$$u_i^{(3)} \sim N(0, \tau_3^2), \quad u_{ij}^{(2)} \sim N(0, \tau_2^2), \quad \epsilon_{ijk} \sim N(0, \sigma^2)$$

This is a simple example of a three-level model (see Bryk and Raudenbush, 1992, Goldstein 1995, Kreft and De Leeuw, 1998, or Snijders and Bosker, 1999, for detailed treatments of multilevel models). Observations (level 1) are nested in methods (level 2) that in turn are nested in subjects (level 3). A likelihood ratio test indicates that this model provides a better fit than does the 'two-level' model considered in the previous section (with constant variance σ^2), $p = 0.002$. The results from fitting the three-level model are given in Table 12.4.

TABLE 12.4. Three-level model for peak flow measurement

```
Linear mixed-effects model fit by REML
 Data: pefr2
    AIC   BIC logLik
  685.6 696.5 -337.8

Random effects:
 Formula:  ~ 1 | id
        (Intercept)
StdDev:          112

 Formula:  ~ 1 | meth %in% id
          (Intercept) Residual
StdDev:        19.84    17.76

Fixed effects: y ~ meth
             Value Std.Error DF t-value p-value
(Intercept) 441.9     30.00 34   14.73  <.0001
       meth   6.0      8.05 16    0.75  0.4649
 Correlation:
     (Intr)
meth -0.403

Standardized Within-Group Residuals:
    Min      Q1      Med      Q3    Max
 -2.781 -0.3281 -0.01353 0.3715 2.625

Number of Observations: 68
Number of Groups:
```

The level 3 (between subjects) standard deviation is estimated as 112. The level 2 (between methods within subjects) standard deviation is estimated as 19.84, and the level 1 standard deviation (within method within subjects), or residual standard deviation, is estimated as 17.76. The within-subject correlation between measurements using the same instrument is therefore estimated as $19.84^2/(19.84^2 + 17.76^2) = 0.56$. The level 2 error term can be interpreted as a method by subject interaction or as subject-specific bias (see, for example, Dunn, 1992).

As another example of a three-level data set, we now consider part of the data from a WHO study on psychological problems in general health care (Üstün and Sartorius, 1995). All subjects were screened using a 12-item version of the 'General Health Questionnaire' (GHQ) to assess distress. Patients were then selected to enter into a second phase based on these GHQ screen scores. This is an example of a two-phase study (see, for example, Dunn 2000). The individuals in the second phase were followed up soon after screening, after three months and one year later. Different versions of the GHQ (with different subsets of a total of 34 questions) were administered during these follow-up interviews. We will analyze the logarithm of the total score on six questions asked on all occasions. We will restrict the analysis to the data from Paris. In addition to observations (level 1) being clustered in subjects (level 2), subjects are also clustered in clinics (level 3). There were a total of 2,094 subjects from 42 clinics at phase 1, reducing to 382 subjects in phase 2. Only 187 patients had measurements on all occasions. A sample of the data is shown in Table 12.5. In this table, many subjects only have a single observation at time 0, one subject has two observations at time 0 (screen and first assessment in phase 2) and one at three months and two subjects have a single observation at time 0 and observations at three months and 12 months.

We will model changes in GHQ over time, taking into account the hierarchical nature of the data. By including all subjects in the analysis, including those who were only measured once, we should obtain consistent parameter estimates if the data are missing at random. Note that most of the data are missing at random by design because the second phase sample was randomly selected based on the initial GHQ scores.

Assuming a linear relationship between log GHQ score and time with random intercepts at levels 2 and 3 gives the output shown in Table 12.6. The standard deviation of the random intercept for clinics is estimated as 0.08 compared with the standard deviation of the random intercept for subjects of 0.22 and a within subject residual standard deviation of 0.33.

The confidence intervals for the parameter estimates are given in Table 12.7. It appears as if there is significant heterogeneity between clinics. This is confirmed by a likelihood ratio test comparing the three-level model with a two-level model that ignores clinics, as shown in Table 12.8. Allowing the slopes to vary between subjects does not significantly improve model fit with a likelihood ratio of 1.78 and a p-value of 0.41 (see Table 12.9).

TABLE 12.5. Sample of the GHQ data

id	clinic	lghq	time
2010797	20001	1.9459	0
2017059	20001	2.3026	0
2017062	20001	2.3026	0
2017062	20001	1.9459	0
2017062	20001	2.3026	3
2017075	20001	1.7918	0
2014744	20002	2.1972	0
2014760	20002	2.3026	0
2014760	20002	2.3026	3
2014760	20002	2.0794	12
2014786	20002	1.6094	0
2014799	20002	2.5649	0
2014799	20002	2.4849	3
2014799	20002	2.1972	12
2014803	20002	2.3026	0
2014816	20002	2.0794	0
2014829	20002	1.6094	0
2014845	20002	2.0794	0
2014962	20002	1.7918	0

If this test had been significant, we could also have considered adding a random slope at level 3 to allow 'average' changes over time to vary between clinics.

There are too many subjects to present the model fit in a single graph. Figure 12.2 shows the observed (circles) and predicted (crosses) values for one of the clinics, clinic 20024. Only three subjects in the clinic had observations at three time points. The model appears to fit reasonably well.

12.5   Assessing model assumptions

The assumptions of linear mixed models are that the level 1 residuals ϵ_{ijk} are normally distributed with constant variance (unless a different variance function is specified) and that the random effects at each level are normally distributed.

For the GHQ data, we can assess the assumptions of normality by plotting normal quantile plots of the the level 1 residuals and the BLUP estimates of the level 2 and level 3 random effects. These are shown in Figures 12.3, 12.4 and 12.5. Whereas the level 1 residuals appear to be slightly skewed, those corresponding to levels 2 and 3 appear to be close to normal.

TABLE 12.6. Three-level model for GHQ data with random intercepts only

```
Linear mixed-effects model fit by REML
 Data: ghq
   AIC  BIC logLik
  2929 2959  -1459

Random effects:
 Formula:  ~ 1 | clinic
         (Intercept)
 StdDev:     0.07615

 Formula:  ~ 1 | id %in% clinic
         (Intercept) Residual
 StdDev:      0.2214   0.3328

Fixed effects: lghq ~ time
            Value Std.Error   DF t-value p-value
(Intercept) 1.944   0.01571 2052   123.8  <.0001
       time -0.021   0.00201  878   -10.6  <.0001
 Correlation:
     (Intr)
time -0.112

Standardized Within-Group Residuals:
    Min       Q1      Med      Q3    Max
 -6.019  -0.5327  0.04707  0.5526  3.241

Number of Observations: 2973
Number of Groups:
 clinic id %in% clinic
     42           2094
```

TABLE 12.7. Confidence intervals for parameter estimates

```
Approximate 95% confidence intervals

Fixed effects:
                  lower       est.    upper
(Intercept)    1.91364   1.94445   1.97526
       time  -0.02519  -0.02125  -0.01731

Random Effects:
 Level: clinic
                      lower      est.   upper
sd((Intercept))    0.04415   0.07615  0.1313
 Level: id
                    lower     est.  upper
sd((Intercept))    0.1936   0.2214  0.2533

Within-group standard error:
 lower    est.   upper
0.3146  0.3328  0.3521
```

TABLE 12.8. Likelihood ratio test comparing three level and two level random intercept models

	Model	df	AIC	BIC	logLik	Test	L.Ratio	p-value
ghq.lme	1	5	2929	2959	−1459			
ghq.lme0	2	4	3071	3095	−1532	1 vs 2	144.7	<.0001

TABLE 12.9. Likelihood ratio test for random slope of time at level 3

	Model	df	AIC	BIC	logLik	Test	L.Ratio	p-value
ghq.lme1	1	7	2931	2973	−1458			
ghq.lme	2	5	2929	2959	−1459	1 vs 2	1.779	0.4109

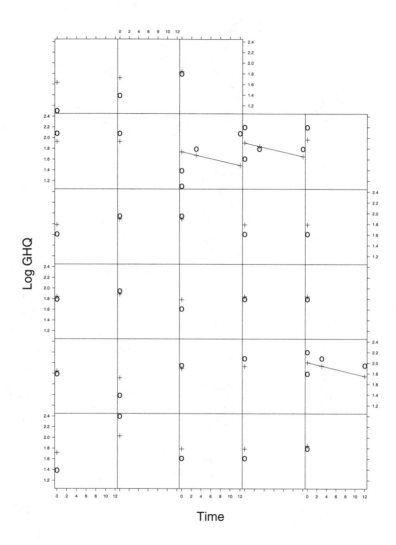

FIGURE 12.2. Observed (circles) and predicted (crosses) values of log GHQ in clinic 20024 by subject.

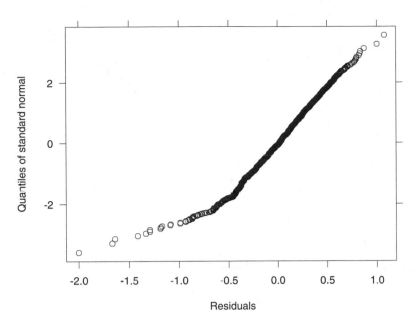

FIGURE 12.3. Normal quantile plot of level 1 residuals.

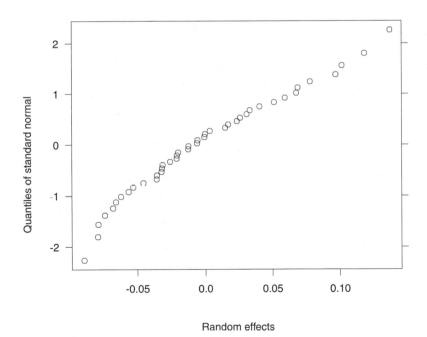

FIGURE 12.4. Normal quantile plot of level 3 random effects estimates.

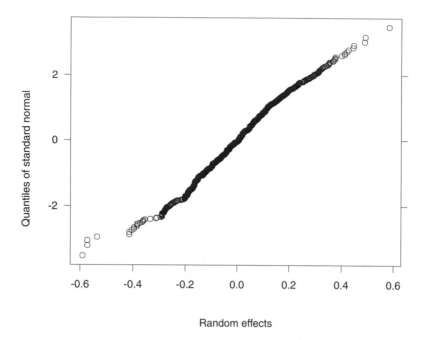

FIGURE 12.5. Normal quantile plot of level 2 random effects estimates.

12.6 Summary

In this chapter, we extended the simple linear mixed models in several ways. For longitudinal data, the simple linear mixed model will often be inadequate because it assumes a compound symmetric structure of the within-subject covariances. Including subject heterogeneity as well as serial autocorrelations is likely to provide a better model for the data. Heteroscedasticity is often a problem, not just in mixed models, and we have shown how models can be exended to allow the level 1 residual variance to depend on covariates. Finally, many medical data sets include more than one level of clustering. Such data can be analyzed using multilevel models. Further extensions to linear mixed models and their implementation in S-PLUS are covered in Pinheiro and Bates (2000) .

12.7   Using S-PLUS

Section 12.2

In this section, the `correlation` option is used in `lme()` to specify a first-order autoregressive model. The `anova()` function is used to compare nested mixed effects models. The `unique()` function used here to extract the values of the clustering variable is very useful for clustered data.

Script for Section 12.2

```
# Read in babies data, and refit model used in Chapter 11
babies<-data.frame(babies,linsp=log(babies$inspirat))
new<-babies[!is.na(babies$maxp),]
new<-data.frame(new,maxp2=new$maxp^2)
new<-data.frame(new,maxp3=new$maxp^3)
maxp.lme<-lme(fixed=linsp~maxp+maxp2+maxp3+squeezen,
    random=~maxp|baby,data=new)

# Introduce serial correlations
maxp.lme2<-update(maxp.lme,
    correlation=corAR1(form=~squeezen|baby))
# This gives error message that covariate must have
# unique values within groups

# find out where several observations within baby have
# the same value of squeezen
for (i in unique(new$baby)){
    l<-length(new$squeezen[new$baby==i])
    # number of values of squeezen for baby i
    l2<-length(unique(new$squeezen[new$baby==i]))
    # number of unique values of squeezen for baby i
    if( l2<l){
        cat("baby ",i," has ",l," values and only ", l2,
            " are unique")
    }
}
new$squeezen[new$baby==21]

# create sequ to be same as squeezen except first
# 1 for baby 21 is a 2
sequ<-new$squeezen
cbind(new$squeezen[new$baby==21],(1:length(sequ))[new$baby==21])
# this lists the values of squeezen for baby 21
# together with the observation numbers
sequ[429]<-2
```

```
new<-data.frame(new,sequ)

# Fit model with AR(1) model for level 1 residuals
maxp.lme2<-lme(fixed=linsp~maxp+maxp2+maxp3+squeezen,
    random=~maxp|test,
    correlation=corAR1(form=~sequ|baby),data=new)

# Test significance of serial autocorrelations
anova(maxp.lme,maxp.lme2)

# Display model output
summary(maxp.lme2)
```

$\Longrightarrow$ Table 12.1

Section 12.3

In this section, the **weights** option is used in **lme()** to specify a variance function for the level 1 residuals. Here, the variance function **varIdent** is selected, which allows the variance to depend on a grouping variable. See Pinheiro and Bates (2000) for other variance functions.

Script for Section 12.3

```
# Prepare the data as in Section 11.2
pefr<-read.table("pefr.dat",header=T)
y<-as.vector(as.matrix(pefr[,2:5]))
meth<-c(rep(1,34),rep(2,34))
occ<-rep(c(rep(1,17),rep(2,17)),2)
id<-rep(pefr[,1],4)
pefr2<-data.frame(id=id,y=y,meth=meth,odd=occ)

# Fit basic linear mixed model
pefr.lme<-lme(fixed=y~meth,random=~1|id,data=pefr2)
summary(pefr.lme)
```
$\Longrightarrow$ ⌐Table 12.2⌐

```
# Allow measurement errors to differ between methods
pefr.lme2<-lme(fixed=y~meth,random=~1|id,
    weights=varIdent(form=~1|meth),data=pefr2)
summary(pefr.lme2)
```
$\Longrightarrow$ ⌐Table 12.3⌐

```
# Test significance of heteroscadisticity
anova(pefr.lme,pefr.lme2)

# Plot measurement of both instruments
win.graph()
attach(pefr2)
plot(id,y,type="n",xlab="Subject id",
    ylab="Peak expiratory flow")
points(id[meth==1],y[meth==1],pch=1)
points(id[meth==2],y[meth==2],pch=3)
legend(2,300,legend=c("Wright peak flow","Mini Wright"),
    marks=c(1,3))
mn<-mean(y)
abline(mn,0)
```
$\Longrightarrow$ ⌐Figure 12.1⌐

Section 12.4

The **random** argument in **lme()** is used to specify three-level models. Two different syntaxes are used, the more general being **random=list(lev3= 1, lev2= 1)**, where **lev3** and **lev2** are the variables that define levels 3 and 2, respectively. Here, a model formula is specified for each level, the highest level being specified first. The **predict()** function is used to obtain predicted values of the dependent variable. The **level=2** option specifies that the random effects at levels 2 and 3 are both to be included in the predictions. In S-PLUS, levels are counted from outermost (highest level in our terminology) to innermost so that for three-level models, S-PLUS refers to our level 3 as level 1 and our level 2 as level 2. Level 0 denotes fixed effects only. (This is consistent with the order in which the levels are specified in the random option.)

The trellis graphics function xyplot() is used to plot observed and predicted values.

Script for Section 12.4

```
# Include a random effect for method within subjects
meth2<-meth-1
pefr.lme3<-lme(fixed=y~meth,random=~1|id/meth,data=pefr2)
# id/meth specifies that meth is nested in id
summary(pefr.lme3)                              ==> Table 12.4

# Test significance of random effect for method
anova(pefr.lme,pefr.lme3)

# Read GHQ data
ghq<-read.table("ghqp.dat",header=T)

# Fit three-level model
ghq.lme<-lme(lghq~time,random=list(clinic=~1,id=~1),data=ghq)
# this is the same as random=~1|clinic/id
summary(ghq.lme)                                ==> Table 12.6

# Confidence intervals for parameters
intervals(ghq.lme)                              ==> Table 12.7

# Two-level model
ghq.lme0<-lme(lghq~time,random=list(clinic=~1),data=ghq)
anova(ghq.lme,ghq.lme0)                         ==> Table 12.8

# Include a random slope at level 2
ghq.lme1<-lme(lghq~time,random=list(clinic=~1,id=~time),data=ghq)
summary(ghq.lme1)
anova(ghq.lme1,ghq.lme)                         ==> Table 12.9

# Graph the data and predicted curves for one of the clinics
pred<-predict(ghq.lme,level=2)
# predicts GHQ using fixed effects and both random effects

# Select clinic 20024
ghq24<-ghq[ghq$clinic==20024,]
pred24<-pred[ghq$clinic==20024]

# Plot observed and predicted values by subject using trellis
```

```
trellis.device(win.graph)
xyplot(lghq~time|id,data=ghq24,subscripts=T,
   xlab=list("Time",cex=1.3),
   ylab=list("Log GHQ",cex=1.3),
     strip=F,
   panel=function(x,y,subscripts){
     points(x,y)
     p<-pred24[subscripts]
     lines(x,p)
     points(x,p,pch=3)
   }
)
```
$\Longrightarrow$ | Figure 12.2 |

Section 12.5

The level 1 residuals can be computed using the `resid()` function. Here, the predicted values, including random effects at levels 2 and 3, need to be subtracted from the observed values, and this is achieved by specifying the `level=2` option. The `ranef()` function is used to produce the random effects estimtas at levels 2 and 3 (referred to in S-PLUS as levels 2 and 1). The `qqnorm()` function is used with the syntax `qqnorm(object, formula)`. Within the formula, the symbol "." refers to the fitted object specified as the first argument.

Script for Section 12.5

```
# Plot Q-Q plot of residuals after removing fixed effects and
# both random effects
qqnorm(ghq.lme,~resid(.,level=2))
```
$\Longrightarrow$ | Figure 12.3 |

```
# Plot Q-Q plot of clinic random effects
qqnorm(ghq.lme,~ranef(.,level=1),strip=F)
# level 1 refers to clinics, level 2 refers to subjects
```
$\Longrightarrow$ | Figure 12.4 |

```
# Plot Q-Q plot of subject random effects
qqnorm(ghq.lme,~ranef(.,level=2),strip=F)
```
$\Longrightarrow$ | Figure 12.5 |

12.8 Exercises

12.1 For the postnatal depression data of Chapter 6, is there any evidence of serial autocorrelations of the within-subject residuals? As in Exercise 11.5, use the mean baseline measure as a covariate and include baseline, group and time as fixed effects.

TABLE 12.10. Sample of the data in *hear.dat* (taken from Jackson (1991) with permission of the publisher, John Wiley & Sons)

id	l500	l1000	l2000	l4000	r500	r1000	r2000	r4000
1	0	5	10	15	0	5	5	15
2	-5	0	-10	0	0	5	5	15
3	-5	0	15	15	0	0	5	15
4	-5	0	-10	-10	-10	-5	-10	10
5	-5	-5	-10	10	0	-10	-10	50
6	5	5	5	-10	0	5	0	20
7	0	0	0	20	5	5	5	10
8	-10	-10	-10	-5	-10	-5	0	5
9	0	0	0	40	0	0	-10	10
10	-5	-5	-10	20	-10	-5	-10	15
11	-10	-5	-5	5	5	0	-10	5
12	5	5	10	25	-5	-5	5	15
13	0	0	-10	15	-10	-10	-10	10
14	5	15	5	60	5	5	0	50
15	5	0	5	15	5	-5	0	25
16	-5	-5	5	30	5	5	5	25
17	0	-10	0	20	0	-10	-10	25
18	5	0	0	50	10	10	5	65
19	-10	0	0	15	-10	-5	5	15
20	-10	-10	-5	0	-10	-5	-5	5

Test for serial autocorrelations with and without a random co-efficient of time.

12.2 Check the distributional assumptions for the linear mixed effects model for the postnatal depression data.

12.3 Analyze the data in the file *hear.dat* relating to hearing loss. A sample of the data is given in Table 12.10. Individuals were exposed to a sound of a given frequency with increasing intensity until the sound was heard. The lowest intensity at which the signal is perceived is a measure of hearing loss, calibrated in units referred to as *decibel loss* in comparison to a reference standard for that particular instrument. Observations are obtained one ear at a time for a number of frequencies. The data can be viewed as a three-level data set with measurements at different frequencies nested in ears nested in individuals. We will use the log of the hearing loss as the response variable (add 11 to the hearing loss before taking the logarithm) and frequency, coded as 1,2,3,4 as explanatory variables.

1. Use trellis graphics to plot log hearing loss against frequency for the first 20 subjects, connecting the points with different line styles for each ear.

2. Fit a three-level random intercept model to the data assuming that log hearing loss depends linearly on frequency.

3. Compare this model with a model treating frequency as a factor.

4. Treating frequency as a factor in the fixed part of the model, test if a random slope for frequency (as a continuous variable) at the subject level improves the fit of the model.

5. Produce another trellis graph for the first 20 subjects including the fitted curves.

13
Generalized Additive Models

13.1 Introduction

The multiple linear regression model discussed in Chapter 8 and the generalized linear model covered in Chapters 9 and 10 accommodate nonlinear relationships between the response variable (or the link function of its mean) and one or more of the explanatory variables by using polynomial terms or parametric transformations. (The predictor remains linear in the parameters, of course; nonlinear models are nonlinear in their parameters and are the subject of Chapter 14.) In this chapter, however, we consider some more flexible models in which the relationship between the response variable and one or more of the explanatory variables is modeled by using some type of *scatterplot smoother* (these were introduced informally in earlier chapters—see, for example, Chapter 4); their use here allows the data to suggest the form of the relationship involved, and indirectly to suggest whether the data might be better modeled by a linear or generalized linear model which included polynomial terms of a particular degree for some, or all, of the explanatory variables.

(The models to be described in this chapter are probably best used as a tool for suggesting parametric transformations or alternative forms for terms in the model. Once these transformations have been uncovered, subsequent fitting and testing can then be based on them via the more routine multiple regression or generalized linear model.)

13.2   Additive models

In a linear regression model as described in Chapter 8, we have a dependent variable y and a set of predictor variables $x_1, x_2, \cdots, x_p$ and the model assumed is

$$y = \alpha + \sum_{j=1}^{p} \beta_j x_j + \epsilon \qquad (13.1)$$

Additive models replace the linear function by a smooth non-parametric function to give

$$y = \alpha + \sum_{j=1}^{p} f_j(x_j) + \epsilon \qquad (13.2)$$

The function is estimated in a flexible way using a *scatterplot smoother* (see the next section). The estimated function $\hat{f}_j(x_j)$ can reveal possible nonlinearities in the effect of x_j. (The investigator can, of course, choose to have particular variables entered linearly in an additive model.)

A *generalized additive model* arises from (13.2) in the same way as a generalized linear model arises from the usual multiple regression model; namely, some function of the expectation of the response variable is now modeled by a sum of nonparametric functions. So, for example, the logistic additive model is

$$\mathrm{logit}(\pi) = \alpha + \sum_{j=1}^{p} f_j(x_j) \qquad (13.3)$$

13.3   Fitting additive models

Fitting a smooth curve $f(x)$ that summarizes the dependence of a response variable y on a single explanatory variable x can be done in a variety of ways; one, locally weighted regression, was described briefly in Chapter 4. Another, the *cubic spline smoother*, is described briefly in Display 13.1.

When there are multiple explanatory variables to consider, the fitting process involves what is known as a *backfitting algorithm*. This cycles through the individual terms in the additive model and updates each using an appropriate smoother. It does this by smoothing suitably defined partial residuals. The cycle continues until none of the functions change from one interaction to the next. Any linear terms in the model are fitted by least squares. Full details are given in Chambers and Hastie (1993).

Various tests are available to assess the nonlinear contributions of the fitted smoothers, and generalized additive models can be compared with say, linear models fitted to the same data, by means of an F-test on the residual sums of squares of the competing models. In this process the fitted smooth curve is assigned an estimated equivalent number of degrees of freedom. For full details again see Chambers and Hastie (1993).

Display 13.1 Fitting a cubic spline scatterplot smoother

- The smooth curve $f(x)$ that summarizes the dependence of a response variable y on an explanatory variable x is fitted by minimizing

$$\sum_{i=1}^{n} [(y_i - f(x_i)]^2 + \lambda \int f''(x)^2 dx \qquad (1)$$

  where $f''(x)$ is the second derivative of $f(x)$ with respect to x.

- The first term represents the sum of squares criterion used in least squares. The integral in the second term, $\int f''(x)^2 dx$, measures the departure from linearity of f (for linear f, the term is zero), and λ is a nonnegative smoothing parameter. It governs the tradeoff between the goodness-of-fit to the data and the degree of smoothness of f. Larger values of λ force f to be smoother.

- For any value of λ, the solution to (1) is a cubic spline—a piecewise cubic polynomial with pieces joined at the unique observed values x_i of the explanatory variable.

- The 'effective number of parameters' (analogous to the number of parameters in a parametric fit) or degrees of freedom of a cubic spline smoother is generally used to specify its smoothness rather than λ directly. A numerical search is then used to determine the value of λ corresponding to the required degrees of freedom.

- Roughly, the complexity of a cubic spline is about the same as a polynomial of degree one less than the degrees of freedom. But the cubic spline smoother 'spreads out' its parameters in a more even way and, hence, is much more flexible than is polynomial regression.

  (The above account follows that given in Hastie and Tibshirani, 1990).

13.4   Some examples of the use of additive models

In this section, we look at a number of examples of the possible application of additive models, beginning with two data sets introduced in Chapter 4, each involving a response variable and a single explanatory variable.

13.4.1   Heights and resting pulse and oxygen uptake and expired ventilation

The two data sets to be used in this section were given previously in Chapter 4 (Tables 4.1 and 4.2). Scatterplots of the two sets of observations also appear in Chapter 4 (Figures 4.1 and 4.2). Here, we shall consider some additive models for both data sets.

The results of fitting a cubic spline to the height/resting pulse data are shown in Table 13.1. The smoothed curve for height is graphed in Figure 13.1. In this case, comparing the additive model and the linear model suggests that the former provides no improvement in fit over the latter—see also Table 13.1.

The corresponding results for the oxygen uptake/expired ventilation data are shown in Table 13.2 and Figure 13.2. Here, there is overwhelming evidence that the additive model leads to a far better fit than does the linear model. The form of the smoothed curve suggests that fitting a quadratic in oxygen uptake to the data might be appropriate. Such a model is compared with the additive cubic spline model in Table 13.3. There remains some evidence that the smoothed curve has modeled oxygen uptake more flexibly.

13.4.2   Maximal static expiratory pressure for patients with cystic fibrosis

In Chapter 8 multiple regression was applied to a set of data obtained from 25 patients with cystic fibrosis (Table 8.3). Nine explanatory variables were

TABLE 13.1. Results of fitting an additive models to height/resting pulse data and comparison with linear model

DF for Terms and F-values for Nonparametric Effects				
	Df	Npar Df	Npar F	Pr(F)
(Intercept)	1			
s(Height)	1	3	1.645255	0.1922873

	Terms	Resid. Df	RSS	Test	Df	Sum of Sq	F Value	Pr(F)
1	Height	48.00000	2750.512					
2	s(Height)	44.99865	2478.527	1 vs. 2	3.00135	271.9845	1.645255	0.1922873

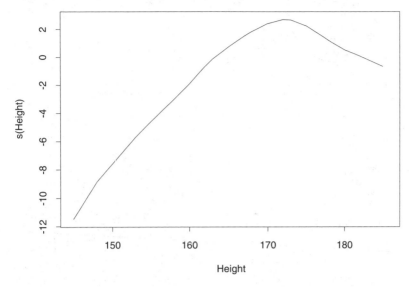

FIGURE 13.1. Fitted generalized additive model for height/resting pulse data.

TABLE 13.2. Results of fitting an additive models to oxygen uptake data and comparison with linear model

DF for Terms and F-values for Nonparametric Effects

	Df	Npar Df	Npar F	Pr(F)
(Intercept)	1			
s(Oxygen)	1	3	244.9107	0

	Terms	Resid. Df	RSS	Test	Df	Sum of Sq	F Value	Pr(F)
1	Oxygen	51.00000	7292.381					
2	s(Oxygen)	47.99798	446.895	1 vs. 2	3.002023	6845.486	244.9107	0

TABLE 13.3. Comparison of quadratic model with GAM for oxygen uptake data

	Terms	Resid. Df	RSS	Test	Df	Sum of Sq	F Value
1	Oxygen + O2	50.00000	507.6565				
2	s(Oxygen)	47.99798	446.8949	1 vs. 2	2.002023	60.76156	3.259698

	Pr(F)
1	
2	0.04700431

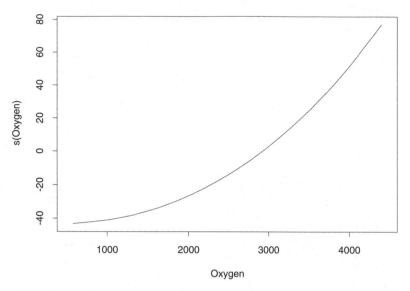

FIGURE 13.2. Fitted generalized additive model for oxygen uptake data.

examined in respect to their ability to predict maximal static expiratory pressure (PEmax). Stepwise regression identified four variables as the most informative about the response, BMP, FEV, RV and Weight. Here, generalized additive models linking PEmax to these four explanatory variables will be considered.

The results of fitting a GAM with cubic spline smoothers for each of the four variables, is compared with the corresponding linear model in Table 13.4. There is little evidence that the smoothed curves for any of the explanatory variables fit better than do the linear terms for the variables. The form of the smoothed curves for each variable and confidence bands for the curves are shown in Figure 13.3.

13.5   Using a logistic additive model

To illustrate the application of a logistic additive model, we shall use some data given originally by Collett and Jemain (1985), concerning the erythrocyte sedimentation rate (ESR), i.e., the rate at which red blood cells (erythrocytes) settle out of suspension in blood plasma, when measured under standard conditions. The ESR increases if levels of certain proteins in the blood rise, such as in rheumatic diseases, chronic infections and malignant diseases; this makes the determination of the ESR one of the most commonly used screening tests performed on samples of blood. The data are shown in Table 13.5 and relate to an investigation of how ESR is related to two plasma proteins, fibrinogen and γ-globulin, both mesured in gm/l, for a sample of 32 individuals. The ESR for a 'healthy' individual should be less than 20 mm/h, and here the response variable denotes whether this

TABLE 13.4. Results of fitting an additive model to cystic fibrosis data and comparison with linear model

	Df	Npar Df	Npar F	Pr(F)
(Intercept)	1			
s(Weight)	1	3	2.163373	0.1703504
s(BMP)	1	3	0.883252	0.4897322
s(FEV)	1	3	1.012321	0.4363152
s(RV)	1	3	1.099613	0.4039473

	Terms	Resid. Df	RSS	Test	Df
1	Weight + BMP + FEV + RV	20.00000	10335.58		
2	s(Weight) + s(BMP) + s(FEV) + s(RV)	7.99631	3629.10	1 vs. 2	12.00369

	Sum of Sq	F Value	Pr(F)
1			
2	6706.475	1.231032	0.394417

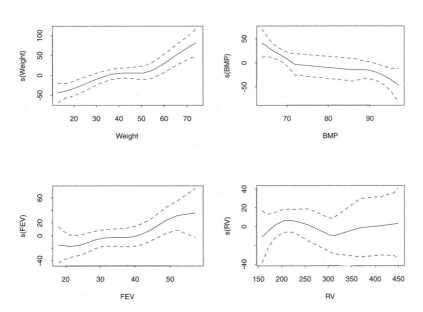

FIGURE 13.3. Smoothed curves for cystic fibrosis predictors and confidence bands.

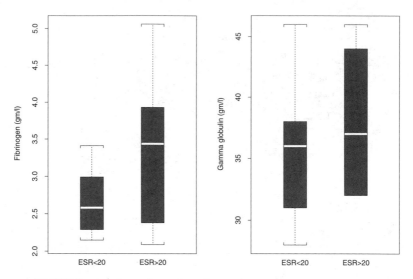

FIGURE 13.4. Box plots of explanatory variables for ESR data.

is the case (0 = less than 20, 1 = greater than 20). The question of interest is how the probability of an ESR reading greater than 20 depends on the levels of the two proteins.

Before undertaking the modeling process, it is helpful to look at some box plots of the two variables for the two levels of the response variable—see Figure 13.4. There are no obvious outliers.

We can compare the fit of an additive model for these data with the routine logistic regression model that would usually be fitted. The results are shown in Table 13.6. There is no strong evidence that the additive model is preferable here, which is also supported by the wide confidence intervals for the fitted smooth curves shown in Figure 13.5.

13.6   Summary

Generalized additive models can be used in virtually any setting in which linear models are used. They provide a flexible alternative to say fitting polynomials for investigating and identifying possible nonlinear relationships between a response variable and explanatory variables. They compliment rather than replace the more conventional, generalized linear model.

TABLE 13.5. Erythrocyte sedimentation rate (ESR) and fibrinogen and γ-globulin (gamma)

Fibrinogen	Gamma	ESR
2.52	38	0
2.56	31	0
2.19	33	0
2.18	31	0
3.41	37	0
2.46	36	0
3.22	38	0
2.21	37	0
3.15	39	0
2.60	41	0
2.29	36	0
2.35	29	0
5.06	37	1
3.34	32	1
2.38	37	1
3.15	36	0
3.53	46	1
2.68	34	0
2.60	38	0
2.23	37	0
2.88	30	0
2.65	46	0
2.09	44	1
2.28	36	0
2.67	39	0
2.29	31	0
2.15	31	0
2.54	28	0
3.93	32	1
3.34	30	0
2.99	36	0
3.32	35	0

TABLE 13.6. Results of fitting a logistic additive model to ESR data and comparison with linear logistic model

	Df	Npar Df	Npar Chisq	P(Chi)
(Intercept)	1			
s(Fibrinogen)	1	2.9	4.310233	0.2140778
s(Gamma)	1	2.9	2.610255	0.4286487

	Terms	Resid. Df	Resid. Dev	Test	Df	Deviance
1	Fibrinogen + Gamma	29.00000	22.97111			
2	s(Fibrinogen) + s(Gamma)	23.27291	11.09298	1 vs. 2	5.727087	11.87814

	Pr(Chi)
1	
2	0.05592989

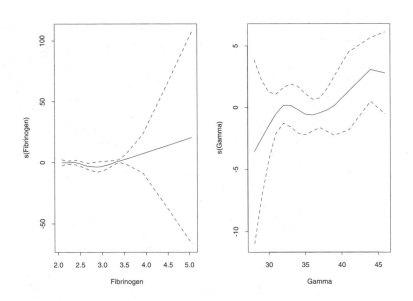

FIGURE 13.5. Fitted curves of logistic gam model for ESR data.

13.7   Using S-PLUS

13.7.1   Using the S language

Section 13.4

The `gam()` function is used for fitting generalized additive models, and `anova()` is used to compare competing models.

Script for Section 13.4

```
# Read in height and resting pulse data
rest<-read.table("resting.dat",header=T)

# Attach data frame
attach(rest)

# Fit a generalized additive model using a cubic spline
rest.gam<-gam(Pulse~s(Height))
summary(rest.gam)

# Plot GAM
win.graph()
plot(rest.gam)                              ==> Figure 13.1


# Compare with linear model
rest.lm<-lm(Pulse~Height)
anova(rest.lm,rest.gam)                     ==> Table 13.1


# Read in expired volume and oxygen uptake data
uptake<-read.table("anaerob.dat",header=T)
attach(uptake)

# Fit gam
uptake.gam<-gam(Ventilation~s(Oxygen))
summary(uptake.gam)

# Compare gam and linear model
uptake.lm<-lm(Ventilation~Oxygen)
anova(uptake.lm,uptake.gam)                 ==> Table 13.2


win.graph()
plot(uptake.gam)                            ==> Figure 13.2


# Now fit linear model with a quadratic in oxygen uptake,
```

```
# and compare fit with cubic spline model
uptake1.lm<-lm(Ventilation~Oxygen+I(Oxygen*Oxygen))
# Note use of I() to 'protect' quadratic effect of oxygen

anova(uptake1.lm,uptake.gam)
```
$\Longrightarrow$ Table 13.3

```
# Read in cystic fibrosis data
cystic<-read.table("cystic.dat",header=T)
attach(cystic)

# Fit a generalized additive model using four
# of the explanatory variables
cystic.gam<-gam(PEmax~s(Weight)+s(BMP)+s(FEV)+s(RV),
   bf.maxit=50)
# Note that the number of iterations of the back fitting
# algorithm has been increased from its default of 10 to 50.

# Compare model with linear model.
cystic.lm<-lm(PEmax~Weight+BMP+FEV+RV)
summary(cystic.gam)
anova(cystic.lm,cystic.gam)
```
$\Longrightarrow$ Table 13.4

```
# Plot form of smoothed curves
win.graph()
par(mfrow=c(2,2))
plot(cystic.gam,se=T)
```
$\Longrightarrow$ Figure 13.3

Section 13.5

In this section, gam() is used to fit an additive logistic model by specifying the binomial family.

Script for Section 13.5

```
# Read in blood test data, and store the ESR variable as a factor.
plasma<-read.table("plasma.dat",header=T)
plasma$ESR<-as.factor(plasma$ESR)
attach(plasma)

# Get box plots to check for outliers
win.graph()
par(mfrow=c(1,2))
boxplot(Fibrinogen[ESR==0],Fibrinogen[ESR==1],
   names=c("ESR<20","ESR>20"),ylab="Fibrinogen (gm/l)")
boxplot(Gamma[ESR==0],Gamma[ESR==1],names=c("ESR<20","ESR>20"),
ylab="Gamma globulin (gm/l)")
```
$\Longrightarrow$ Figure 13.4

```
# Fit an additive logistic model
plasma.gam<-gam(ESR==1~s(Fibrinogen)+s(Gamma),binomial)
summary(plasma.gam)

# Fit a logistic regression model
plasma.lm<-glm(ESR==1~Fibrinogen+Gamma,binomial)

# Compare fits of the two models using a chi-squared statistic.
anova(plasma.lm,plasma.gam,test="Chi")
```
$\implies$ ⌑Table 13.6⌑

```
# Plot smoothed curves for Fibrinogen and Gamma
win.graph()
par(mfrow=c(1,2))
plot(plasma.gam,se=T)
```
$\implies$ ⌑Figure 13.5⌑

13.8   Exercises

13.1 As an alternative to the cubic spline smoother s, the lowess smoother, lo, can be used when fitting GAMs. Investigate this possibility for both the heights/resting pulse data and the oxygen uptake/expired volume data.

13.2 For the oxygen uptake/expired volume data, produce a scatterplot showing the data and fitted linear regression for both

$$\text{Ventilation} = \beta_0 + \beta_1 \text{Oxygen}$$

$$\text{Ventilation} = \beta_0 + \beta_1 \text{Oxygen} + \beta_2 \text{Oxygen}^2$$

Add the predictions made by fitted generalized linear additive models with both locally weighted and cubic spline smoothers.

13.3 Again, investigate the use of the lowess smoother in modeling the ESR data. In particular, assess whether an additive surface is sufficient or whether an interaction surface might be necessary.

13.4 Investigate the use of GAM models on the cystic fibrosis data using all explanatory variables.

14
Nonlinear models

14.1   Introduction

In several previous chapters, we have considered a number of models for
different types of responses. We have generalized the linear model by allowing different links and distributions (generalized linear models) and by
estimating nonlinear transformations of the explanatory variables (generalized additive models). In all of these models, the explanatory variables,
or transformations of these variables, are combined *linearly* to form a linear predictor. In this chapter, we will consider more complex, *nonlinear
models* and methods for estimating their parameters. Here, the mean of
the (continuous) response variable is modeled as a nonlinear function of
explanatory variables. As in the linear model, the response is typically assumed to have a normal distribution and a constant variance. In addition
to nonlinear models, we will also consider maximum likelihood estimation
in situations when the likelihood equations cannot be solved analytically,
because the same S-PLUS functions are often involved.

14.2   Nonlinear models

Two examples of models that are nonlinear in their parameters are

$$y = \beta_1 e^{\beta_2 x_1} + \beta_3 e^{\beta_4 x_2} + \epsilon \qquad (14.1)$$

TABLE 14.1. Concentration of bound and free ligand in an assay of human mammmary tumour

Free	Bound
84.6	12.1
83.9	12.5
148.2	17.2
147.8	16.7
463.9	28.3
463.8	26.9
964.1	37.6
967.6	35.8
1926.0	38.5
1900.0	39.9

$$y = \beta_1 e^{-\beta_2 x} + \epsilon \tag{14.2}$$

Some nonlinear models can be converted into linear form relatively simply. The model in (14.2), for example, becomes linear after taking logarithms. Examples in which this is not possible, e.g., the model in (14.1), are often referred to as *intrinsicially nonlinear models*. Parameters in intrinsically nonlinear models usually have to be estimated by some form of numerical optimization—see Display 14.1. In these nonlinear models, *linear parameters* are those for which the second partial derivative of the model function with respect to the parameter is zero (β_1 and β_2 in 14.1); when this is not the case (β_2 and β_4 in 14.2), they are referred to as *nonlinear parameters*.

14.3   Two examples of nonlinear models

As a relatively simple introduction to the fitting of nonlinear models, we shall use the data shown in Table 14.1, taken from Cressie and Keightly (1981). The data arise from a hormone-receptor assay of a human mammary tumour. In such an assay the concentration of a receptor is determined *in vitro* by exposing a given cell or tissue homogenate to varying concentrations of radioactivity labelled ligand until near-saturation of the receptor is obtained. Concentration of bound (B) and free (F) ligand at equilibrium is measured for each replicate.

The relationship between the concentration of bound and free ligand in a receptor assay is described by the Michaelis-Menten equation

$$B_i = \frac{B_{\max} F_i}{K_D + F_i} + \epsilon_i \tag{14.3}$$

Display 14.1 Estimating nonlinear models

- Assume the model to be fitted is $y_i = f(\mathbf{x}_i; \boldsymbol{\theta}) + \epsilon_i$, where $\mathbf{x}_i' = [x_{i1}, x_{i2}, \cdots x_{ip}]$ is the vector of explanatory variable values for the ith observation, y_i is the corresponding response, $\boldsymbol{\theta}' = [\theta_1, \theta_2, \cdots \theta_k]$ is a vector of parameters and ϵ_i is a residual term generally assumed to be independent of other error terms and to have a $N(0, \sigma^2)$ distribution.

- The sum of squares function, S, given by

$$S = \sum_{i=1}^{n} [y_i - f(\mathbf{x}_i; \boldsymbol{\theta})]^2 \tag{1}$$

provides the basis of estimation and the least-squares estimator of $\boldsymbol{\theta}$ is the value of $\boldsymbol{\theta}$ minimizing S.

- One way of finding such an estimator directly is to use a minimization technique such as steepest descent, Gauss-Newton or Mardquart's method (see Everitt, 1987) to minimize S numerically with respect to $\boldsymbol{\theta}$.

- Alternatively, differentiating S with respect to each of the θ_i in turn and setting the resulting expressions to zero yields the set of simultaneous equations

$$\sum_{i=1}^{n} \left[\{y_i - f(\mathbf{x}_i; \boldsymbol{\theta})\} \left(\frac{\partial f}{\partial \theta_j} \right)_{\boldsymbol{\theta} = \hat{\boldsymbol{\theta}}} \right] = 0 \quad (j = 1, \cdots, k) \tag{2}$$

In general, an iterative numerical method is needed to solve these equations.

- The optimisation procedures used to find parameter estimates in nonlinear models require initial values. Two possibilities listed by Krzanowski (1998) are as follows:

  1. Use knowledge of the parameters to estimate initial values from a plot of the data.

  2. Fit a regression to the nearest 'linear' approximation of the model, and use the resulting parameter estimates as initial values.

- In nonlinear models, the parameter estimates will not in general be linear combinations of the observations y_i, so even assuming normality of the y_i will not ensure the normality of the $\hat{\theta}_i$. Also, the covariance matrix of $\boldsymbol{\theta}$ will no longer be $(\mathbf{X'X})^{-1}\sigma^2$ (see Chapter 8).

- If we assume normality of the y_i, then the least-squares estimators are also maximum likelihood ones; so we can obtain approximate standard errors of the $\hat{\theta}_i$ from asymptotic properties of maximum likelihood estimators, i.e., from the matrix of second derivatives of the log-likelihood.

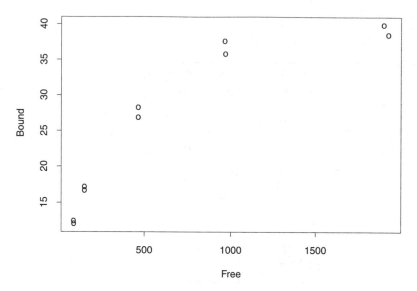

FIGURE 14.1. Scatterplot of concentration of bound ligand versus concentration of free ligand.

TABLE 14.2. Parameter estimates for assay data

	Value	Std. Error	t value
Bmax	44.3776	1.1290	39.3071
KD	241.6870	20.9458	11.5387

where $B_{\max}$ and K_D are parameters known as *capacity* and *affinity*. (It is possible to linearize the Michaelis-Menten equation—see Exercise 14.1—but here we shall deal directly with the model as specified in 14.3.)

Application of a Gauss-Newton procedure to minimize the relevant sum of squares for (14.3) leads to the parameter estimates and standard errors shown in Table 14.2. The initial values used in this case were $B_{\max} = 4.0$ and $K_D = 250$. These were choosen from a plot of the data (see Figure 14.1) as the likely maximum of the bound values and the free value corresponding to half the maximum bound. Here, other initial values lead to identical final values for the two parameters.

For some nonlinear regression problems, the standard error may be an inadequate summary of the uncertainty of a parameter estimate, and an alternative way to explore the distribution of the parameter estimates is to use the bootstrap. Here, this leads to the results shown in Table 14.3. The distributions of the bootstrap estimates of the two parameters are shown in Figure 14.2.

The standard errors calculated by the bootstrap procedure are similar to the standard errors in Table 14.2. The confidence intervals obtained from the bootstrap distributions of each parameter are also similar to those that

TABLE 14.3. Results of bootstrapping the parameter estimates

```
Number of Replications: 1000

Summary Statistics:
        Observed    Bias    Mean      SE
Bmax      44.38  0.09596  44.47   1.163
  KD     241.69  2.28581 243.97  18.025

Empirical Percentiles:
         2.5%      5%      95%   97.5%
Bmax    42.24   42.68   46.26   46.81
  KD   217.43  220.30  276.89  284.56

BCa Confidence Limits:
         2.5%      5%      95%  97.5%
Bmax    42.17   42.58   46.15   46.7
  KD   216.51  220.08  275.11  283.7

Correlation of Replicates:
       Bmax      KD
Bmax  1.000   0.756
  KD  0.756   1.000
```

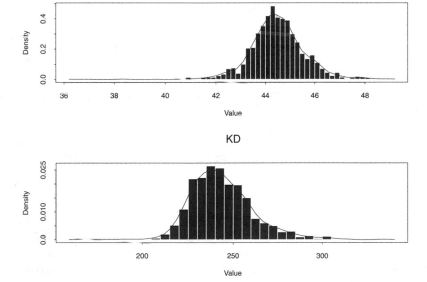

FIGURE 14.2. Bootstrap distribution of parameter estimates.

TABLE 14.4. Results of radioimmunoassay experiment

Concentration	Absorbance
10000	0.880
10000	0.784
5000	0.776
5000	0.769
2500	0.622
2500	0.614
1250	0.500
1250	0.488
625	0.347
625	0.356
312	0.263
312	0.260
156	0.192
156	0.173
78	0.125
78	0.138
39	0.070
39	0.064
20	0.050
20	0.044
10	0.029
10	0.029
5	0.018
5	0.018

would be obtained in the usual way from the parameter's standard error, although that for K_D is now asymmetric about the estimated value of K_D.

As a further, more complex example of the application of a nonlinear model, we shall use the data shown in Table 14.4 taken from Krzanowski (1998). These data were obtained from a radioimmunoassay experiment in which a standard solution was diluted to a number of concentrations and the absorbance was measured at each concentration. A model used widely in radioimmunoassay work is the four-parameter logistic model given by

$$y_i = \alpha + \frac{\beta - \alpha}{1 + (x_i/\gamma)^{-\delta}} + \epsilon \quad (i = 1 \cdots n) \tag{14.4}$$

where α, β, γ and δ are the four parameters. Initial values for α, β and γ can be found from a plot of absorbance against log (concentration) - see Figure 14.3. The initial value for α is the intercept, 0.0, that for β the asymptote, 0.9, and γ is the value of concentration when $y = \frac{1}{2}(\alpha + \beta)$, leading to the value 1096. An initial estimate of δ can be found from the slope of the approximate straight line of the plot of

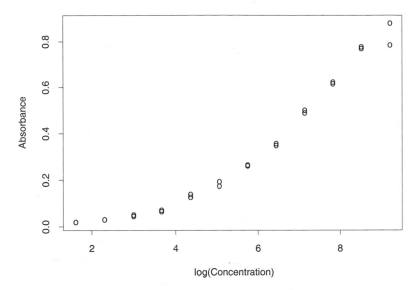

FIGURE 14.3. Plot of absorbance against log concentration.

TABLE 14.5. Parameter estimates for radioimmunoassay data

	Value	Std. Error	t value
alpha	2.519e-003	0.01397	0.1803
beta	1.074e+000	0.06973	15.3979
gamma	1.579e+003	308.61500	5.1152
delta	7.106e-001	0.06452	11.0141

$$\log\left[\frac{\text{absorption} - \alpha}{\beta - \text{absorption}}\right] \text{ against } \log(\text{concentration}) \qquad (14.5)$$

using the initial values of α and β found previously. This plot is given in Figure 14.4 and leads to an intial value of δ of 0.7.

The least-squares estimates of the four parameters and their standard errors are shown in Table 14.5. The fitted curve and the observed values are graphed in Figure 14.5. Clearly, the model provides an excellent fit for these data.

Again, the bootstrap might be used to investigate parameter uncertainty further. The results are shown in Table 14.6, and the distributions of the bootstrap estimates of the four parameters are given in Figure 14.6.

Here, there are considerable differences in the evaluation of parameter uncertainty using the standard errors in Table 14.5 and the bootstrap results given in Table 14.6. The parameter γ seems particularly poorly determined by the data.

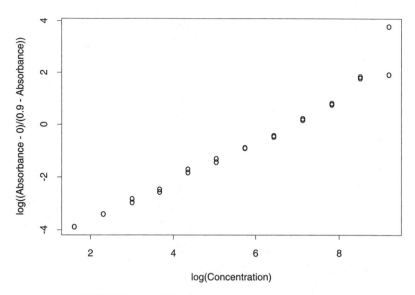

FIGURE 14.4. Plot for finding initial value of δ.

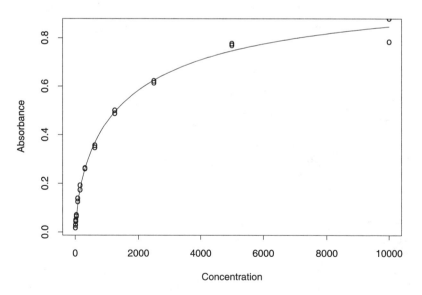

FIGURE 14.5. Observed and fitted radioimmunoassay data.

TABLE 14.6. Bootstrap results for radioimmunoassay data

Number of Replications: 1000

Summary Statistics:

	Observed	Bias	Mean	SE
alpha	2.519e-003	-0.002288	2.311e-004	0.01080
beta	1.074e+000	0.052480	1.126e+000	0.17988
gamma	1.579e+003	426.892170	2.006e+003	1506.72578
delta	7.106e-001	-0.009706	7.009e-001	0.07714

Empirical Percentiles:

	2.5%	5%	95%	97.5%
alpha	-0.02173	-0.01895	0.01491	0.01846
beta	0.92385	0.93648	1.45472	1.54832
gamma	1052.57327	1088.08135	3928.70267	4804.83603
delta	0.55587	0.57431	0.81827	0.83997

BCa Confidence Limits:

	2.5%	5%	95%	97.5%
alpha	-0.01785	-0.01484	0.01945	0.02503
beta	0.91086	0.92151	1.35644	1.44235
gamma	958.58450	1019.40592	3064.93440	3621.62728
delta	0.57515	0.58876	0.84030	0.87211

Correlation of Replicates:

	alpha	beta	gamma	delta
alpha	1.0000	-0.8733	-0.7066	0.9583
beta	-0.8733	1.0000	0.8949	-0.8983
gamma	-0.7066	0.8949	1.0000	-0.6894
delta	0.9583	-0.8983	-0.6894	1.0000

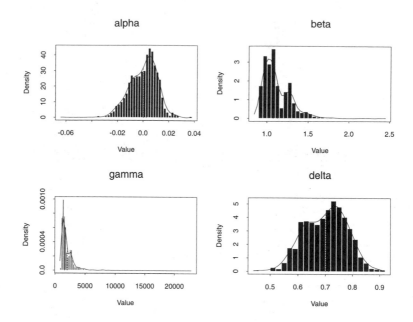

FIGURE 14.6. Distributions of bootsrap estimates for radioimmunoassay data.

14.4 Age of onset of schizophrenia

We now consider a different type of problem, that of estimating the parameters of a model that does not fit into any of the modeling frameworks discussed so far, namely, a *finite mixture model*. We shall use such a model in an investigation of the age of onset of schizophrenia.

A sex difference in the age of onset of schizophrenia was noted by Kraepelin (1919). Subsequently, it has been one of the most consistent findings in the epidemiology of the disorder. Lewine (1981) collated the results of seven studies on the age of onset of the illness, and 13 studies on age at first admission, and showed that all of these studies were consistent in reporting an earlier onset of schizophrenia in men that in women. Lewine suggested two competing models to explain these data:

- *The timing model*: Schizophrenia is essentially the same disorder in the two sexes but has an early onset in men and a late onset in women.

- *The subtype model*: Posits two types of schizophrenia. One is characterized by early onset, typical symptoms, and poor premorbid competence, and the other by late onset, atypical symptoms and good premorbid competence. The early onset typical schizophrenia is more common among men, and the late onset atypical schizophrenia, is more common among women.

TABLE 14.7. Age of onset of schizophrenia

Women					Men				
20	30	21	23	30	21	18	23	21	27
25	13	19	16	25	24	20	12	15	19
20	25	27	43	6	21	22	19	24	9
21	15	26	23	21	19	18	17	23	17
23	23	34	14	17	23	19	37	26	22
18	21	16	35	32	24	19	22	19	16
48	53	51	48	29	16	18	16	33	22
25	44	23	36	58	23	10	14	15	20
28	51	40	43	21	11	25	9	22	25
48	17	23	28	44	20	19	22	23	24
28	21	31	22	56	29	24	22	26	20
60	15	21	30	26	25	17	25	28	22
28	23	21	20	43	22	23	35	16	29
39	40	26	50	17	33	15	29	20	29
17	23	44	30	35	24	39	10	20	23
20	41	18	39	27	15	18	20	21	30
28	30	34	33	30	21	18	19	15	19
29	46	36	58	28	18	25	17	15	42
30	28	37	31	29	27	18	43	20	17
32	48	49	30		21	5	27	25	18
					24	33	32	29	34
					20	21	31	22	15
					27	26	23	47	17
					21	16	21	19	31
					34	23	23	20	21
					18	26	30	17	21
					19	22	52	19	24
					19	19	33	32	29
					58	39	42	32	32
					46	38	44	35	45
					41	31			

A possible way to investigate these models is to apply *finite mixture distributions* to some age of onset data. The finite mixture distribution to be used here is described in Display 14.2. Age of onset data (determined by age on first admission to a psychiatric hospital) of 99 female and 152 male schizophrenics are given in Table 14.7. Initial values for the five parameters of the distribution in Display 14.2 can be 'guessed' by examining histograms of the data—see Figure 14.7. Here, we use the same initial values for both men and women, namely, $p = 0.5$, $\mu_1 = 25$, $\mu_2 = 45$, $\sigma_1 = 3$ and $\sigma_1 = 5$. The maximum likelihood estimates of the five parameters are shown in Table 14.8.

The parameter estimates are given in Table 14.8, and the results are graphed in Figure 14.8 (women) and Figure 14.9 (men). In each diagram,

TABLE 14.8. Maximum likelihood parameter estimates

WOMEN	p = 0.738	mu1 = 24.798	sigma1 = 6.54	mu2 = 46.447	sigma2 = 7.064
MEN	p = 0.512	mu1 = 20.249	sigma1 = 3.07	mu2 = 27.757	sigma2 = 10.594

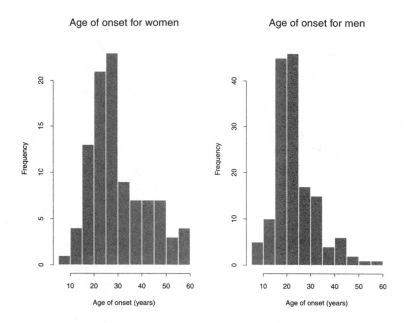

FIGURE 14.7. Histograms of age of onset data for men and women.

Display 14.2 A finite mixture distribution

- If the data are thought to consist of two subpopulations, in each of which a variable of interest has a normal distribution, then a suitable model for the distribution of the variable in the population is

$$f(x) = pN(\mu_1, \sigma_1) + (1 - p)N(\mu_2, \sigma_2) \qquad (1)$$

where p is known as the mixing proportion and $\mu_1, \sigma_1, \mu_2, \sigma_2$ are the means and standard deviations of the two component densities.

- Given a sample of observations $x_1, \cdots, x_n$ from the mixture, the log-likelihood can be written as

$$l(p, \mu_i, \sigma_1, \mu_2, \sigma_2) = \Sigma_{i=1}^{n} \log\left[pN(\mu_i, \sigma_1) + (1 - p)N(\mu_1, \sigma_2)\right] \qquad (2)$$

- Minimizing $-l$ will give estimates of the five parameters.

WOMEN

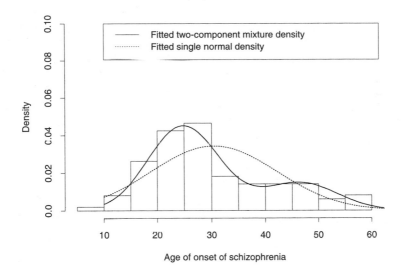

FIGURE 14.8. Histogram and fitted density for women.

a histogram of the relevant data is drawn, and superimposed on this histogram are the fitted mixture distribution and a fitted normal distribution.

The two-component mixture seems to be required to describe adequately the distribution of the women's data but perhaps not the men's. A likelihood ratio test could be applied in each case to formally assess whether the mixture provides a better fit than does a normal distribution (see Exercise 14.2). Clearly, larger data sets are needed to give convincing evidence for or against the subtype model in either men or women, although here it seems to be more applicable to women.

Again, the bootstrap approach is convenient for exploring the uncertainty in each of the five parameters. The results for women and men are shown in Tables 14.9 and 14.10. Plots of the bootstrap distributions are given in Figure 14.10 (women) and Figure 14.11 (men). The very large confidence intervals for some of the parameters reflect the uncertainty in the estimates because of the small sample size.

14.5 Summary

Nonlinear models often occur in particular areas of medicine. Parameter estimation is generally more difficult than for their nonlinear cousins, and most often involves the use of some numerical optimization procedure. Parameter uncertainty in such models is often best investigated by using a bootstrap approach. The same methods can be used to estimate parameters of any models by maximum likelihood.

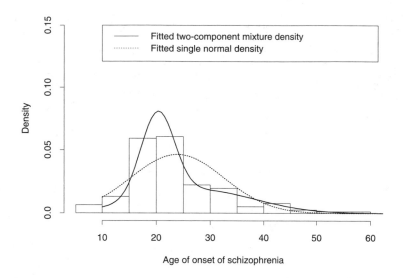

FIGURE 14.9. Histogram and fitted density for men.

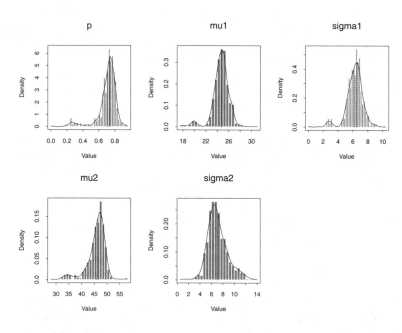

FIGURE 14.10. Bootstrap results for women.

TABLE 14.9. Bootstrap results for women
Number of Replications: 500

Summary Statistics:
	Observed	Bias	Mean	SE
p	0.7378	-0.03191	0.7059	0.125
mu1	24.7977	-0.20276	24.5950	1.541
sigma1	6.5384	-0.30742	6.2310	1.172
mu2	46.4468	-0.70719	45.7396	3.844
sigma2	7.0640	0.01811	7.0821	1.776

Empirical Percentiles:
	2.5%	5%	95%	97.5%
p	0.2736	0.4049	0.8293	0.8543
mu1	19.9727	22.4335	26.6128	26.9384
sigma1	2.7970	4.5032	7.8311	8.1916
mu2	34.4794	37.0781	49.8662	50.6218
sigma2	4.4270	4.8342	10.6245	11.3852

BCa Confidence Limits:
	2.5%	5%	95%	97.5%
p	0.3698	0.575	0.8489	0.8874
mu1	20.2599	22.888	26.7251	27.1563
sigma1	5.0972	5.319	8.9369	9.3516
mu2	34.4108	36.053	49.8517	50.4990
sigma2	4.9050	5.179	11.4322	11.9475

Correlation of Replicates:
	p	mu1	sigma1	mu2	sigma2
p	1.0000	0.7320	0.7760	0.8488	-0.7389
mu1	0.7320	1.0000	0.7191	0.7175	-0.6299
sigma1	0.7760	0.7191	1.0000	0.7630	-0.6231
mu2	0.8488	0.7175	0.7630	1.0000	-0.7875
sigma2	-0.7389	-0.6299	-0.6231	-0.7875	1.0000

TABLE 14.10. Bootstrap results for men

Number of Replications: 500

Summary Statistics:

	Observed	Bias	Mean	SE
p	0.5117	0.1359	0.6476	0.1698
mu1	20.2486	0.3211	20.5697	0.7773
sigma1	3.0700	0.8213	3.8913	1.2616
mu2	27.7568	4.6527	32.4095	5.7491
sigma2	10.5943	-1.3277	9.2666	2.3235

Empirical Percentiles:

	2.5%	5%	95%	97.5%
p	0.3892	0.4155	0.9211	0.9301
mu1	19.4076	19.5164	22.1147	22.3739
sigma1	2.2564	2.3752	6.0581	6.3506
mu2	25.5403	26.1319	43.8845	44.8744
sigma2	3.4245	4.4378	11.9689	12.4764

BCa Confidence Limits:

	2.5%	5%	95%	97.5%
p	0.301	0.3089	0.7569	0.809
mu1	19.039	19.2235	21.4286	21.767
sigma1	1.980	2.1745	5.5472	5.759
mu2	23.553	23.5692	31.4211	34.604
sigma2	6.868	8.3889	13.2479	13.640

Correlation of Replicates:

	p	mu1	sigma1	mu2	sigma2
p	1.0000	0.6660	0.9319	0.9116	-0.6175
mu1	0.6660	1.0000	0.6875	0.6828	-0.4278
sigma1	0.9319	0.6875	1.0000	0.9063	-0.6417
mu2	0.9116	0.6828	0.9063	1.0000	-0.7107
sigma2	-0.6175	-0.4278	-0.6417	-0.7107	1.0000

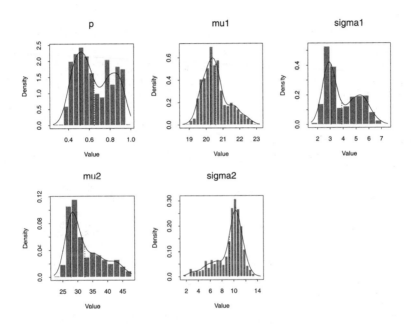

FIGURE 14.11. Bootstrap results for men.

14.6   Using S-PLUS

14.6.1   Using the S language

Section 14.3

In this section, parameter values are added to a data frame using the `param()` function, and the use of the nonlinear least-squares function `nls()` is illustrated. The `bootstrap()` function is used to explore parameter uncertainty. Before running `bootstrap()`, the random number seed is set to an arbitrary value using the `set.seed()` function to allow replication of the results.

Script for Section 14.3

```
# Store assay results
assay<-c(84.6,83.9,148.2,147.8,463.9,463.8,964.1,967.6,
    1926.0,1900.0,12.1,12.5,17.2,16.7,28.3,26.9,37.6,
    35.8,38.5,39.9)
assay<-matrix(assay,ncol=2)

dimnames(assay)<-list(NULL,c("Free","Bound"))
assay<-as.data.frame(assay)
attach(assay)

# Plot the data
win.graph()
plot(Free,Bound)                              ⟹ ┌──────────────┐
                                                │ Figure 14.1  │
                                                └──────────────┘

# Attach initial values for the two parameters
param(assay,"Bmax")<-40
param(assay,"KD")<-250

# Use least squares to estimate the two parameters
# and their standard error
assay.fit<-nls(Bound~Bmax*Free/(KD+Free),assay)
summary(assay.fit)                            ⟹ ┌──────────────┐
                                                │ Table 14.2   │
                                                └──────────────┘

# Get boostrap results and plots of parameters, distributions
set.seed(1345124371)
assay.boot<-bootstrap(assay,nls(Bound~Bmax*Free/(KD+Free),
    assay)$parameters)

summary(assay.boot)                           ⟹ ┌──────────────┐
                                                │ Table 14.3   │
                                                └──────────────┘
plot(assay.boot)                              ⟹ ┌──────────────┐
                                                │ Figure 14.2  │
                                                └──────────────┘

# Read in radioimmunoassay data
radioim<-read.table("radioim.dat",header=T)
```

```
attach(radioim)

# Plot absorbance against concentration to get initial
# parameter estimates
win.graph()
plot(log(Concentration),Absorbance)
```
$\implies$ ⟦Figure 14.3⟧

```
# Make plot to get initial value for delta
win.graph()
plot(log(Concentration),
   log((Absorbance-0.0)/(0.9-Absorbance)))
```
$\implies$ ⟦Figure 14.4⟧

```
# Set initial values of parameters
param(radioim,"alpha")<-0.0
param(radioim,"beta")<-0.9
param(radioim,"gamma")<-1096
param(radioim,"delta")<-0.7

# Estimate parameters in the model
radioim.fit<-nls(Absorbance~alpha+(beta-alpha)/
   (1+(Concentration/gamma)^(-delta)),radioim)
summary(radioim.fit)
```
$\implies$ ⟦Table 14.5⟧

```
# Plot fitted curve and observations
x<-seq(range(Concentration)[1],range(Concentration)[2],
   length=100)
alpha<-radioim.fit$parameters[1]
beta<-radioim.fit$parameters[2]
gamma<-radioim.fit$parameters[3]
delta<-radioim.fit$parameters[4]
y<-alpha+(beta-alpha)/(1+(x/gamma)^(-delta))
win.graph()
plot(x,y,xlab="Concentration",ylab="Absorbance",type="l")
points(Concentration,Absorbance)
```
$\implies$ ⟦Figure 14.5⟧

```
# Use bootstrap to explore further parameter uncertainty
set.seed(135421)
radioim.boot<-bootstrap(radioim,nls(Absorbance~alpha
   +(beta-alpha)/(1+(Concentration/gamma)^(-delta)),
   radioim)$parameters)
summary(radioim.boot)
```
$\implies$ ⟦Table 14.6⟧

```
plot(radioim.boot)
```
$\implies$ ⟦Figure 14.6⟧

Section 14.3

This section uses the ms() function to minimize the log-likelihood function for a mixture of two normal distributions. Again, the bootstrap() function is used to investigate parameter uncertainty. A for loop is used to repeat the same sequence of commands for men and for women. The cat() function is used to print out the parameter estimates.

Script for Section 14.4

```
# Read in age of onset data for women
onsetw<-scan("onsetw.dat")
onsetm<-scan("onsetm.dat")

# Examine histograms to help in selecting initial values
win.graph()
par(mfrow=c(1,2))

hist(onsetw,xlab="Age of onset (years)",ylab="Frequency")
title("Age of onset for women")
hist(onsetm,xlab="Age of onset (years)",ylab="Frequency")
title("Age of onset for men")
```
$\Longrightarrow$ Figure 14.7

```
# Loop through code for the two data sets
sex<-c("WOMEN","MEN")

transf<-function(x) {
    x1<-exp(x[1])/(1+exp(x[1]))
    x2<-x[2]
    x3<-exp(x[3])
    x4<-x[4]
    x5<-exp(x[5])
    X<-c(x1,x2,x3,x4,x5)
    names(X)<-c("p","mu1","sigma1","mu2","sigma2")
    X
}

for(i in 1:2) {
    # beginning of loop
    if(i==1) onset<-onsetw else onset<-onsetm

    # Store as suitable data frame
    onset<-matrix(onset,ncol=1)
    dimnames(onset)<-list(NULL,c("Onsetage"))
    onset<-as.data.frame(onset)
    attach(onset)

    # Set initial parameter values
    param(onset,"w")<-log(0.5/0.5)
```

```
param(onset,"mu1")<-25
param(onset,"w1")<-log(3)
param(onset,"mu2")<-45
param(onset,"w2")<-log(5)

# Now minimize -log-likelihood to get parameter estimates
onset.fit<-ms(~-log(exp(w)/(1+exp(w))
   *dnorm(Onsetage,mu1,exp(w1))
   +1/(1+exp(w))*dnorm(Onsetage,mu2,exp(w2))),onset)
summary(onset.fit)

# Plot fitted mixture
# Get correct parameter values
p<-exp(onset.fit$parameters["w"])/
   (1+exp(onset.fit$parameters["w"]))
mu1<-onset.fit$parameters["mu1"]
sigma1<-exp(onset.fit$parameters["w1"])
mu2<-onset.fit$parameters["mu2"]
sigma2<-exp(onset.fit$parameters["w2"])

# Print values
cat(sex[i]," p = ",round(p,digits=3)," mu1 = ",
   round(mu1,digits=3)," sigma1 = ", round(sigma1,digits=2),
   " mu2 = ", round(mu2,digits=3)," sigma2 = ",
   round(sigma2,digits=3))
```
$\implies$ Table 14.8
```
win.graph()
x<-seq(10,70,length=100)
f1<-dnorm(x,mu1,sigma1)
f2<-dnorm(x,mu2,sigma2)
f<-p*f1+(1-p)*f2
hist(onset[,1],probability=T,col=0,ylab="Density",
   ylim=c(0,0.15),xlab="Age of onset of schizophrenia")
lines(x,f,lwd=2)

# superimpose single component density
mu<-mean(onset[,1])
sig<-var(onset[,1],unbiased=F)
f<-dnorm(x,mu,sqrt(sig))
lines(x,f,lwd=2,lty=2)
legend(locator(1),c("Fitted two component mixture density",
   "Fitted single normal density"),lty=1:2)

title(sex[i])
```
$\implies$ Figures 14.8 and 14.9
```
# Bootstrap-need to transform parameters back to p,mu1,
# sigma1,mu2,sigma2 and rename using transf() defined above
```

```
set.seed(13471)
onset.boot<-bootstrap(onset,transf(ms(~-log(exp(w)/(1+exp(w))
   *dnorm(Onsetage,mu1,exp(w1))+1/(1+exp(w))
   *dnorm(Onsetage,mu2,exp(w2))),onset)$parameters),B=500)

win.graph()
print(summary(onset.boot))
```

$\implies$ | Tables 14.9 and 14.10 |

```
plot(onset.boot)
```

$\implies$ | Figures 14.10 and 14.11 |

```
} # end of loop
```

14.7   Exercises

14.1 Show how the Michaelis-Menten equation can be linearised, and when put in this form, estimate the two parameters for the data in Table 14.1 from simple linear regression.

14.2 Calculate the likelihood ratio test for comparing the fit of a mixture of two normals with the fit of a single normal for both the male and female age of onset data.

14.3 Because the usual chi-square distribution for the likelihood ratio test does not strictly apply when fitting mixtures (see Everitt and Hand, 1981), use the bootstrap approach to finding a more convincing p-value for the test.

15
Regression Trees

15.1 Introduction

Previous chapters have dealt with a number of regression type models, linear and multiple regression (Chapters 4 and 8), generalized linear models (Chapters 9 and 10), mixed-effects regression for longitudinal data (Chapters 11 and 12) and generalized additive and nonlinear models (Chapters 13 and 14). These parametric regression methods are widely used, but they may not give faithful data descriptions when the assumptions on which they are based are not met, or in the presence of higher order interactions among some of the explanatory variables.

A method of nonparametric regression that evolved to overcome these potential difficulties is the *classification and regression tree* approach (CART). The central theme of such tree techniques is the extraction of subgroups of observations. Within these subgroups, covariates are homogeneous and between subgroups outcomes are distinct. Interpretation in terms of prognostic group identification is frequently possible. Creation of subgroups takes place according to a tree structure, in essence a series of binary splits. The basic ideas are illustrated in Figure 15.1 taken from Zhang and Singer (1999). Here, the tree is formed by two variables, and the tree has three layers of nodes. The first layer is the unique root node, namely, the circle on the top. One internal (the circle) node is in the second layer, and the three terminal (the boxes) nodes are, respectively, in the second and third layers. Both the root node and the internal nodes are partitioned into two nodes in the next layer that are called left and right daughter nodes. By definition, however, the terminal nodes do not have offspring nodes. How parent nodes are split into two daughter nodes and when a terminal node declared are questions that will be taken up in the next section.

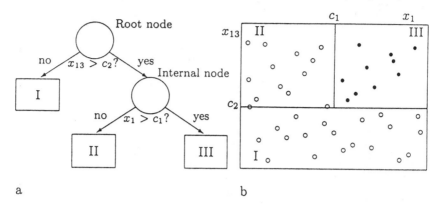

a   b

FIGURE 15.1. An illustrative tree structure. Circles and dots are different outcomes (Zhang and Singer, 1999).

15.2   Tree-based models

The central thrust of tree techniques is the elicitation of subgroups. So, for example, if we have a single continuous response variable y and a set of explanatory variables $x_1 \cdots x_p$, application of a tree-modeling procedure might lead to a 'rule' such as

if $(x_2 < 413)$ and $(x_9 \in \{C, D, E\})$ and $(x_5 < 3.5)$
then the predicted value of y is 4.75.

A regression tree is a collection of many such rules determined by a procedure known as *recursive partitioning*. Brief details of the procedure are given in Display 15.1.

A crucial aspect of tree-structured regression is determination of tree size; i.e., how many splits should be made? Simple 'stopping' rules are as follows:

- Node size—stop when this drops below a threshold value.

- Improvement as measured by the split function ϕ, as defined in Display 15.1—stop when this is below a threshold.

Neither of those is particularly attractive because they have to be judged relative to preset thresholds, mispecification of which can result in overfitting or underfitting. These difficulties can be overcome by use of a *pruning algorithm* that operates as follows:

Display 15.1 Finding a regression tree using recursive partitioning.

- A series of binary splits is made based on the answers to questions of the type, 'Is observation or case $x_i \epsilon A$?', where A is a region of the covariate space.

- Answering such a question induces a partition, or split, of the covariate space; cases for which the answer is yes are assigned to one group, and those for which the answer is no to an alternative group.

- Most implementations of tree-modeling proceed by imposing the following constraints.

  1. Each split depends on the value of only a single covariate.

  2. For ordered (continuous or categorical) covariates X_j, only splits resulting from the questions of the form 'Is $X_j < C$?' are considered. Thus, ordering is preserved.

  3. For categorical explanatory variables, all possible splits into disjoint subsets of the categories are allowed.

- A tree is grown as follows:

  1. Examine every allowable split on each explanatory variable.

  2. Select and execute (i.e., create left and right 'daughter' nodes) from the best of these splits.

- The initial or root node of the tree comprises the whole sample. Steps (1) and (2) above are then reapplied to each of the daughter nodes. Various procedures are used to control tree size, as described in the text.

- The best split is determined by the value of the split function $\phi(s, g)$ that can be evaluated for any split s of node g. Most commonly, the split function used is essentially the sum of squares.

  - g designates a node of the tree—g contains a subsample of cases $\{x_i', y_i\}$, where $x_i' = [x_{i1}, x_{i2}, \cdots, x_{ip}]$ is the vector of observed covariate values and y_i is the observed outcome for the ith case.

  - Let N_g be the total number of cases in g, and let $\bar{y}(g) = (1/N_g)\Sigma_{i\epsilon g}y_i$ be the response average for node g.

  - The within-node sum of squares for node g is given by

$$SS(g) = \Sigma_{i\epsilon g}[y_i - \bar{y}(g)]^2 \qquad (1)$$

  Now, suppose a split s partitions g into left and right daughter nodes g_L and g_R. The least-squares split function is

$$\phi(s, g) = SS(g) - SS(g_L) - SS(g_R) \qquad (2)$$

  - The best split s^* of g is the split such that

$$\phi(s^*, g) = \max_{s\epsilon\Omega} \phi(s, g) \qquad (3)$$

  where Ω is the set of all allowable splits s of g.

- A least-squares regression tree is constructed by recursively splitting nodes to maximize the above ϕ function.

- The function is such that we create smaller and smaller nodes of progressively increased homogeneity.

- Grow a very large tree initially to capture all potentially important splits.

- Collapse this back up using *cost complexity pruning*, as described in Display 15.2, creating a nested sequence of trees.

- Having arrived at such a sequence, we are left with the problem of selecting a 'best' tree from the sequence.

- If a separate validation sample is available, we can predict on that set of observations and calculate the sum of squares (often referred to in this context as *deviance*) versus α for the pruned trees. This will often have a minimum, and so the smallest tree whose sum of squares is close to the minimum can be chosen.

- If no validation set is available, one can be constructed from the observations used in constructing the tree, by splitting the observations into a number of (roughly) equally sized subsets. If n subsets are formed this way, $n - 1$ can be used to grow the tree and it can be tested on the remaining subset. This can be done n ways, and the results averaged.

15.3   Birthweight of babies

In this chapter,the use of CART will be illustrated on a data set given by Hosmer and Lemeshow (1989) involving 189 births at a hospital in the USA. The following information is recorded about each birth (see Table 15.1).

low—a binary variable indicating whether birthweight was below 2.5 kg.

age—age of mother in years.

lwt—weight of mother (lbs) at last menstrual period.

race—white/black/other.

smoke—a binary variable indicating smoking status during pregnancy.

ptl—number of previous premature labours.

ht—a binary variable indicating history of hypertension.

ui—a binary variable indicating whether mother has uterine irritability.

ftv—number of physician visits in the first trimester.

bwt—actual birthweight (grams).

Interest centres on deriving a procedure for predicting whether a pregnant woman is at risk of having a low birthweight baby.

Display 15.2 Cost complexity pruning

- Pruning successfully snips off the least important splits. The importance of a subtree is assessed by a measure of within-node homogeneity or *cost*, and pruning is accomplished using a *cost-complexity algorithm*.

- We will let $R(g)$ be the cost of node g. For example, for least-squares splitting, we take $R(g) = SS(g)$.

- Now, define $R(G)$ as the cost of the entire tree G, where

$$R(G) = \Sigma_{g \epsilon \tilde{G}} R(g) \qquad (1)$$

  where $\tilde{G}$ is the collection of terminal nodes of G.

- Also, define the *complexity* of G as $|\tilde{G}|$, the number of terminal nodes of G.

- The cost-complexity of G is

$$R_\alpha(G) = R(G) + \alpha|\tilde{G}| \qquad (2)$$

  where $\alpha \geq 0$ is called the *complexity parameter*.

- The aim is to minimize simultaneously both cost and complexity; large trees will have small cost but high complexity and the reverse is the case for small trees. Solely minimizing cost will err on the side of overfitting; for example, with $R(g) = SS(g)$, we can achieve zero cost by splitting to a point where each terminal node contains only one observation.

- Initially, a large tree $G_{\max}$ is grown using the split function. The size of this tree is not critical. Following this, the strategy adopted is as follows: For each value of α, we find the subtree $G(\alpha)$ of $G_{\max}$ that minimizes $R_\alpha(G)$.

- The following points should be noted about this strategy.

  1. If α is small, the penalty for large $|\tilde{G}|$ will also be small and, hence, $G(\alpha)$ will be large.

  2. As α increases, $|\tilde{G}|$ decreases.

  3. For α sufficiently large, $|\tilde{G}| = 1$ and the minimal cost-complexity tree is the root node (the entire original sample) because any splitting will increase the cost complexity.

TABLE 15.1. Sample of birthweight data

Low	Age	Lwt	Race	Smoke	Ptl	Ht	Ui	Ftv	Bwt
0	19	182	black	no	0	absent	present	0	2523
0	33	155	other	no	0	absent	absent	3	2551
0	20	105	white	yes	0	absent	absent	1	2557
0	21	108	white	yes	0	absent	present	2	2594
0	18	107	white	yes	0	absent	present	0	2600
0	21	124	other	no	0	absent	absent	0	2622
0	22	118	white	no	0	absent	absent	1	2637
0	17	103	other	no	0	absent	absent	1	2637
0	29	123	white	yes	0	absent	absent	1	2663
0	26	113	white	yes	0	absent	absent	0	2665
0	19	95	other	no	0	absent	absent	0	2722
0	19	150	other	no	0	absent	absent	1	2733
0	22	95	other	no	0	present	absent	0	2751
0	30	107	other	no	1	absent	present	2	2750

TABLE 15.2. Simple tree to predict birthweight from mother's smoking status
node), split, n, deviance, yval
* denotes terminal node

```
1) root 189 99970000 2945
  2) smoke:yes 74 31760000 2772 *
  3) smoke:no 115 64580000 3056 *
```

15.3.1 Some simple examples of regression trees for the birthweight data

To illustrate the process of finding a regression tree as described in Display 15.1, we shall construct some simple trees for the birthweight data. The simplest tree results from using a binary variable such as smoke to predict actual birthweight. The details of the regression tree for birthweight using only a single explanatory variable smoke is shown in Table 15.2. The root node contains all 189 subjects; it is from this node that the tree is grown. Thereafter, nodes of the tree contain subsets of the root node sample. Here, the only possible partition is into smokers ($n = 74$) and non-smokers ($n = 115$). The average birthweight for babies of smokers is 2771.9 gm, and for nonsmokers, it is 3055.7 gm. The deviance shown is simply the corrected sum of squares for the birthweights of the subjects in a node, i.e., the within-node sum of squares for birthweight.

A slightly more interesting tree results from using race with three unordered categories. Here, the allowable splits from the root mode are {white: black and other}, {black: white and other}, and {other: white and black}. These three splits are considered, and the one that maximizes ϕ as defined in Display 15.1, is selected. This leads to the tree shown in Table 15.3. A graphic representation of the tree helps here— see Figure 15.2. From the root node, the first split is white: black, other, and then a further split

TABLE 15.3. Simple tree to predict birthweight from ethnicity

```
node), split, n, deviance, yval
     * denotes terminal node

1) root 189 99970000 2945
  2) race:black,other 93 44760000 2781
    4) race:black 26 10200000 2720 *
    5) race:other 67 34420000 2805 *
  3) race:white 96 50330000 3103 *
```

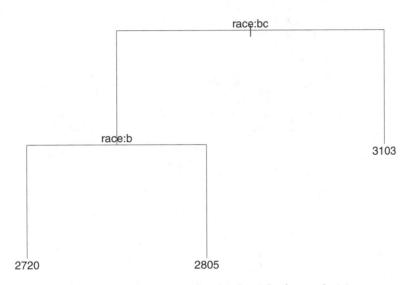

FIGURE 15.2. Tree to predict birthweight from ethnicity.

of the black/other node is made. Here, the regression tree simply orders average birthweights: black 2719.7 gm, other 2805.3 gm, white, 3102.7 gm.

Now, consider the regression tree for the continuous variable age. Age has 23 distinct values in the range 14 to 36. Hence, it may result in $23 - 1 = 22$ allowable splits. For example, one split can be whether age is more than 20 years. In general, for an ordinal or a continuous explanatory variable, the number of allowable splits is one fewer than the number of its distinctly observed values. The regression tree for birthweight on age is shown in Table 15.4 and in graphical form in Figure 15.3. Things have now become a little more complicated! The first split is into mothers less than 35 years of age and those 35 years and older. There are only five women in the second group, and so it is not split any further; the average birthweight for this group is 3709.6 gm. The larger group is then split into finer and finer partitions.

Finally, in this section, let us examine the regression tree approach for birthweight and two explanatory variables, smoke and race. Details of the tree are given in Table 15.5 and the tree is displayed graphically in Fig-

TABLE 15.4. Tree to predict birthweight from mother's age

```
node), split, n, deviance, yval
      * denotes terminal node

  1) root 189 99970000 2945
    2) age<34.5 184 93750000 2924
      4) age<29.5 162 82460000 2905
        8) age<24.5 120 51930000 2944
         16) age<15.5 6  1857000 2736 *
         17) age>15.5 114 49800000 2955
           34) age<16.5 7  2899000 3332 *
           35) age>16.5 107 45840000 2930
             70) age<21.5 68 26740000 2884
              140) age<20.5 56 21010000 2918
                280) age<17.5 12  2162000 2758 *
                281) age>17.5 44 18460000 2961
                  562) age<19.5 26  9955000 3031
                    1124) age<18.5 10  2961000 2998 *
                    1125) age>18.5 16  6976000 3052 *
                  563) age>19.5 18  8191000 2860 *
              141) age>20.5 12  5366000 2724 *
             71) age>21.5 39 18700000 3011
              142) age<22.5 13  3653000 3150 *
              143) age>22.5 26 14670000 2941
                286) age<23.5 13  4920000 2952 *
                287) age>23.5 13  9742000 2930 *
        9) age>24.5 42 29840000 2795
         18) age<27.5 26 16170000 2709
           36) age<25.5 15 11710000 2767 *
           37) age>25.5 11  4331000 2628 *
         19) age>27.5 16 13170000 2934
           38) age<28.5 9  7497000 2909 *
           39) age>28.5 7  5658000 2967 *
      5) age>29.5 22 10810000 3062
       10) age<31.5 12  3392000 3186
         20) age<30.5 7  1552000 3222 *
         21) age>30.5 5  1818000 3136 *
       11) age>31.5 10  7015000 2913 *
    3) age>34.5 5  3210000 3710 *
```

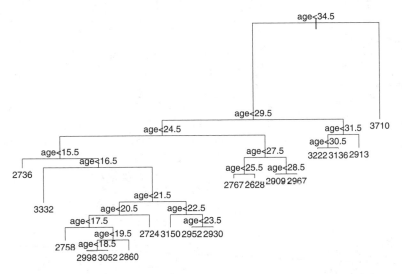

FIGURE 15.3. Tree to predict birthweight from mother's age.

ure 15.4. Here, the first split is on race into white and black/other. Each of the new nodes is then further split on the smoke variable into smokers and nonsmokers, and then, in the left-hand side of the tree, further nodes are introduced by spitting race into black and other. The six terminal nodes and their average birthweights are as follows:

1. black, smokers: 2504, $n = 10$.

2. other, smokers: 2757, $n = 12$.

3. other, non-smokers: 2816, $n = 55$.

4. black, non-smokers: 2854, $n = 16$.

5. white, smokers: 2827, $n = 52$.

6. white, non-smokers: 3429, $n = 44$.

Here, there is evidence of a race $\times$ smoke interaction, at least for black and other women. Among smokers, black women produce babies with lower average birthweight than do 'other' women. But for nonsmokers, the reverse is the case.

15.4   More complex trees for the birthweight data

Using all explanatory variables, the initial regression tree for birthweight is as shown in Table 15.6. The tree is graphed in Figure 15.5. The tree is complex, and we shall try to find a simplified version using the cost-complexity primary algorithm and cross-validation on the original data using a 10-fold split. The deviance against size diagram shown in Figure 15.6 suggests that

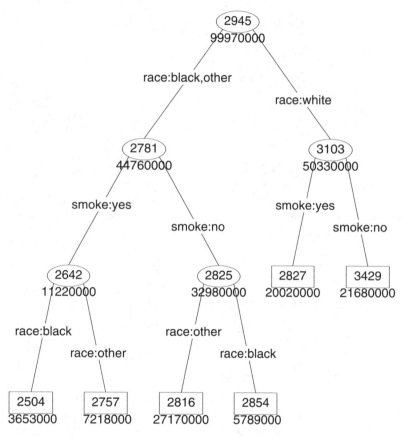

FIGURE 15.4. Tree to predict birthweight from ethnicity and smoking.

TABLE 15.5. Simple tree to predict birthweight from ethnicity and smoking

```
node), split, n, deviance, yval
       * denotes terminal node
 1) root 189 99970000 2945
   2) race:black,other 93 44760000 2781
     4) smoke:yes 22 11220000 2642
       8) race:black 10  3653000 2504 *
       9) race:other 12  7218000 2757 *
     5) smoke:no 71 32980000 2825
       10) race:other 55 27170000 2816 *
       11) race:black 16  5789000 2854 *
   3) race:white 96 50330000 3103
     6) smoke:yes 52 20020000 2827 *
     7) smoke:no 44 21680000 3429 *
```

a tree of size 5 should be selected. The optimal tree of this size is shown in Figure 15.7. Here, the first split involves the weight of the mother. Mothers with weights at last menstrual period below 110 lbs produce babies with very low birthweights, the average being 2,549 gm. Mothers of 110 lbs and above are next split according to whether they had suffered uterine irritability, those who had forming a terminal node with average birthweight of 2,410 gm. Next, women who had not suffered uterine irritability are split into smokers and nonsmokers, and finally, the resulting nonsmokers are split by race into black/other and white. The final five subgroups are ordered by average birthweight of their babies.

15.5 Summary

The use of tree-based models is relatively unfamiliar to many statisticians, although researchers in other fields have found trees to be an attractive way to express knowledge and decision-making. Examples of their use in medicine are to be found in Goldman *et al.* (1982, 1996), Levy *et al.* (1985), McConnochie *et al.* (1993), Choi *et al.* (1991) and Temkin *et al.* (1995). The increasing availability of suitable software such as that found in S-PLUS will hopefully lead to more statisticians considering these methods and uncovering both their strengths and their weaknesses.

TABLE 15.6. Tree for birthweight on all explanatory variables

```
node), split, n, deviance, yval
      * denotes terminal node

 1) root 189 99970000 2945
   2) lwt<109.5 42 12920000 2549
     4) age<18.5 10  1803000 2864
       8) age<17.5 5  1637000 2875 *
       9) age>17.5 5   165500 2852 *
     5) age>18.5 32  9816000 2451
      10) lwt<93 7  2068000 2227 *
      11) lwt>93 25  7300000 2514
        22) lwt<95.5 6  1005000 2870 *
        23) lwt>95.5 19  5294000 2401
          46) age<20.5 6  1688000 2684 *
          47) age>20.5 13  2904000 2271
            94) ftv<0.5 5   727500 1965 *
            95) ftv>0.5 8  1416000 2462 *
   3) lwt>109.5 147 78610000 3058
     6) ui:present 17 10320000 2405
      12) smoke:yes 6  3198000 2101 *
      13) smoke:no 11  6266000 2571
        26) lwt<127.5 5  1973000 2806 *
        27) lwt>127.5 6  3786000 2375 *
     7) ui:absent 130 60100000 3143
      14) smoke:yes 47 20150000 2920
        28) age<19.5 14  5157000 3299
          56) age<18.5 8  3051000 3036 *
          57) age>18.5 6   810400 3650 *
        29) age>19.5 33 12130000 2759
          58) lwt<141 20  4381000 2875
           116) age<28.5 15  2838000 2773
             232) ftv<0.5 9  1846000 2848 *
             233) ftv>0.5 6   865900 2661 *
           117) age>28.5 5   920400 3180 *
          59) lwt>141 13  7070000 2582
           118) ftv<1.5 8  4828000 2370 *
           119) ftv>1.5 5  1314000 2920 *
      15) smoke:no 83 36300000 3269
        30) race:black,other 44 18200000 3037
          60) lwt<156.5 39 15440000 2954
           120) lwt<138 32 12020000 3060
             240) age<26.5 27  9962000 2991
               480) lwt<127.5 20  4707000 3127
                 960) age<20.5 11  1631000 3236
                  1920) lwt<117 5   150300 3113 *
                  1921) lwt>117 6  1342000 3338 *
                 961) age>20.5 9  2788000 2995 *
               481) lwt>127.5 7  3825000 2602 *
             241) age>26.5 5  1240000 3430 *
           121) lwt>138 7  1428000 2471 *
          61) lwt>156.5 5   393300 3685 *
        31) race:white 39 13070000 3531
          62) lwt<137.5 22  7479000 3690
           124) age<22.5 8  3043000 3409 *
           125) age>22.5 14  3444000 3850
             250) lwt<126.5 8  2354000 4015 *
             251) lwt>126.5 6   583400 3630 *
          63) lwt>137.5 17  4313000 3325
           126) lwt<156.5 6  1454000 3050 *
           127) lwt>156.5 11  2156000 3475
             254) age<30 6  1042000 3381 *
             255) age>30 5   996300 3589 *
```

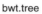

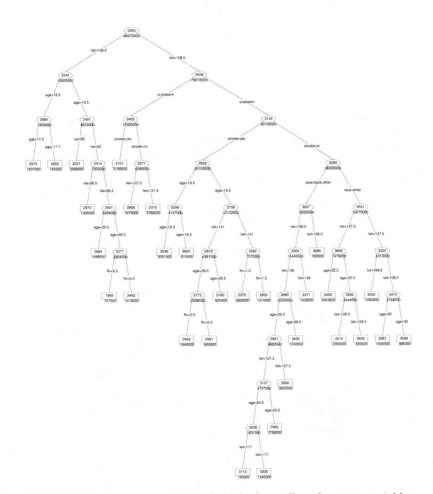

FIGURE 15.5. Tree to predict birthweight from all explanatory variables.

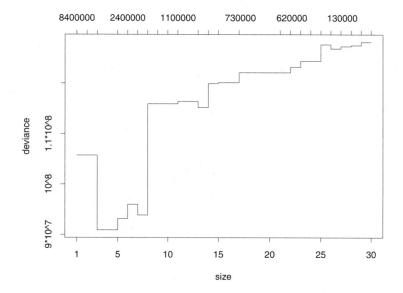

FIGURE 15.6. Deviance against size for cost-complexity pruning and cross-validation applied to tree for birthweight data in Figure 15.5.

bwt.best

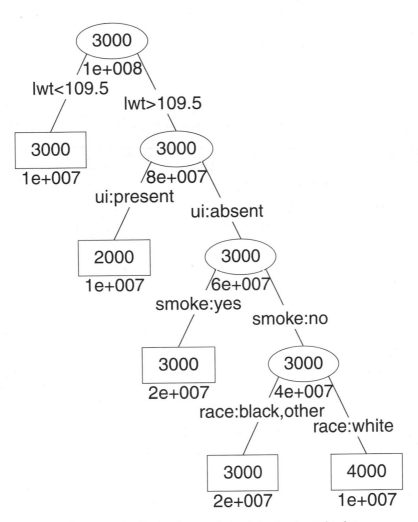

FIGURE 15.7. Optimal tree of size 5 for birthweight data.

15.6   Using S-PLUS

15.6.1   Using the S language

Section 15.3

Here, the `tree()` function is used to produce some simple classification trees for the birthweight data. The function `post.tree()` is used to generate a postscript file that can be used to obtain a 'pretty' tree diagram.

Script for Section 15.3

```
# Read attach birthweight data
birthwt<-read.table(file="birthwt.dat")
birthwt$smoke<-factor(birthwt$smoke,levels=0:1,
    labels=c("no","yes"))
birthwt$race<-factor(birthwt$race,levels=1:3,
    labels=c("white","black","other"))
birthwt$ht<-factor(birthwt$ht,levels=0:1,
    labels=c("absent","present"))
birthwt$ui<-factor(birthwt$ui,levels=0:1,
    labels=c("absent","present"))
attach(birthwt)

# Use the tree() function to produce a number of simple trees
bwt.trees<-tree(bwt~smoke)
bwt.trees
```
$\implies$ Table 15.2

```
# Tree for ethnicity
bwt.treer<-tree(bwt~race)
bwt.treer
```
$\implies$ Table 15.3

```
win.graph()
plot(bwt.treer,type="u")
# uses uniform spacing
text(bwt.treer)
```
$\implies$ Figure 15.2

```
# Tree for age
bwt.treea<-tree(bwt~age)
bwt.treea
```
$\implies$ Table 15.4

```
win.graph()
plot(bwt.treea)
text(bwt.treea,cex=0.8)
```
$\implies$ Figure 15.3

```
# Now use race and smoke
bwt.treesr<-tree(bwt~smoke+race)
bwt.treesr
```
⟹ Table 15.5

```
# post.tree() produces a postscript file for a better graph
post.tree(bwt.treesr,file="birthwt.ps")
```
⟹ Figure 15.4

Section 15.4

In this section, the function cv.tree() is used for cross-validation in asso
ciation with the function prune.tree(), which applies the cost-complexity
algorithm described in the text. The rand option in cv.tree() is used to
generate a 10-fold split via the sample() function. In order to obtain the
same results when this procedure is repeated, the random number seed is
set using set.seed().

Script for Section 15.4

```
# Now use all explanatory variables
bwt.tree<-tree(bwt~age+lwt+race+smoke+ptl+ht+ui+ftv)
win.graph()
plot(bwt.tree)
text(bwt.tree,cex=0.7)

# Need to produce a readable tree from a postscript file
post.tree(bwt.tree,file="bwt.ps")
```
⟹ Figure 15.5

```
# Use cross-validation and the cost-complexity algorithm
# to try to find an optimal smaller tree

# Set random number seed so that same results each time
# use rand option in cv.tree() to generate a 10-fold
# permutation of data
set.seed(148975)

bwt.cv<-cv.tree(bwt.tree, FUN=prune.tree,
    rand=sample(10,189,T))

# Plot deviance against size
win.graph()
plot(bwt.cv)
```
⟹ Figure 15.6

```
# Find best-fitting tree of size 5
bwt.best<-prune.tree(bwt.tree,best=5)
```

```
# Generate corresponding postscript file
post.tree(bwt.best,file="best.ps")
```

$\Longrightarrow$ Figure 15.7

15.7   Exercises

15.1 The trees constructed in this chapter have all involved the continuous response variable bwt, actual birthweight in grams. How are the results affected if the binary variable low is used as the response instead?

15.2 Compare the results obtained in the chapter using regression trees with those obtained from a multiple regression of bwt on the explanatory variables.

15.3 Perform an analysis of variance of bwt on the two factors smoke and race, and assess whether a smoke × race interaction is needed as suggested by the results from the tree regression in Section 15.3.1.

16
Survival Analysis I

16.1 Introduction

In many medical studies, the main outcome variable is the time to the occurrence of a particular event. In a randomized controlled trial of cancer, for example, surgery, radiation and chemotherapy might be compared with respect to time from randomization and the start of therapy until death. In this case, the event of interest is the death of a patient, but in other situations, it might be remission from a disease, relief from symptoms, or the recurrence of a particular condition. Such observations are generally referred to by the generic term *survival data* even when the endpoint or event being considered is not death but something else. Such data generally require special techniques for analysis for two main reasons:

1. Survival data are generally not symmetrically distributed—they will often appear positively skewed, with a few people surviving a very long time compared with the majority; so assuming a normal distribution will not be reasonable.

2. At the completion of the study, some patients may not have reached the endpoint of interest (death, relapse, etc.). Consequently, the exact survival times are not known. All that is known is that the survival times are greater than the amount of time the individual has been in the study. The survival times of these individuals are said to be *censored* (precisely, they are right-censored).

16.2   The survivor function

We will first consider the data set on the survival of leukaemia patients previously analysed in Chapter 9 using logistic regression. This is a rare example of survival data in which right-censoring has not occurred and we actually know the survival times of all individuals. One way of describing the survival experiences is to report the median survival time, the time beyond which 50% of subjects survived. Other percentiles are also of interest. A full description is given by plotting the percentage of subjects surviving for at least time t against t. This function is known as the *survivor function*, $S(t)$. When there is no censoring, the survivor function can be estimated as

$$\hat{S}(t) = \frac{\text{Number of individuals with survival times} \geq t}{\text{Number of individuals in the dataset}}$$

Because this is simply a proportion, confidence intervals can be obtained for each time t by using the variance estimate

$$\hat{S}(t)(1 - \hat{S}(t))/n$$

where n is the total number of subjects. Figure 16.1 shows the survivor function for the leukaemia data with 95% confidence intervals.

The median survival was 22 weeks with a 95% confidence interval from 7 to 56 weeks. The mean survival was 40.9 months with a standard error of 8.01 weeks.

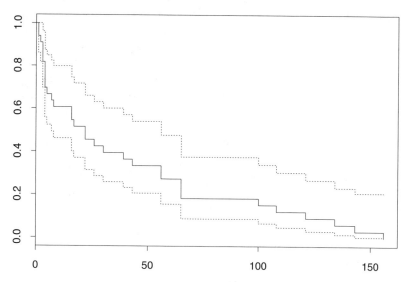

FIGURE 16.1. Survivor function for leukaemia data with 95% confidence intervals.

A more typical example of survival data, in which censoring occurs, is the data set in Table 16.1. These data arise from a randomized, controlled clinical trial to compare two treatments for prostate cancer. The full data set is given in Andrews and Herzberg (1985), and this subset of the data is discussed in Collett (1994) as well as in Everitt and Pickles (2000).

The groups took 1 mg of diethylstilbestrol (DES) or placebo daily by mouth, and their survival was recorded in months. The variable Treatment indicates which treatment was received, Time is the time from the beginning of the trial to death or the end of the trial, whichever happened first, and Status indicates whether the subject died or whether the subject's survival time is right-censored. (The other variables in Table 16.1 will be described and used in the next chapter.) The main question of interest is whether survival differed between the two groups. An obvious graphical display for comparing the survival experiences of the two groups is a graph of the two survivor functions. In the presence of censoring, the survivor functions can be estimated using the Kaplan-Meier estimator described in Display 16.1.

Display 16.1 Kaplan-Meier estimate of survivor functions

- First, order the survival times such that $t_{(1)} \leq t_{(2)} \cdots \leq t_{(n)}$, where $t_{(j)}$ is the jth largest unique failure time. An example is shown in Table 16.2.

- The Kaplan-Meier estimate of the survival function is obtained by applying the following formula:

$$\hat{S}(t) = \prod_{j|t_{(j)} \leq t} \left(1 - \frac{d_j}{r_j}\right) \tag{1}$$

   where r_j is the number of individuals at risk just before $t_{(j)}$ (including those censored at $t_{(j)}$) and d_j is the number who experience the event of interest at $t_{(j)}$.

   For example, the survivor function at the second death time $t_{(2)}$ is equal to the estimated probability of not dying at time $t_{(1)}$ times the estimated probability, given that the individual is still at risk at time $t_{(2)}$, of not dying at time $t_{(2)}$.

- The variance of the Kaplan-Meier estimator is given by

$$\mathrm{var}[\hat{S}(t)] = [\hat{S}(t)]^2 \sum_{j|t_{(j)} \leq t} \frac{d_j}{r_j(r_j - d_j)} \tag{2}$$

Figure 16.2 shows the survivor functions for both treatment groups. The data on which the survival curve for the Placebo group is based are shown in Table 16.2. Here, $t_{(j)}$ is the jth largest survival time, d_j is the number of deaths at time $t_{(j)}$, r_j is the number of subjects still alive and under observation, and c_j is the number censored at time $t_{(j)}$. A step in the survival curve occurs every time at least one death occurs; i.e., $d_j > 0$, and crosses in the figure indicate that an individual's survival time was censored at that point ($c_j > 0$).

There is approximately a difference of 20% in the proportion surviving for at least 50 to 60 months between the two groups.

TABLE 16.1. Prostate cancer trial data

Treatment	Time	Status	Age	Haem	Size	Gleason
1	65	0	67	13.4	34	8
2	61	0	60	14.6	4	10
2	60	0	77	15.6	3	8
1	58	0	64	16.2	6	9
2	51	0	65	14.1	21	9
1	51	0	61	13.5	8	8
1	14	1	73	12.4	18	11
1	43	0	60	13.6	7	9
2	16	0	73	13.8	8	9
1	52	0	73	11.7	5	9
1	59	0	77	12.0	7	10
2	55	0	74	14.3	7	10
2	68	0	71	14.5	19	9
2	51	0	65	14.4	10	9
1	2	0	76	10.7	8	9
1	67	0	70	14.7	7	9
2	66	0	70	16.0	8	9
2	66	0	70	14.5	15	11
2	28	0	75	13.7	19	10
2	50	1	68	12.0	20	11
1	69	1	60	16.1	26	9
1	67	0	71	15.6	8	8
2	65	0	51	11.8	2	6
1	24	0	71	13.7	10	9
2	45	0	72	11.0	4	8
2	64	0	74	14.2	4	6
1	61	0	75	13.7	10	12
1	26	1	72	15.3	37	11
1	42	1	57	13.9	24	12
2	57	0	72	14.6	8	10
2	70	0	72	13.8	3	9
2	5	0	74	15.1	3	9
2	54	0	51	15.8	7	8
1	36	1	72	16.4	4	9
2	70	0	71	13.6	2	10
2	67	0	73	13.8	7	8
1	23	0	68	12.5	2	8
1	62	0	63	13.2	3	8

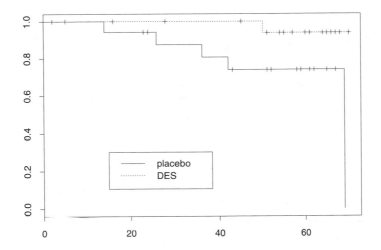

FIGURE 16.2. Survivor functions for the two treatment groups in the prostate cancer trial.

TABLE 16.2. Failure times, number of deaths, number at risk, and number censored in Placebo group of prostate cancer trial

j	$t_{(j)}$	d_j	r_j	c_j
1	2	0	18	1
2	14	1	17	0
3	23	0	16	1
4	24	0	15	1
5	26	1	14	0
6	36	1	13	0
7	42	1	12	0
8	43	0	11	1
9	51	0	10	1
10	52	0	9	1
11	58	0	8	1
12	59	0	7	1
13	61	0	6	1
14	62	0	5	1
15	65	0	4	1
16	67	0	3	1
17	69	1	1	0

TABLE 16.3. Log-rank test for comparing survival in prostate cancer treatment groups

	N	Observed	Expected	(O-E)^2/E	(O-E)^2/V
Treatment=1	18	5	2.47	2.58	4.42
Treatment=2	20	1	3.53	1.81	4.42

Chisq= 4.4 on 1 degrees of freedom, p = 0.0355

TABLE 16.4. Peto-Wilcoxon test for comparing survival in prostate cancer treatment groups

	N	Observed	Expected	(O-E)^2/E	(O-E)^2/V
Treatment=1	18	4.670	2.30	2.43	4.51
Treatment=2	20	0.879	3.25	1.73	4.51

Chisq= 4.5 on 1 degrees of freedom, p = 0.0337

16.3   The log-rank test

In addition to comparing the survivor functions graphically, we often wish to test for a difference in the survival experience of the groups. In the absence of censoring (e.g., for the leukaemia data), we could use a nonparametric test, like the Mann-Whitney U-test to compare the survival times. In the presence of censoring, the *long-rank* test is most commonly used. First, the expected number of deaths is computed for each unique death time, or *failure time* (survival time with Status=1) in the data set, assuming that the chances of dying, given that subjects are at risk, is the same for both groups. The total number of expected deaths is then computed for each group by adding the expected number of deaths for each failure time. The test then compares the observed number of deaths in each group with the expected number of deaths using a χ^2-test (see Display 16.2).

The results of applying the log-rank test to the prostate data are shown in Table 16.3. There is a significant difference in the survival experience between the two groups. The test weights the contributions from all failure times equally, regardless of when they occurred. However, we have more precise information at the beginning when a large proportion of subjects are still alive. Various tests have been proposed to give greater weight to earlier survival times. The Peto-Wilcoxon method weights observation by the Kaplan-Meyer estimate of the proportion of subjects still alive at each failure time. Applying this method gives the results shown in Table 16.4, which are very similar to the results of the log-rank test.

Display 16.2 Log-rank test

- The log-rank or Mantel-Haenszel test can be used to compare survival between K groups.

- For each failure time $t_{(j)}$ and group $k = 1, \cdots K$, let r_{kj} denote the number of subjects at risk and d_{kj} the number of deaths. The total number of individuals at risk at time $t_{(j)}$ is $r_j = \sum_k r_{kj}$, and the total number of deaths is $d_j = \sum_k d_{kj}$.

- If the survival experience is the same in all groups, the estimated probability of a person in group k dying at time $t_{(j)}$ given that the individual is still alive is d_j/r_j, and the expected number of deaths in each group is

$$E_{kj} = \frac{r_{kj}d_j}{r_j}, k = 1, \cdots K \tag{1}$$

- The difference between the total number of observed deaths and the total number of expected deaths in the kth group is

$$U_k = \sum_j E_{kj} - d_{kj} \tag{2}$$

with variance

$$\mathrm{var}(U_k) = \sum_j v_{kj} \tag{3}$$

where v_{kj} is the variance of d_{kj} from the hyperbolic distribution. (This assumes that the r_j and d_j are fixed.) The test-statistic is

$$X^2 = \sum_k \frac{\left(\sum_j E_{kj} - d_{kj}\right)^2}{\sum_j v_{kj}} \tag{4}$$

Under the null hypothesis, this statistic has an approximate χ^2 distribution with $K - 1$ degrees of freedom.

- Here, contributions from all failure times are weighted equally. Several alternative test-statistics have been proposed of the form

$$X^2 = \sum_k \frac{\left(\sum_j w_{kj}(E_{kj} - d_{kj})\right)^2}{\sum_j w_{kj}^2 v_{kj}} \tag{5}$$

where the w_{kj} are weights. The Gehan-Wilcoxon test uses $w_{kj} = r_{kj}$, and the Peto modification of the Wilcoxon test uses $w_{kj} = \hat{S}(t_j)$.

16.4   The hazard function

In the analysis of survival data, it is often of interest to assess which periods have high or low chances of the event (e.g., death), among those still alive at the time. A suitable approach to assessing such risks is the *hazard function*, $h(t)$, defined as the probability that an individual experiences the event in a small time interval s, given that the individual has survived up to the beginning of the interval, when the size of the time interval approaches zero; i.e.,

$$h(t) = \lim_{s \to 0} \Pr(t \leq T < t + s | T \geq t) \tag{16.1}$$

where T is an individual's survival time. The conditioning is very important. For example, the probability of dying at age 100 is very small because most people die before that age, but the probability of a person dying at age 100 who has reached that age is much greater. Display 16.3 outlines the relationship between the survivor and hazard functions, and Display 16.4 describes methods of estimating the hazard and integrated hazard functions. The Nelson-Aalen estimate of the integrated hazard to the data for the placebo group in the prostate cancer trial is shown in Figure 16.3.

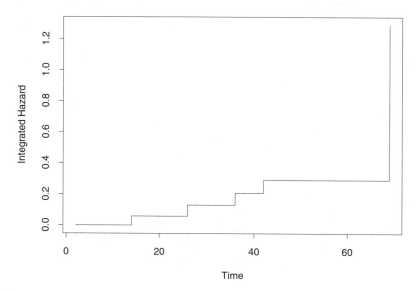

FIGURE 16.3. Integrated hazard for placebo group in the prostate cancer trial.

The hazard is the slope of the integrated hazard. It appears to be approximately constant and then close to zero betwen 43 and 67 months. However, due to censoring, the risk set decreases from 11 to 1 during that time with only one person at risk at 69 months, explaining the large increase in integrated hazard associated with a single death at 69 months.

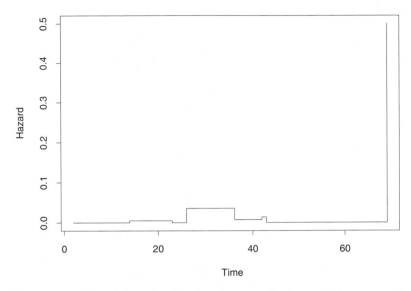

FIGURE 16.4. Hazard function for placebo group in the prostate cancer trial.

The Kaplan-Meier type estimate of the hazard function is shown in Figure 16.4. In practice, the hazard function is rarely plotted because it is too 'noisy', the integrated hazard being a preferred option.

16.5 Summary

Time to event data cannot be analyzed by any of the methods discussed in previous chapters because the times are typically censored for some of the subjects. The survivor function, hazard and integrated hazard functions can be used to describe survival experiences, and the log-rank test can be used to compare survival between groups.

Display 16.3 Survivor function, hazard rate and cumulative hazard

- The survival time T may be regarded as a random variable with a probability distribution $F(t)$ and probability density function $f(t)$. The survivor function $S(t)$ is defined as

$$S(t) = P(T \geq t) = 1 - F(t) \tag{1}$$

- The hazard function is the probability that an individual experiences the event of interest at a time point, given that the event has not yet occurred. It is given by

$$h(t) = \frac{f(t)}{S(t)} \tag{2}$$

the instantaneous probability of failure at time t divided by the probability of surviving up to time t. It follows from (1) and (2) that

$$\frac{-d\log(S(t))}{dt} = h(t) \tag{3}$$

so that

$$S(t) = \exp(-H(t)) \tag{4}$$

where $H(t)$ is the *integrated hazard function*, also known as the *cumulative hazard* function,

$$H(t) = \int_0^t h(u)du \tag{5}$$

Display 16.4 Estimating the hazard and integrated hazard

- Using the Kaplan-Meier approach, we can estimate the hazard function in the intervals between failure times, $t_{(j)} \leq t < t_{(j+1)}$, using the ratio

$$\hat{h}(t) = \frac{d_j}{n_j(t_{(j+1)} - t_{(j)})} \tag{1}$$

- Using the relationship that $H(t) = -\log S(t)$ (see Display 16.3), the Kaplan-Meier estimate of the integrated hazard is

$$\hat{H}_{KM}(t) = -\sum_j \log\left(\frac{n_j - d_j}{n_j}\right) \tag{2}$$

Because, using a Taylor expansion, $\log(1 - d_j/n_j) \approx -d_j/n_j$ for small d_j/n_j,

$$\hat{H}_{KM}(t) \approx \sum_j d_j/n_j \tag{3}$$

- The Nelson-Aalen estimate of the integrated hazard is

$$\hat{H}_{NA}(t) = \sum_j d_j/n_j \tag{4}$$

- The hazard function is just the slope of the cumulative hazard.

- The Breslow estimator of the survival function is just the exponential of the Nelson-Aalen estimator of the cumulative hazard

$$\hat{S}_B(t) = \exp(\hat{H}_{NA}(t)) \tag{5}$$

16.6   Using S-PLUS

16.6.1   Using the S language

Section 16.2

In this section, the survivor function for an uncensored data set is initially estimated "by hand". This illustrates the use of the `unique()` function to find the unique failure times, the `table()` and `cumsum()` functions to compute the cumulative probability and `type="s"` option in the `plot()` function for plotting step functions. This is purely an illustration. In practice, the `survfit()` function would always be used to estimate survivor functions. A graph of the survivor function(s) can be obtained by simply passing the object returned by `survfit()` as the only argument to the `plot()` function.

Script for Section 16.2

```
# Read leukaemia data
leuk<-matrix(scan("leuk.dat"),ncol=3,byrow=T)
leuk<-as.data.frame(list(wbc=leuk[,1],ag=leuk[,2],
    surv=leuk[,3]))

# Sort leukaemia data in ascending order of survival times
leuk<-leuk[order(leuk$surv),]

# Work out survivor function "by hand"
# Extract unique survival times using unique() function
t<-unique(leuk$surv)
# these are in the same order as in leuk$surv and therefore
# ascending

# Compute frequencies of survival times
f<-table(leuk$surv)

# Obtain number of subjects
n<-dim(leuk)[1]

# Compute proportion of subjects suriving longer than t
surv1<-1-cumsum(f)/n
# cumsum() takes the cumulative sum of the elements in a vector

# Compute proportion of subjects surving at least for time t
surv2<-c(1,surv1[-length(surv1)])
# This is the survivor function

# Plot survivor function
win.graph()
```

```
plot(t,surv2, type="s")
# type = "s" causes points to be connected using steps

# Use survfit() to produce the same graph including confidence
# intervals
win.graph()
attach(leuk)
leuk.surv<-survfit(Surv(surv))
plot(leuk.surv)
leuk.surv
summary(leuk.surv)
```
$\implies$ Figure 16.1

```
# Read prostate data
prostate<-read.table(file="prostate.dat",header=T)

# Plot survivor functions
win.graph()
plot(survfit(Surv(Time,Status)~Treatment,data=prostate),lty=1:2)
legend(15,0.3,legend=c("placebo","DES"),lty=1:2)
```
$\implies$ Figure 16.2

Section 16.3

Here, the `survdiff()` function is used to apply the log-rank test. The `rho` option is used to change the weighting of contributions from different risk sets.

Script for Section 16.3

```
# Compare treatment groups using log-rank test
survdiff(Surv(Time,Status)~Treatment,data=prostate)
```
$\implies$ Table 16.3

```
# Peto-Peto modification of Wilcoxon test
survdiff(Surv(Time,Status)~Treatment,data=prostate,rho=1)
```
$\implies$ Table 16.4

Section 16.4

The hazard and cumulative hazard functions are computed by using information returned form the `survfit()` function

Script for Section 16.4

```
# Nelson-Aalen cumulative hazard in placebo group
nasurv<-survfit(Surv(Time,Status),type="fl",
   data=prostate,subset=Treatment==1)
# type="fl" gives Breslow estimate of survival function based on
# Nelson-Aalen estimate of cumulative hazard

# Compute Nelson-Aalen estimate of integrated hazard
ih<- -log(nasurv$surv)

# Check if ih is correct
ih2<-cumsum(nasurv$n.event/nasurv$n.risk)
cbind(nasurv$time,nasurv$n.event,nasurv$n.risk,ih,ih2)

# Plot hazard and integrated hazard
time<-nasurv$time
plot(time,ih, type="s",ylab="Integrated Hazard",xlab="Time")
```
$\implies$ Figure 16.3

```
# Compute hazard
haz<-nasurv$n.event/nasurv$n.risk
time0<-c(0,time[-length(time)])
haz<-haz/(time-time0)

# Plot hazard
plot(time, haz,type="s",ylab="Hazard",xlab="Time")
```
$\implies$ Figure 16.4

16.7   Exercises

16.1 For the leukaemia data in Chapter 9, test for a difference in survival between patients with AG absent and AG present.

16.2 Plot the integrated hazard functions for both groups as well as for the logarithm of the integrated hazards. Are the logarithms of the cumulative hazards parallel?

16.3 Table 16.5 below gives length of survival after mastectomy of women with breast cancer. The cancers were classified as having metastized or not based on a histochemical marker.

Censoring is indicated by an asterix. The file containing these data is called *breast.dat*, where `time` is the suvival time, `status` is the censoring indicator and `stain` indicates whether the tumor has metastized (1 = yes, 0 = no).

1. Plot the survivor functions estimated using both the Kaplan-Meier and Breslow estimates on the same graph for both groups. Are there substantial differences?

TABLE 16.5. Table for Exercise 16.3

Not metastized

23	47	69	70*	71*	100*	101*	148
181	198*	208*	212*	224*			

Metastized

5	8	10	13	18	24	26	26
31	35	40	41	48	50	59	61
68	71	76*	105*	107*	109*	113	116*
118	143	154*	162*	188*	212*	217*	225*

2. Use a log-rank test to compare surival between the two groups.

17
Survival Analysis II: Cox's Regression

17.1 Introduction

In Chapter 13 we looked at ways of summarizing and plotting survival data as well as simple tests for comparing groups. In this chapter, we will discuss modeling survival using several explanatory variables simultaneously analogously to linear regression or generalized linear models. The most popular, and in many cases most useful, regression model for survival data in medicine is Cox's regression model.

17.2 Cox's regression

In Cox's regression, it is assumed that the hazard functions for different individuals are proportional and that the effects of covariates are constant over time. The assumption of a constant hazard ratio is called the *proportional hazards* assumption. The model can be written as

$$h(t) = h_0(t) \exp(\boldsymbol{\beta}'\mathbf{x}) \tag{17.1}$$

where $h_0(t)$ is the *baseline hazard* function. The ratio of the hazards of any two individuals i and j is $\exp(\boldsymbol{\beta}'(\mathbf{x}_i - \mathbf{x}_j))$, the *hazard ratio* or incidence rate ratio. The baseline hazard function $h_0(t)$ is left unspecified; a different paramater is essentially included for each unique survival time. These parameters can be thought of as nuisance parameters whose purpose is

TABLE 17.1. Cox regression model for prostate cancer data

n= 38

	coef	exp(coef)	se(coef)	z	p
Treatment	-1.801	0.165	1.131	-1.59	0.110
Gleason	0.734	2.083	0.314	2.34	0.019

	exp(coef)	exp(-coef)	lower .95	upper .95
Treatment	0.165	6.05	0.018	1.52
Gleason	2.083	0.48	1.127	3.85

Rsquare= 0.242   (max possible= 0.616)
Likelihood ratio test= 10.5 on 2 df,   p=0.00519
Wald test   = 9.08 on 2 df,   p=0.0107
Score (logrank) test = 10.9 on 2 df,   p=0.00432

merely to control the parameters of interest β for any changes in the hazard over time. Display 17.1 outlines the main features of Cox's regression. Cox's regression is a *semi-parametric* approach to survival analysis. Unlike parametric methods, Cox's regression does not require specification of the probability distribution of the survival times. Unlike most nonparametric methods, however, the effects of covariates are estimated in much the same way as in parametric methods, such as generalized linear models. For more information on Cox's regression, see Therneau and Grambsch (2000) and Collett (1994).

We will now fit a Cox regression model to the prostate data looked at in the previous chapter. Initially, we will examine the effect of a single explanatory variable, treatment group. The result of fitting a Cox's regression model is given in Table 17.1. A graph of the fitted survival curves is given in Figure 17.1.

The coefficient of Treatment is estimated as −1.80, and its exponential is 0.165. Therefore, the hazard in the treatment group is only about 16.5% that in the placebo group. Three different tests are reported, the likelihood ratio test, Wald test and the score test. The score test for Cox's proportional hazards model is identical to the log-rank test described in Chapter 16. The three tests are asymptotically equivalent but differ in finite samples. The likelihood ratio test is generally considered the most reliable, and the Wald test the least (see Therneau and Grambsch, 2000).

The prostate data contains other prognostic variables, including

1. Age: Age at trial entry

2. Haem: Serum haemoglobin level ingm/100 ml

3. Size: Size of primary tumor in centimeters squared

4. Gleason: the value of a combined index of tumour stage and grade (the larger the index, the more advanced the tumour).

Display 17.1 Cox's proportional hazards model

- In Cox's regression, the hazard function is modeled as

$$h(t) = h_0(t) \exp(\boldsymbol{\beta}' \mathbf{x}) \tag{1}$$

  where $h_0(t)$ is the *baseline hazard*.

- The hazards depend multiplicatively on the covariates, and $\exp(\beta_1)$ is the ratio of the hazards between two individuals whose value of x_1 differ by one unit if all other covariates are the same. This ratio is assumed to be constant over time, making the model a *proportional hazards* model.

- The form of the baseline hazard function $h_0(t)$ is left unspecified. The model therefore has a parametric part for the effects of covariates on the hazard and a nonparametric part for the hazard function and is therefore known as a *semiparametric* model.

- The regression parameters are estimated by maximizing the *partial log-likelihood* given by

$$\sum_f \log \left(\frac{\exp(\boldsymbol{\beta}' \mathbf{x}_f)}{\sum_{r(f)} \exp(\boldsymbol{\beta}' \mathbf{x}_r)} \right) \tag{2}$$

  where the first summation is over all deaths or failures f and the second summation is over all subjects $r(f)$ still alive (and therefore "at risk") at the time of failure. The subjects contributing to the denominator are referred to as the *risk set*. The partial log-likelihood can be interpreted as the log profile likelihood for $\boldsymbol{\beta}$ after eliminating $h_0(t)$, i.e., the log-likelihood, where the $h_0(t)$ have been replaced by functions of $\boldsymbol{\beta}$ that maximize the likelihood with respect to $h_0(t)$ for fixed $\boldsymbol{\beta}$.

- Once the regression coefficients $\boldsymbol{\beta}$ have been estimated, the baseline hazard can be estimated by maximum profile likelihood, keeping $\boldsymbol{\beta}$ fixed (see, for example, Collett, 1994, pp. 95–97). It is then possible to derive the cumulative hazard and survivor functions for different values of the covariates.

- If we do not wish to assume proportionality among groups of individuals defined by a certain predictor, we can estimate a *stratified Cox model* with distinct baseline hazards for the groups but common values of the coefficient vector $\boldsymbol{\beta}$.

  This is achieved by confining the contributions to the denominator in (2) (i.e., the risk sets) to only those subjects belonging to the same stratum as the subject who died.

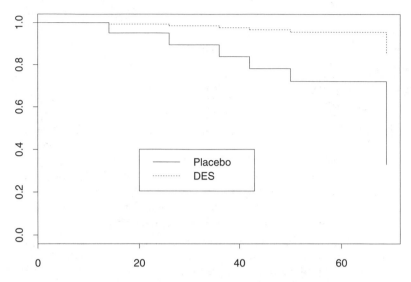

FIGURE 17.1. Fitted survival curves for prostate data.

We can test if adding any of these covariates significantly improves the fit of the model by using likelihood ratio tests. Adding the Gleason index, for example, increases the log-likelihood from -15.8997 to -12.9135, giving a likelihood ratio statistic of 5.97 and a p-value of 0.015. (Note that if there were missing values for the Gleason index, these observations would have to be excluded from both models because the likelihood ratio test is only valid if both models use the same observations.)

Details of the model, including treatment group and Gleason index, are given in Table 17.2. The coefficient of the Gleason index is 0.71, and its exponential is 2.03. For each increase in Gleason index by one unit, the hazard approximately doubles within the treatment groups. For anyone unfamiliar with the Gleason index, this is a meaningless statement because changes by one unit may never occur (this would be the case if we measured age in centuries). We obtain a meaningful effect size if we divide the Gleason index by its standard deviation and refit the model. The standard deviation of the Gleason index is 1.34, and the hazard ratio associated with an increase in Gleason index by one standard deviation is 2.67 with a 95% confidence interval from 1.17 to 6.10.

There are some ties in the survival times. For example, three subjects died after 51 months. Three common methods of dealing with ties in Cox regression are outlined in Display 17.2. The default method we have used so far is Efron's method. Using the exact method yields identical estimates here, but this would not be true in general.

17.3   Left truncation

The Cox model is estimated by maximizing the partial log-likelihood given in Display 17.1. The partial likelihood is a product of terms, one for each

TABLE 17.2. Cox regression for prostate data using treatment group and Gleason index as predictors

	coef	exp(coef)	se(coef)	z	p
Treatment	-1.1128	0.329	1.2031	-0.925	0.360
Size	0.0826	1.086	0.0475	1.740	0.082
Gleason	0.7102	2.034	0.3379	2.102	0.036

	exp(coef)	exp(-coef)	lower .95	upper .95
Treatment	0.329	3.043	0.0311	3.47
Size	1.086	0.921	0.9896	1.19
Gleason	2.034	0.492	1.0491	3.95

```
Rsquare= 0.304    (max possible= 0.616 )
Likelihood ratio test= 13.8  on 3 df,    p=0.00323
Wald test             = 10.3  on 3 df,    p=0.0163
Score (logrank) test = 14.9  on 3 df,    p=0.0019
```

Display 17.2 Handling ties in Cox's regression

- The partial likelihood is derived by assuming continuous survival times. However, in reality, survival times are measured in discrete units and there are often ties. There are three common methods for dealing with ties:

  - *Breslow approximation*: There is a contribution to the partial log-likelihood from each of the tied failure times (as in in Display 17.1, equation (2)). For each failure time, the risk set comprises all subjects failing *at or* after the failure time. This includes all subjects whose failure times are tied with that of the subject contributing to the numerator.

  - *Efron approximation*: In the Breslow approximation, if m subjects share the same survival time, they all contribute to the risk set for each of the m failures as if each time one of the m subjects failed, all others were still alive. In the Efron approximation, the contribution to the denominator from the m subjects with tied survival times is weighted down by a factor $(m - k)/m$ for the kth term.

  - *Exact partial likelihood*: Assuming that no two subjects ever died simulateneously (we would see this if we had survival times in miliseconds!), there is a true (unkown) unique ordering of the tied survival times. The exact partial likelihood can be obtained by taking the sum (or average) of the partial likelihoods for all possible orderings of the tied survival times because this represents the probability of *any* of the orders having occurred that are consistent with the data. This method is computationally intensive.

failure time. The subjects contributing to each term are those subjects who are still "at risk" at the time of the failure; i.e., they have not yet died and are still under observation.

In the prostate trial, the time scale used in the Cox regression was the time since randomization. An alternative time scale would be age or time since diagnosis. The effect of selecting a different time scale is to change the relative "alignment" of different people's histories and this affects the risk sets. For example, suppose a man age 70 is alive when his father dies at age 95. If the time scale is calendar time, the son would contribute to his father's risk set. However, if the time scale is age, the son does not contribute to his father's risk set if he dies before he is 95.

A person can contribute to a risk set from the time when observation begins. As in the prostate trial, time since observation began is often also the time scale of interest. If the origin of the time scale of interest is earlier than the time when observation began, the data are said to be *left truncated* because people who experience the event before observation begins are not included in the sample. An example is when the time scale of interest is time since diagnosis but subjects enter the trial some time after diagnosis (*delayed entry*). In order to ensure that the subjects are correctly aligned, we have to specify how long after diagnosis each person entered the trial. Two times are therefore specified per subject; entry time (time when person starts being at risk) and exit time, or event time (time when person dies or is censored), in which both times are measured from the origin of the time scale of interest.

For left truncated data, we can only model the conditional hazard rates, given that the event time exceeds entry time (otherwise subjects would not be included in the sample). If event time and entry time are conditionally independent given the covariates, then this conditional hazard rate is equivalent to the unconditional hazard rate and no biases are introduced by the left truncation.

As an example of left truncation, we will consider bone marrow transplant data, a subset of which is given in Table 17.3. The data derive from a multicenter trial of different preparatory regimens before bone marrow transplant on patients with myeloctic leukemia (AML) and lymphoblastic leukemia (ALL) and are discussed in Klein and Moeschberger (1997). Several events postsurgery can change the patient's prognosis for recovery, an important one being the return of platelet count to normal levels. We are interested in disease-free survival (time to death or relapse) since bone marrow transplant in only those patients whose platet counts have recovered to a self-sustaining level. Although the patients are under observation from the time of the transplant, they start being at risk only after platelet recovery. Entry time is therefore time of platelet recovery (since transplant) and exit time is time of death (since transplant).

Potential explanatory variables are disease group (ALL, AML low risk, AML high risk), the age of the patient, the age of the donor, whether MTX was used as a graft-versus-host-prophylactic, and FAB (morphological classification). The data are presented and discussed in Klein and Moeschberger (1997).

TABLE 17.3. Subset of bone marrow transplant data

group	time to platelet recovery (PR)	status (PR)	time to death or relapse (DR)	status (DR)	fab fab	age of donor	age of patient	MTX
1	13	1	2081	0	0	33	26	0
1	18	1	1602	0	0	37	21	0
1	12	1	1496	0	0	35	26	0
1	13	1	1462	0	0	21	17	0
1	12	1	1433	0	0	36	32	0
1	12	1	1377	0	0	31	22	0
1	17	1	1330	0	0	17	20	0
1	12	1	996	0	0	24	22	0
1	10	1	226	0	0	21	18	0
1	29	1	1199	0	0	40	24	1
1	22	1	1111	0	0	28	19	1
1	34	1	530	0	0	28	17	1
1	22	1	1182	0	0	23	24	1
1	1167	0	1167	0	0	22	27	1
1	21	1	418	1	0	14	18	0
1	16	1	383	1	0	20	15	0
1	21	1	276	1	0	5	18	0
1	20	1	104	1	0	33	20	0
1	26	1	609	1	0	27	27	0
1	37	1	172	1	0	37	40	0

TABLE 17.4. Effect of patient's and donor's age on survival after bone marrow transplant

```
                  coef exp(coef) se(coef)      z       p
agepat        -0.08097     0.922  0.04124  -1.96  0.0500
agedon        -0.10038     0.904  0.03717  -2.70  0.0069
agepat:agedon  0.00323     1.003  0.00114   2.83  0.0047

Likelihood ratio test=8.18  on 3 df, p=0.0424  n= 120
```

Only patients whose platelets recovered (status PR $= 1$) are used in the analysis. Entry time is time to platelet recovery, and exit time is time to death or relapse. Initially, we test for the effect of the patient's age and donor's age (both centred at 28 years) and the interaction giving the estimates shown in Table 17.4.

There is a significant interaction between the patient's age and the donor's age according to the Wald test. Increasing age of the donor has a positive effect on survival when the patient is 28, with every increase in donor's age being associated with an 8% decrease in the hazard. However, the benefit of donor's age decreases as the patient gets older.

17.4   Stratification

In addition to the explanatory variables whose effects on survival we wish to estimate, there may be groupings or strata in the data that also need to be adjusted for but whose effect is of little interest. In addition, we may not wish to assume proportional hazard between strata. A typical example is a multicentre trial in which the aim is to estimate a common treatment effect across centres, but in which it may be unrealistic to assume common baseline survival curves. As explained in Display 17.1, a stratified Cox model can be used that allows separate baseline hazards but common coefficients between strata. In the bone marrow transplant example, we can stratify on the use of MTX as a graft-versus-host-prophylactic. We repeat the analysis of Klein and Moeschberger (1997) here with covariates group, FAB, and main effects and interaction of age of patient and age of donor. In order to obtain the same estimates, we use Breslow's method of handling ties. The output is given in Table 17.5.

A graph of the predicted survival curves with all covariates equal to their mean values is given in Figure 17.2. Although evaluating predictors at their mean does not make much sense for categorical variables such as group, the graph still gives an impression of how different the shapes of the survival curves are in the two strata. The difference in survival functions between

TABLE 17.5. Cox's regression model for bone marrow transplant data stratified on MTX

	coef	exp(coef)	se(coef)	z	p
g2	-1.75212	0.173	0.43761	-4.00	0.000062
g3	-0.75036	0.472	0.40769	-1.84	0.066000
fab	1.27753	3.588	0.32494	3.93	0.000084
agepat	0.04174	1.043	0.02229	1.87	0.061000
agedon	-0.03460	0.966	0.02068	-1.67	0.094000
agepat:agedon	0.00228	1.002	0.00122	1.87	0.062000

```
Likelihood ratio test=37.2  on 6 df, p=1.62e-006  n= 120
```

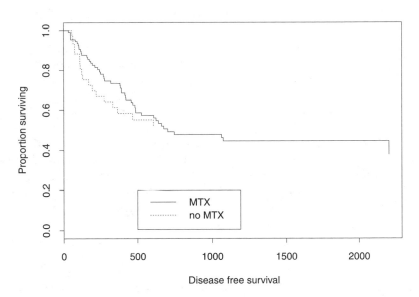

FIGURE 17.2. Fitted survival curves bone marrow transplant data where covariates are evaluated at the mean.

patients with and without MTX increases early on and then decreases again.

17.5   Diagnostics and assessing the proportional hazards assumption

The Cox model assumes that the estimated hazard ratios are constant over time or that the hazards are proportional. If we have two independently estimated survival curves, we can assess graphically whether the hazards appear to be proportional by plotting the logarithm of the integrated hazards (where the integrated hazards are given by $H(t) = -\log(S(t))$. This can be seen as follows: if $h_1(t) = ah_2(t)$, then the same is true of the integrated hazards; i.e., $H_1(t) = aH_2(t)$. Taking logarithms, the log cumulative hazards are parallel, $\log(H_1(t)) = \log(a) + \log(H_2(t))$.

For grouping variables, we can therefore test the proportionality of the hazard function by plotting the log-integrated hazard functions. If there are other predictors, we can obtain the integrated hazard functions by fitting a Cox regression model to the whole set of predictors but stratifying on the grouping variable.

We can apply this method to the variable MTX for the heart transplant data. To obtain a clearer picture, we will only consider survival to 1,000 days by replacing all survival times that are larger than 1,000 by 1,000 and the corresponding status variable by 0. The survival curves and log-integrated hazard curves are shown in Figure 17.3. The log-integrated hazard curves are not parallel, and it is therefore appropriate to stratify on MTX instead of using MTX as a covariate.

A number of residuals have been suggested for survival data. These are described in Display 17.3. Figure 17.4 shows a graph of deviance residuals against the index (observation number), with label 1 if the observation was censored and 0 otherwise. Because of the way the residuals are defined, the residuals for censored observations tend to be negative. The apparent pattern along the X-axis of the graph is due to the nonrandom order of the observations in the data set. None of the deviance residuals are large; so the model appears to fit all observations well.

Figure 17.5 shows the change in each regression coefficient when each observation is removed from the data. The changes are scaled in units of standard errors. The largest change caused by a single observation is about 0.1 standard error. Therefore, removing these observations is unlikely to have a large effect on the statistical significance of the coefficients.

Figure 17.6 shows plots of the scaled Schoenfeld residuals against time for each coefficient. The fitted curves can be interpreted as estimates of $\beta(t)$ if the coefficients were allowed to vary over time. A flat line indicates that the hazards are proportional for different values of the corresponding covariate. The only variable where there is some doubt is FAB.

We can test the proportional hazards assumption for each variable using a test proposed by Grambsch and Therneau (1994) based on the scaled

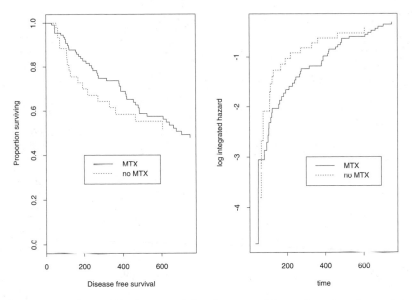

FIGURE 17.3. Survival curves and log integrated hazard curves for surivival times up to 1000 days.

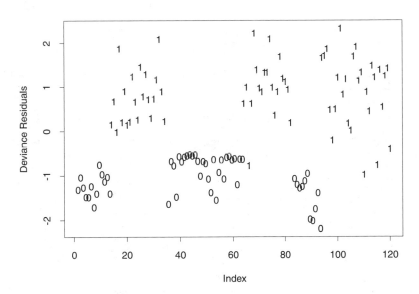

FIGURE 17.4. Deviance residuals for bone marrow transplant data with status as label.

Display 17.3 Diagnostics for Cox regression

- The *Cox-Snell residual* is defined as

$$r_{Ci} = \exp(\hat{\boldsymbol{\beta}}' \hat{H}_0(t_i)$$

where $\hat{H}_0(t_i)$ is the estimated integrated hazard function at time t_i, the observed surivival time of subject i. If the model is correct, r_{Ci} follows an exponential distribution with mean 1.

- The *martingale residual* is the difference between the event indicator δ_i (equal to 1 if the person died and 0 otherwise) and the Cox-Snell residual:

$$r_{Mi} = \delta_i - r_{Ci}$$

- The *deviance residual* is defined as

$$r_{Di} = \text{sign}(r_{Mi} \sqrt{-2[r_{Mi} + \delta_i \log(\delta_i - r_{Mi})]}$$

Subjects with large positive or negative deviance residuals are poorly predicted by the model.

- The partial score residual, also known as *Schoenfeld residual* or *efficient score residual*, is defined as the first derivative of the partial log-likelihood function with respect to an explanatory variable. For the jth explanatory variable,

$$r_{Sij} = \frac{x_{ij} - \sum_{r(i)} x_{rj} \exp(\boldsymbol{\beta}' \mathbf{x}_r)}{\sum_{r(i)} x_{rj} \exp(\boldsymbol{\beta}' \mathbf{x}_r)}$$

The score residual is large in absolute value if a case's explanatory variable differs substantially from the the explanatory variables of subjects whose estimated risk of failure is large at the case's time of failure or censoring.

This residual can be used to detect potentially influential points.

- For each explanatory variable, there is one score residual for each event. A rescaled score residual can be defined whose expected value is equal to the corresponding regression coefficient (Grambsch and Therneau, 1994). If the hazards are proportional, the regression coefficient is constant over time and the plot of the rescaled Schoenfeld residuals against time should form a horizontal line. Grambsch and Therneau (1994) proposed a test of proportional hazards based on these rescaled residuals.

- Influence statistics are defined as for linear regression. For example, we can compute the change in scaled coefficient associated with the removal of each observation from the data set.

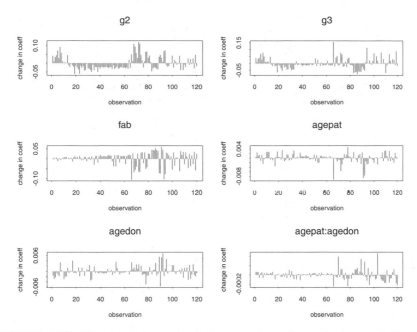

FIGURE 17.5. Change in beta (scaled as number of standard errors) for all covariates used in bone marrow transplant data.

Schoenfeld residuals. The results in Table 17.6 indicate that there is no evidence of nonproportionality for any of the variables.

17.6   Summary

Cox's regression can be used to investigate the relationship between explanatory variables and survival without making any distributional assumptions regarding the survival times. The model assumes that the hazards of different individuals are proportional and that the explanatory variables affect the hazard rate multiplicatively, although this assumption can be relaxed for some variables using stratification. Cox's regression can be used when there is left truncation. The model can be extended further by

TABLE 17.6. Tests of proportional hazards

	rho	chisq	p
g2	0.1852	2.3796	0.123
g3	−0.0194	0.0262	0.871
fab	−0.0976	0.6320	0.427
agepat	−0.0153	0.0133	0.908
agedon	−0.0282	0.0483	0.826
agepat:agedon	0.0545	0.2680	0.605

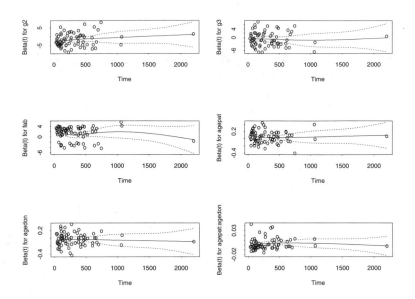

FIGURE 17.6. Scaled Schoenfeld residuals versus time for all covariates used in bone marrow transplant data.

including time-varying covariates. We refer interested readers to Therneau and Grambsch (2000) for the implementation in S-PLUS.

17.7 Using S-PLUS

17.7.1 Using the S language

Section 17.2

In this section, the coxph() function is used to fit Cox's proportional hazards model. The method="exact" option causes S-PLUS to use the exact method of dealing with ties. The I() function is used in the model formula to include functions of explanatory variables. The function survfit() is used to obtain predicted survival curves for subgroups.

Script for Section 17.2

```
# Read prostate data
prostate<-read.table(file="prostate.dat",header=T)

# Fit Cox model
pros.cox<-coxph(Surv(Time,Status)~Treatment,data=prostate)
summary(pros.cox)                                       ⟹  Table 17.1

# Plot fitted survival curves
win.graph()
plot(survfit(pros.cox))
surv0<-survfit(pros.cox,newdata=data.frame(Treatment=1),se=F)
surv1<-survfit(pros.cox,newdata=data.frame(Treatment=2),se=F)
plot(surv0, type="l")
lines(surv1,lty=2)
legend(20,0.4,legend=c("Placebo","DES"),lty=1:2)
                                                        ⟹  Figure 17.1

# Add Gleason index
pros.cox2<-coxph(Surv(Time,Status)~Treatment + Gleason,data=prostate)

# Carry out likelihood ratio test
x2<-2*(pros.cox2$loglik[2]-pros.cox$loglik[2])
1-pchisq(x2,1)

# Results of Cox regression
summary(pros.cox2)                                      ⟹  Table 17.2

# Effect of standard deviation increase in Gleason index
sd<-sqrt(var(prostate$Gleason))
summary(coxph(Surv(Time,Status)~Treatment +
   I(Gleason/sd),data=prostate))
```

```
# Try exact method of handling ties
summary(coxph(Surv(Time,Status)~Treatment +
   I(Gleason/sd),data=prostate,method="exact"))
```

Section 17.3

The `contrasts()` and `contr.treatment()` functions are used to obtain the required coefficients for the effect of a grouping variable. The `Surv()` function is used to specify entry time, exit time and censoring. The `plot()` function is used with the object returned from `coxph()` as the only argument to plot survival functions evaluated at the means of the covariates.

Script for Section 17.3

```
# Read bone marrow transplant data
bmt<-as.matrix(read.table("bmt.dat"))
dimnames(bmt)  <-list(NULL,c("g", "td", "trel", "cd", "crel",
   "cdf", "tac", "cac", "tchr", "cchr", "tplate", "cplate",
   "agepat", "agedon","sexpat", "sexdon", "cmvpat", "cmvdon",
   "wait", "fab", "hospital", "mtx"))
bmt<-as.data.frame(bmt)
bmt$g<-factor(bmt$g,levels=1:3,labels=c("all","low","high"))
contrasts(bmt$g)<-contr.treatment(3)
bmt$agepat<-bmt$agepat-28
bmt$agedon<-bmt$agedon-28

# Exclude patients whose platelet count did not return to normal
bmt1<-bmt[bmt$cplate>0,]

# Specify tplate as entry time and trel as exit time
bmt.cox<-coxph(Surv(tplate,trel,cdf)~ agepat*agedon,data=bmt1)
bmt.cox                                              ⟹ | Table 17.4 |
```

Section 17.4

The `strata()` function is used within the model formula to fit a stratified Cox regression model.

Script for Section 17.4

```
# Fit Cox model stratified on MTX
bmt.cox<-coxph(Surv(tplate,trel,cdf)~ g + fab + agepat*agedon +
   strata(mtx), method="breslow",data=bmt1)

bmt.cox
```

$\Longrightarrow$ Table 17.5

```
plot(survfit(bmt.cox),lty=1:2,xlab="Disease free survival",
    ylab="Proportion surviving")
legend(500,.2,legend=c("MTX","no MTX"),lty=1:2)
```
$\Longrightarrow$ Figure 17.2

Section 17.3

The resid() function is used to compute different types of residuals and influence statistics. The cox.zph() function is used to plot scaled Schoenfeld
residuals against time and to test the proportional hazards assumtpion.

Script for Section 17.3

```
Restrict analysis to survival times up to 1,000 days
bmt2<-bmt1
bmt2$cdf[bmt1$trel>1000]<-0
bmt2$trel[bmt1$trel>1000]<-1000
bmt.cox<-coxph(Surv(tplate,trel,cdf)~ g + fab + agepat*agedon +
    strata(mtx), method="breslow",data=bmt2)
win.graph()
par(mfrow=c(1,2))
fit<-survfit(bmt.cox)
plot(fit,lty=1:2,xlab="Disease free survival",
    ylab="Proportion surviving")
legend(200,0.4,legend=c("MTX","no MTX"),lty=1:2)

# Find out which observations refer to which stratum
fit$strata
# stratum 1: 1 to 43
# stratum 2: 43 + 1:17
lniha<-log(-log(fit$surv[1:43]))
lnihb<-log(-log(fit$surv[43 + (1:17)]))
timea<-fit$time[1:43]
timeb<-fit$time[43 + (1:17)]

# Plot integrated hazards
plot(c(timea,timeb),c(lniha,lnihb),type="n",xlab="time",
    ylab="log integrated hazard")
lines(timea,lniha,type="s")
lines(timeb,lnihb,type="s",lty=2)
legend(300,-3,legend=c("MTX","no MTX"),lty=1:2)
```
$\Longrightarrow$ Figure 17.3

```
# Use full range of survival times again
bmt.cox<-coxph(Surv(tplate,trel,cdf)~ g + fab + agepat*agedon +
```

```
    strata(mtx),method="breslow",data=bmt1)

# Plot deviance residuals with status indicator
plot(resid(bmt.cox,type="deviance"),
    ylab="Deviance Residuals",type="n")
text(resid(bmt.cox,type="deviance"), labels=bmt1$cdf)
```
$\Longrightarrow$ Figure 17.4

```
# Plot influence statistics
bresid<-resid(bmt.cox,type="dfbeta")

# Use a loop to plot six graphs in one figure
par(mfrow=c(3,2))
expl<-c("g2","g3","fab","agepat","agedon","agepat:agedon")
for (i in 1:6){
    plot(1:120,bresid[,i],type="h",xlab="observation",
        ylab="change in coeff")
    # type="h" causes vertical lines to be plotted
    title(expl[i])
}
```
$\Longrightarrow$ Figure 17.5

```
# Scaled Schoenfeld residual plots for assessing
# proportional hazards
par(mfrow=c(3,2))
plot(cox.zph(bmt.cox))
```
$\Longrightarrow$ Figure 17.6

```
# Tests of proportional hazards
cox.zph(bmt.cox, global=F)
```
$\Longrightarrow$ Table 17.6

17.8   Exercises

17.1 Use the likelihood ratio test to add other explanatory variables to the survival model for the prostate cancer data.

17.2 For the selected model, plot the deviance residuals against observation number and check the proportional hazards assumption using scaled Schoenfeld residuals (both graphically and using significance tests).

17.3 Fit a Cox's proportional hazards model to the breast cancer data given in Exercise 16.3 of the previous chapter and use a likelihood ratio test to test the significance of whether the cancer has metastized.

17.4 Check the proportional hazards assumption for the model above.

17.5 Plot the (scaled) change in regression coefficient associated with excluding observations against observation number. Are there any influential observations?

18
Principal Components and Factor Analysis

18.1 Introduction

In this chapter, two methods of examining the relationships among a set of variables will be examined. The first, *principal components analysis* (PCA), is essentially a method of data reduction that aims to reduce the dimensionality of multivariate data and, thus, aid in its understanding. The second technique to be discussed is *exploratory factor analysis*, which has somewhat similar aims to principal components analysis, but in addition tries to uncover something more fundamental about the data.

18.2 Principal components analysis

Principal components analysis is among the oldest and most widely used of multivariate techniques. Originally introduced by Pearson (1901) and independently by Hotelling (1933), the basic idea of the method is to describe the variation of a set of multivariate data in terms of a set of uncorrelated variables, each of which is a particular linear combination of the original variables. The new variables are derived in decreasing order of importance so that the first principal component accounts for as much as possible of the variation in the original data, the second for as much of the remaining variation subject to being uncorrelated with the first, and so on. The usual objective of this type of analysis is to see whether the first few components account for a large enough portion of the variation to provide an adequate, simpler description of the data. If they do, then they can be used to summarize the data with little loss of information, thus providing a reduction in the dimensionality of the data. This might be useful in simplifying later analyses. The technique is described in detail in Everitt and Dunn (2001) and more briefly in Displays 18.1 and 18.2.

Display 18.1 Principal components analysis

- The first principal component y_1 is defined as the linear combination of the original variables $x_1, x_2, \cdots, x_p$ that accounts for the maximal amount of the variance of the x variables among all such linear combinations.

- The second principal component y_2 is defined as the linear combination of the original variables that accounts for a maximal amount of the remaining variance subject to being uncorrelated with y_1. Subsequent components are defined similarly.

- So PCA finds new variables $y_1, y_2, \cdots, y_p$ defined as follows:

$$
\begin{aligned}
y_1 &= a_{11}x_1 + a_{12}x_2 + \cdots + a_{1p}x_p \\
y_2 &= a_{21}x_1 + a_{22}x_2 + \cdots + a_{2p}x_p \\
&\vdots \\
y_p &= a_{p1}x_1 + a_{p2}x_2 + \cdots + a_{pp}x_p
\end{aligned}
\tag{1}
$$

with the coefficients $a_{11}, a_{12}, \cdots, a_{pp}$ being chosen so that $y_1, y_2, \cdots, y_p$ account for decreasing proportions of the variance of the x variables and are uncorrelated.

- The sum of squares of the coefficients defining each principal component are set to one so that the total variance of all p components $y_1, y_2, \cdots, y_p$, equals the total variance of the x variables.

- The coefficients are found as the eigenvectors of the sample covariance matrix **S** or, more commonly when the observed variables have different scales, the sample correlation matrix, **R**. The variances of the components are the corresponding eigenvalues of **S** or **R**. It should be noted that there is, in general, no simple relationship between the components found from these two matrices.

- It is often useful to rescale the coefficients defining the components, particularly when they are derived from the correlation matrix. In this case multiplying the coefficients by the square root of the component's variance gives the correlations between variables and components.

18.2.1 Principal components analysis of head lengths

As a first very simple example of applying principal components analysis in practice, we shall use the data shown in Table 18.1, which give the head length (in millimeters) for each of the first two adult sons in 25 families. The results of a principal components analysis of the covariance matrix of these bivariate data are given in Table 18.2. The observations are plotted

---

Display 18.2 Principal component scores and number of components

- Principal components scores are found by applying the appropriate coefficients to the original variable values, usually after subtracting the variable mean so that the component scores for individual i with original variable values $\mathbf{x}_i' = (x_{i1}, x_{i1}, \cdots, x_{ip})$ are

$$y_{i1} \ = \ \mathbf{a}_1'(\mathbf{x}_i - \bar{\mathbf{x}})$$

$$\vdots$$

$$y_{ip} \ = \ \mathbf{a}_p'(\mathbf{x}_i - \bar{\mathbf{x}}) \tag{1}$$

  where the vectors $\mathbf{a}_1, \mathbf{a}_2, \cdots, \mathbf{a}_p$, contain the coefficients defining each component.

- The number of components needed to adequately describe a set of multivariate data may be chosen by any of a variety of ad hoc procedures:

  - Choose that number of components that account for some arbitrary amount of the variance of the original variables—values from 70% to 90% are generally suggested.

  - Plot the eigenvalues, λ_j, against j (this is known as a *screeplot*), and look for an 'elbow' in the curve.

  - Exclude those principal components with eigenvalues below the average. For components calculated from a correlation matrix, this implies excluding components with eigenvalues less than one.

TABLE 18.1. Head length data for first and second sons

First son	Second son	First son	Second son
191	155	185	152
179	145	190	159
195	149	195	157
201	152	188	151
181	148	187	158
185	149	163	137
183	153	161	130
188	149	195	155
176	144	183	158
171	142	186	153
208	157	173	148
192	152	181	145
189	150	182	146
190	149	175	140
197	159	165	137
189	152	192	154
188	152	185	152
197	159	174	143
192	150	178	147
187	151	176	139
179	158	176	143
186	148	197	167
183	147	200	158
174	147	190	163
174	150	187	150

in Figure 18.1 along with the axes corresponding to the principal components. The first of these passes through the mean of the data and has slope $0.548/0.836$. The second also passes through the mean with slope $-0.836/0.548$. This example illustrates that principal components analysis is essentially just a rotation of the axes of the multivariate data scatter.

18.2.2 Principal components analysis of nutrients in foodstuffs

As a second, more complex example of principal components analysis, we shall apply the technique to the data given in Table 18.3, showing the nutrients in different foodstuffs. (The quantity involved is always three ounces.) First, however, it is, as always, good practice to view the data graphically, and here, we shall use a scatterplot matrix, identifying the foodstuffs in each panel—see Figure 18.2. A number of the scatterplots in this figure give strong evidence of outliers that may have a considerable effect when calculating the correlation matrix of the variables and, consequently, may distort the results of the principal components analysis. For the moment,

TABLE 18.2. Principal components analysis of head length data

```
Importance of components:
                              Comp. 1      Comp. 2
        Standard deviation 11.4028946 3.68418174
   Proportion of Variance  0.9054786 0.09452138
   Cumulative Proportion   0.9054786 1.00000000

Loadings:
     Comp. 1 Comp. 2
X1 -0.836    0.548
X2 -0.548   -0.836
```

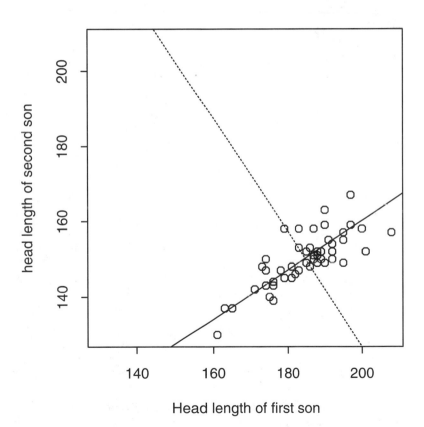

Head length of first son

FIGURE 18.1. Scatterplot of head length data with principal components.

386   18. Principal Components and Factor Analysis

however, we shall ignore this potential problem, and calculate the principal components from the correlation matrix computed in the usual way from the observations. The results are shown in Table 18.4. The first component is essentially an average of the energy and fat content of a food, and the second is essentially a contrast of the protein and iron content of the food. Only the first two components have eigenvalues greater than one, and together these two components account for 67% of the variance of the original five variables. A screeplot of the eigenvalues is shown in Figure 18.3.

TABLE 18.3. Nutrients in food data

		Energy	Protein	Fat	Calcium	Iron
BB	Beef, braised	340	20	28	9	2.6
HR	Hamburger	245	21	17	9	2.7
BR	Beef roast	420	15	39	7	2.0
BS	Beef, steak	375	19	32	9	2.5
BC	Beef, canned	180	22	10	17	3.7
CB	Chicken, broiled	115	20	3	8	1.4
CC	Chicken, canned	170	25	7	12	1.5
BH	Beef heart	160	26	5	14	5.9
LL	Lamb leg, roast	265	20	20	9	2.6
LS	Lamb shoulder, roast	300	18	25	9	2.3
HS	Smoked ham	340	20	28	9	2.5
PR	Pork roast	340	19	29	9	2.5
PS	Pork simmered	355	19	30	9	2.4
BT	Beef tongue	205	18	14	7	2.5
VC	Veal cutlet	185	23	9	9	2.7
FB	Bluefish, baked	135	22	4	25	0.6
AR	Clams, raw	70	11	1	82	6.0
AC	Clams, canned	45	7	1	74	5.4
TC	Crabmeat, canned	90	14	2	38	0.8
HF	Haddock, fried	135	16	5	15	0.5
MB	Mackerel, broiled	200	19	13	5	1.0
MC	Mackerel, canned	155	16	9	157	1.8
PF	Perch, fried	195	16	11	14	1.3
SC	Salmon, canned	120	17	5	159	0.7
DC	Sardines, canned	180	22	9	367	2.5
UC	Tuna, canned	170	25	7	7	1.2
RC	Shrimp, canned	110	23	1	98	2.6

The first two components appear to give a good representation of these five-dimensional data, and we can therefore use the first two principal component scores of each foodstuff to construct a plot of the data; this is shown in Figure 18.4. Foods high in energy and fat appear at the left end of the first dimension, and those low on these two nutrients at the opposite end. Foods high in protein are high on the second dimension and vice versa. Both type of clams are well separated from the remaining foodstuffs—they have very low energy content and high calcium content.

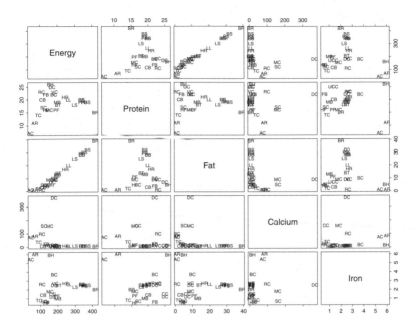

FIGURE 18.2. Scatterplot matrix of nutrients in foods.

TABLE 18.4. Principal components analysis of food data

Importance of components:

	Comp. 1	Comp. 2	Comp. 3	Comp. 4	Comp. 5
Standard deviation	1.4825	1.0697	0.9212	0.8988	0.04000
Proportion of Variance	0.4396	0.2288	0.1697	0.1616	0.00032
Cumulative Proportion	0.4396	0.6684	0.8381	0.9997	1.00000

Loadings:

	Comp. 1	Comp. 2	Comp. 3	Comp. 4	Comp. 5
Energy	-0.654		0.149	-0.199	0.709
Protein	-0.151	0.691	-0.463	-0.525	-0.104
Fat	-0.639	-0.202	0.216	-0.134	-0.697
Calcium	0.355		0.652	-0.670	
Iron	0.122	-0.689	-0.540	-0.468	

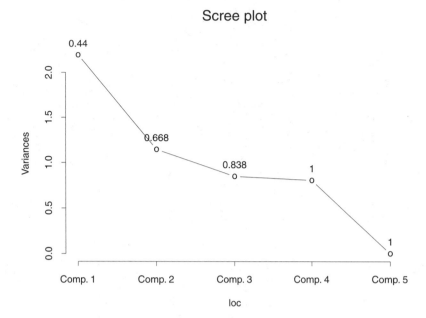

FIGURE 18.3. Screeplot for principal components analysis of food data.

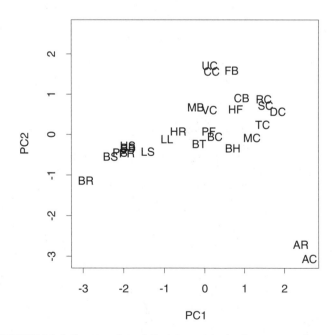

FIGURE 18.4. Scatterplot of first two principal component scores.

TABLE 18.5. Principal components analysis of food data based on robust correlation matrix

```
Importance of components:
                        Comp. 1 Comp. 2 Comp. 3
    Standard deviation   1.7168  1.2176  0.5541
Proportion of Variance  0.5895  0.2965  0.0614
Cumulative Proportion  0.5895  0.8860  0.9474
                        Comp. 4      Comp. 5
    Standard deviation 0.51256 0.01654500
Proportion of Variance 0.05254 0.00005475
Cumulative Proportion 0.99995 1.00000000
```

```
Loadings:
          Comp. 1 Comp. 2 Comp. 3 Comp. 4 Comp. 5
  Energy  -0.503   0.373  -0.349  -0.191   0.670
 Protein   0.518          -0.652  -0.545
     Fat  -0.522   0.344  -0.248          -0.736
 Calcium   0.372   0.545  -0.298   0.690
    Iron   0.260   0.667   0.551  -0.429
```

One of the problems with the foodstuffs data, identified in the scatterplot matrix of the data, is the presence of a number of outliers. One way to deal with this problem is to calculate a *robust* estimate of the correlation matrix and use this as the basis of the principal components analysis. One such estimator is that proposed by Rousseeuw (1985), and known as the *minimum volume ellipsoid estimator*. The results of using this approach on the foodstuffs data are given in Table 18.5. The results are now considerably different from those given previously. The first component is now largely a construct of energy and fat content with protein content, and the second is an average of calcium and iron content. In this analysis, the first two components account for 86% of the variation of the original variables.

18.3   Exploratory factor analysis

Factor analysis is concerned with whether the covariances or correlations between a set of observed variables can be 'explained' in terms of a smaller number of unobservable, latent variables, which it is not possible to measure directly. For example, direct measurement of a concept such as *racial prejudice* is not possible; one could, however, observe whether a person approves or disapproves of a particular piece of government legislation, whether she numbers members of a particular ethnic group among her friends and acquaintances, and so on, and assume that these characteristics are, in some sense, indicators of the underlying latent variable, racial prejudice.

By explanation, in this case, we mean that the correlation between each pair of observed variables results from their mutual association with the latent variables (or *common factors* as these are often called). Consequently, the partial correlations between any pair of observed variables given the values of the latent variables should be close to zero; i.e., the observed variables are independent *given* the latent variables. A brief description of the basic factor analysis model is given in Display 18.3. A more detailed account of the model is given in Everitt and Dunn (2001).

Factor analyis will be illustrated on the data shown in Table 18.6, which arise from a survey of AIDS patients' reactions to their physicians. The 14 items in the survey questionnaire measure patient attitudes about physician personality, demeanour, competence and prescribed treatment using a Likert-type scale of 1 to 5 for each item. Because 7 of the items were stated negatively, they have been recoded (reflected) so that 1 represents most positive and 5 the least positive on all items. The items and the names we shall use for them are as follows:

friend— My doctor treats me in a friendly manner.

doubt—I have some doubts about the ability of my doctor.

cold—My doctor seems cold and impersonal.

reass—My doctor does his/her best to keep me from worrying.

caref—My doctor examines me carefully as necessary.

nores—My doctor should treat me with more respect.

doubttr—I have some doubts about the treatment suggested by my doctor.

comp—My doctor seems very competent and well trained.

inters—My doctor seems to have a genuine interest in me as a person.

unasqu—My doctor leaves me with many unanswered questions about my condition and its treatment.

jargon—My doctor uses words that I do not understand.

confid—I have a great deal of confidence in my doctor.

conf—I feel I can tell my doctor about very personal problems.

notfr—I no not feel free to ask my doctor questions.

Associated with the maximum-likelihood version of factor analysis is a test of the hypothesis that a specified number of factors is adequate to explain the correlations. The test is described in Display 18.4. We shall begin by applying the test to try to determine how many factors are needed to adequately account for the correlations of the five variables in the food nutrients data.

We begin by fitting models with one, two, and three factors and applying the test for the number of factors. The results are as follows:

Display 18.3 Exploratory factor analysis

- The basis of factor analysis is a regression model linking the observed variables to a set of unobserved latent variables.

- For a set of observed variables, $x_1, x_2, \cdots, x_p$ and a set of latent variables $f_1, f_2, \cdots, f_k$ with $k < p$, the factor analysis model is

$$
\begin{aligned}
x_1 &= \lambda_{11}f_1 + \lambda_{12}f_2 + \cdots + \lambda_{1k}f_k + u_1 \\
x_2 &= \lambda_{21}f_1 + \lambda_{22}f_2 + \cdots + \lambda_{2k}f_2 + u_2 \\
&\vdots \\
x_p &= \lambda_{p1}f_1 + \lambda_{p2}f_2 + \cdots + \lambda_{pk}f_k + u_p
\end{aligned}
\tag{1}
$$

- This model can be written more concisely as

$$
\mathbf{x} = \Lambda\mathbf{f} + \mathbf{u} \tag{2}
$$

where

$$
\mathbf{f}' = [f_1, \cdots, f_k], \quad \mathbf{u}' = [u_1, \cdots, u_p] \tag{3}
$$

and

$$
\Lambda = \begin{bmatrix} \lambda_{11} & \cdots & \lambda_{1k} \\ \vdots & \vdots & \vdots \\ \lambda_{p1} & \cdots & \lambda_{pk} \end{bmatrix} \tag{4}
$$

(We have assumed that the $\mathbf{x}$ have been centered so that the mean is the null vector; this is of no practical consequence because we are only interested in the covariance or correlational structure of the variables.)

- We assume that the residual terms, $u_1, u_2, \cdots, u_p$ are uncorrelated with each other and with the factors, $f_1, f_2, \cdots, f_k$. (The u's are also known as *specific variates*.) This implies that given the values of the factors, the observed variables are independent; i.e., the correlations of the observed variables arise from their mutual relationships with the common factors.

- The regression coefficients, the lambdas, in this context, are more usually referred to as factor loadings, and when they are extracted from the correlation matrix, they represent correlations between the observed variables and the factors.

- The model implies the following about the covariance matrix of the observed variables:

$$
\Sigma = \Lambda\Lambda' + \Psi \tag{5}
$$

where $\Psi = \mathrm{diag}(\psi_i)$ and $\psi_i = \mathrm{var}(u_i)$. The variances of the factors are set at one. (We have also assumed that the factors are independent of one another, although this is not necessary.)

- The elements of Ψ are known as *specific variances*.

- In practice, Σ will be estimated by the sample covariance matrix $\mathbf{S}$ (alternatively, the model will be applied to the correlation matrix $\mathbf{R}$), and we will need to obtain estimates of Λ and Ψ so that the observed covariance matrix takes the form required by the model.

- The parameters in the factor analysis model Λ and Ψ can be estimated in a variety of ways, most commonly, by maximum likelihood.

TABLE 18.6. Aids data

1	2	2	3	2	2	4	1	1	2	2	1	2	2
2	3	2	3	2	2	3	2	2	3	3	2	1	2
2	2	3	3	4	4	2	2	4	2	2	4	4	2
2	4	2	2	2	4	4	2	4	4	4	4	4	2
2	2	2	2	2	2	2	2	2	2	2	2	2	2
2	4	2	2	2	2	2	1	2	2	2	2	2	1
2	2	1	5	2	1	1	1	1	2	4	2	2	2
2	2	2	2	2	2	2	2	2	2	2	2	2	5
1	1	2	2	2	1	2	1	1	2	2	2	2	1
2	3	2	3	2	2	3	3	3	4	4	3	2	2
2	2	2	2	2	2	4	2	2	2	2	2	2	2
2	1	4	1	2	1	1	1	3	1	1	1	2	1
2	2	2	2	2	2	2	2	2	2	2	2	2	2
5	2	2	5	4	5	4	3	5	5	2	3	4	4
2	2	2	4	2	3	4	2	2	4	2	2	2	2
1	1	1	1	1	2	2	1	1	1	1	1	1	2
1	1	1	1	1	1	1	1	1	2	3	1	1	1
1	1	2	1	1	2	1	1	1	1	4	1	2	1
1	1	1	1	1	1	3	1	1	1	2	1	1	1
1	1	1	1	1	2	3	1	1	1	1	1	1	1
2	3	1	3	1	2	3	2	3	4	2	2	2	3
1	2	1	1	3	1	3	1	1	3	1	1	1	1
2	2	2	2	2	2	2	2	2	2	2	2	2	2
2	3	3	4	5	3	4	3	4	5	4	4	2	2
1	1	2	1	1	1	1	1	2	1	5	1	1	1
2	3	2	2	2	2	4	2	2	4	4	3	2	3
1	2	1	1	1	2	3	1	1	2	2	2	2	2
1	1	1	1	1	2	2	1	1	2	2	2	1	1
1	1	2	2	1	2	1	1	2	4	1	1	2	1
2	1	1	2	2	1	2	1	2	2	4	2	2	2
1	1	1	2	2	2	2	2	2	2	2	2	2	2
1	1	1	3	3	1	1	1	1	2	1	1	1	1
1	1	1	1	1	1	1	1	1	1	3	1	1	1
2	1	2	2	2	2	2	1	3	2	2	2	3	2
1	1	1	2	2	2	3	2	1	1	4	2	2	1
2	2	2	2	2	2	2	2	2	2	2	3	2	2
4	4	4	4	2	4	2	3	4	2	4	2	3	2
1	1	1	2	2	2	1	1	1	4	1	1	1	1
2	1	1	2	1	3	4	1	1	3	4	2	2	2
2	3	4	2	2	2	2	1	2	2	5	3	2	2
1	1	1	1	1	1	2	1	2	2	2	1	2	2
2	4	3	2	2	2	4	2	2	4	3	2	2	1
1	2	2	1	3	2	2	2	2	2	1	2	2	1
1	3	2	2	2	2	2	2	2	2	2	2	1	2
1	1	1	4	1	1	1	1	1	1	1	1	1	1
1	1	1	1	1	1	1	1	1	1	1	1	1	1
1	1	1	1	1	1	1	1	1	1	2	1	1	1
2	2	2	2	3	4	4	2	2	4	4	2	2	5
1	2	1	2	3	2	2	2	2	2	2	2	2	1
4	4	5	4	4	4	4	3	4	5	4	4	5	4
2	1	1	2	2	2	2	2	1	2	1	1	1	2
2	2	2	2	2	2	2	2	2	2	4	2	2	2
2	2	2	2	2	4	4	2	2	2	2	2	2	2
2	2	2	2	2	2	2	2	2	4	2	2	2	2
2	2	2	2	2	2	2	2	2	3	4	2	2	2
2	2	2	2	2	2	2	2	2	2	2	2	2	2
1	1	1	1	1	2	2	1	1	1	2	1	1	1
2	4	2	2	3	2	2	4	4	4	2	5	1	2
2	3	2	2	2	2	2	2	2	2	2	2	2	2
2	4	2	4	2	3	3	2	3	4	2	4	4	4
1	1	1	1	1	1	1	1	1	1	1	1	1	1
1	1	1	2	1	1	1	1	1	2	2	1	1	1
1	2	1	2	2	2	1	1	1	1	1	2	2	1
1	1	1	1	2	1	1	1	1	2	2	1	1	1

Display 18.4 Test for number of factors

- The test statistic U is given by $U = n' \min(F)$, where $n' = n - 1 - \frac{1}{6}(2p + 5) - \frac{2}{3}k$ and F is given by

$$F = \ln|\mathbf{\Sigma}| + \text{trace}[\mathbf{S}\mathbf{\Sigma}^{-1}] - \ln|\mathbf{S}| - p \qquad (1)$$

- If k common factors are sufficient to describe the data, then U is asymptotically distributed as chi-squared with ν degrees of freedom, where

$$\nu = \frac{1}{2}(p-k)^2 - \frac{1}{2}(p+k) \qquad (2)$$

- The number of variables is 14, and the number of observations is 64. Test of the hypothesis that one factor is sufficient versus the alternative that more are required: $\chi^2(77) = 139.68, p < 0.001$.

- The number of variables is 14, and the number of observations is 64. Test of the hypothesis that two factors are sufficient versus the alternative that more are required: $\chi^2(64) = 101.59, p = 0.002$.

- The number of variables is 14, and the number of observations is 64. Test of the hypothesis that three factors are sufficient versus the alternative that more are required: $\chi^2(52) = 68.96, p = 0.058$.

The three-factor solution is summarized in Table 18.7, but we shall not yet attempt to interpret the factors because this usually becomes simpler after the process of *factor rotation*, which is described briefly in Display 18.5. Factor rotation has often been criticised for possibly allowing researchers to impose their *a priori* prejudices and biases on a factor solution, but in reality, a set of rotated factor loadings merely provides a simpler way of describing a solution. Several methods of rotation are available, the most common of which is the *varimax* method, which has as its rationale to seek for factors with a few large loadings and as many near-zero loadings as possible. This is achieved by iterative maximization of a quadratic function of the loadings—details are given in Mardia *et al.* (1979).

The varimax rotated three-factor solution for the AIDS data is shown in Table 18.8. The rotated factors might, perhaps, be labelled, *trust in doctor*, *confidence in doctor's ability* and *confidence in recommended treatment*. (This can be seen by highlighting loadings greater than or equal to 0.5.)

18.4 Principal components analysis and factor analysis compared

Factor analysis, like principal components analysis, is an attempt to explain a set of data in a smaller number of dimensions than one starts with, but the procedures used to achieve this goal are essentially different in the two methods. Factor analysis is based on a statistical model, whereas principal

TABLE 18.7. Unrotated three factor model for AIDS patient data

Importance of factors:

	Factor1	Factor2	Factor3
SS loadings	3.4125	2.8212	2.5630
Proportion Var	0.2437	0.2015	0.1831
Cumulative Var	0.2437	0.4453	0.6283

The degrees of freedom for the model is 52.

Uniquenesses:

friend	doubt	cold	reass	caref	nores
0.08981	0.4012	0.5208	0.5489	0.5141	0.3188

doubttr	comp	inters	unasqu	jargon	confid
1.291e-006	0.3317	0.2062	0.3626	0.8885	0.1057

conf	notf
0.3914	0.5236

Loadings:

	Factor1	Factor2	Factor3
friend	0.867	0.217	0.333
doubt	0.336	0.596	0.362
cold	0.572	0.348	0.175
reass	0.559	0.285	0.241
caref	0.393	0.511	0.265
nores	0.531	0.331	0.538
doubttr		0.151	0.984
comp	0.397	0.612	0.369
inters	0.699	0.514	0.202
unasqu	0.331	0.475	0.550
jargon	0.215	0.183	0.178
confid	0.308	0.835	0.320
conf	0.577	0.409	0.330
notf	0.482	0.249	0.427

Display 18.5 Factor rotation

- Suppose **M** is an orthogonal matrix of order $k \times k$ and we rewrite the factor analysis model given in Display 18.4, namely,

$$\mathbf{x} = \mathbf{\Lambda f} + \mathbf{u} \tag{1}$$

as

$$\mathbf{x} = (\mathbf{\Lambda M})(\mathbf{M'f}) + \mathbf{u} \tag{2}$$

- This satisfies all of the requirements of a k factor model with new factors $\mathbf{f^*} = \mathbf{M'f}$ and new factor loadings $\mathbf{\Lambda M}$.

- Consequently, the 'new' model implies that

$$\mathbf{\Sigma} = (\mathbf{\Lambda M})(\mathbf{\Lambda M})' + \mathbf{\Psi} \tag{3}$$

- This reduces to

$$\mathbf{\Sigma} = \mathbf{\Lambda \Lambda'} + \mathbf{\Psi} \tag{4}$$

as before, because $\mathbf{MM'} = \mathbf{I}$.

- This implies that if the factors **f** with loadings **Λ** provide an explanation for the observed covariances of the **x** variables, then so also do the factors $\mathbf{f^*}$ with the loading $\mathbf{\Lambda M}$ for any orthogonal matrix **M**.

TABLE 18.8. Loadings of rotated factor solution

Loadings:

	Factor1	Factor2	Factor3
friend	0.893	0.236	0.238
doubt	0.367	0.620	0.283
cold	0.585	0.357	
reass	0.577	0.299	0.168
caref	0.414	0.528	0.189
nores	0.576	0.369	0.462
doubttr	0.183	0.227	0.956
comp	0.428	0.636	0.284
inters	0.714	0.524	
unasqu	0.377	0.514	0.480
jargon	0.230	0.195	0.144
confid	0.335	0.855	0.225
conf	0.603	0.429	0.246
notf	0.517	0.278	0.363

components analysis is just a mathematical transformation of variables. Factor analysis, unlike principal components analysis, begins with a hypothesis about the covariance (or correlational) structure of the variates. Formally, this hypothesis is that a covariance matrix Σ of order and rank p can be partitioned into two matrices $\Lambda\Lambda'$ and Ψ. The first is of order p, but rank k (the number of common factors), whose off-diagonal elements are equal to those of Σ. The second is a diagonal matrix of full rank p, whose elements when added to the diagonal element of $\Lambda\Lambda'$ give the diagonal elements of Σ. In other words, the hypothesis is that a set of k latent variables exists $(k < p)$, and these are adequate to account for the covariances of the variates, although not for their full variances. Principal components analysis, on the other hand, is merely a transformation of the data, and no assumptions are made about the form of the covariance matrix from which the data arise. This type of analysis has no part corresponding to the specific variates of factor analysis. Consequently, if the factor model holds but the specific variances are small we would expect both forms of analysis to give similar results. However, if the specific variances are large, they will be absorbed into all principal components, both retained and rejected, whereas factor analysis makes a special provision for them. Factor analysis also has the advantage that there is a simple relationship between the results obtained by analysing a covariance matrix and those obtained from a correlation matrix. It should be remembered that principal components analysis and factor analysis are similar in one other respect, namely, that they are both pointless if the observed variables are almost uncorrelated— factor analysis because it has nothing to explain, and principal components analysis because it would simply lead to components that are similar to the original variables.

18.5 Summary

Both principal components analysis and factor analysis attempt to find a low-dimensional representation of multivariate data to aid in understanding the structure of the data. Principal components analysis is, however, essentially a simple rotation of the axis of the multivariate data, whereas factor analysis postulates a statistical model to explain the observed correlations or covariances. In many cases in practice, however, both approaches will lead to similar results.

18.6   Using S-PLUS

18.6.1   Using the S language

Section 18.2

Here, the `princomp()` function is used to find the principal components of multivariate data. The function `cov.mve()` provides a robust estimate of the covariance matrix.

Script for Section 18.2

```
# Read in headsize data
head<-matrix(scan("headsize.dat"),ncol=2,byrow=T)

# Find principal components of correlation matrix
head.pc<-princomp(head)
# uses covariance matrix by default

# Print results
summary(head.pc,loadings=T)                          ⟹ Table 18.2


# Plot data and lines representing the two principal components
load<-head.pc$loadings
slope<-load[2,]/load[1,]
mn<-apply(head,2,mean)
intcpt<-mn[2]-(slope*mn[1])

win.graph()
xlim<-range(head[,1],head[,2])
# Get equally scaled axes using the pty="s" option and
# the same limits for the x and y axes
par(pty="s")
plot(head,xlab="Head length of first son",
    ylab="head length of second son",pch=1,lwd=2,
    xlim=xlim,ylim=xlim)
abline(intcpt[1],slope[1],lwd=2)
abline(intcpt[2],slope[2],lwd=2,lty=2)               ⟹ Figure 18.1


# Read in nutrients in food data
food<-read.table("food.dat",header=T)
attach(food)

# Get scatterplot matrix of the data
win.graph()
pairs(food,panel=function(x,y)
    text(x,y,labels=row.names(food),cex=0.5))        ⟹ Figure 18.2
```

```
# Calculate correlation matrix
cor(food)

# Calculate principal components of correlation matrix
food.pc<-princomp(food,cor=T)
summary(food.pc,loadings=T)
```
$\implies$ Table 18.4

```
# Draw screeplot of eigenvalues
win.graph()
plot(food.pc,style="lines",main="Scree plot")
```
$\implies$ Figure 18.3

```
# Plot data in space of first two principal components
win.graph()
par(pty="s")
x<-food.pc$scores[,1]
y<-food.pc$scores[,2]
xlim<-range(c(x,y))
plot(x,y,xlab="PC1",ylab="PC2",xlim=xlim,ylim=xlim,type="n")
text(x,y,labels=row.names(food))
```
$\implies$ Figure 18.4

```
# Calculate principal componets from a robust estimator
# of the correlation matrix
mve.food<-cov.mve(food,cor=T)
mve.food$cor
food.pc1<-princomp(food,covlist=mve.food,cor=T)
summary(food.pc1,loadings=T)
```
$\implies$ Table 18.5

Section 18.3

In this section, the function factanal() is first used to test for number of factors in the survey of AIDS patients and then to find a maximum-likelihood three-factor solution. The function rotate() is used to provide a varimax solution.

Script for Section 18.3

```
# Read in data on AIDS patients
patient<-matrix(scan("patient.dat",width=1),ncol=14,byrow=T)

# Label columns
patient.lab<-c("friend","doubt","cold","reass","caref","nores",
    "doubttr","comp","inters","unasqu","jargon","confid","conf",
    "notf")
```

```
dimnames(patient)<-list(NULL,patient.lab)

# First try to determine the appropriate number of factors
# for the data
patient.fa1<-factanal(patient,factor=1,method="mle")
patient.fa1
patient.fa2<-factanal(patient,factor=2,method="mle")
patient.fa2
patient.fa3<-factanal(patient,factor=3,method="mle")
patient.fa3

# Print out results for three-factor solution
summary(patient.fa3)                                    ⟹  ┃Table 18.7┃

summary(rotate(patient.fa3,rotation="varimax"))         ⟹  ┃Table 18.8┃
```

18.7 Exercises

18.1 The correlation matrix shown below arises from a study of health services systems in which data were obtained for each of 32 counties in New Mexico. The 11 variables used were as follows:

PCENTAG—The percent of the labour force in agriculture.

PCTURBAN—Percent urban.

PCTSPAM—Percent Spanish American.

PCTNOWWH—Percent nonwhite.

NETMIGR—Next migration.

MEDAGE—Median age.

MEDEDUC—Median education.

PCTUNEMP—Percent unemployed.

INCOME—Per Capita income.

HSPBEDS—Hospital beds per 100,000 population.

MORTALITY—Mortality/100,000 population due to accidents, suicide and cirrhosis of the liver.

$\mathbf{R} =$

$$
\begin{bmatrix}
1.00 \\
-0.52 & 1.00 \\
0.13 & -0.49 & 1.00 \\
-0.36 & -0.04 & -0.25 & 1.00 \\
-0.42 & 0.42 & -0.11 & 0.05 & 1.00 \\
0.30 & 0.14 & -0.32 & -0.46 & 0.24 & 1.00 \\
-0.28 & 0.68 & -0.68 & -0.18 & 0.19 & 0.18 & 1.00 \\
-0.01 & -0.45 & 0.75 & 0.18 & -0.22 & -0.55 & -0.71 & 1.00 \\
-0.16 & 0.59 & -0.52 & -0.37 & 0.20 & 0.40 & 0.82 & -0.65 & 1.00 \\
-0.40 & 0.57 & 0.24 & 0.15 & 0.19 & 0.21 & 0.20 & -0.19 & 0.24 & 1.00 \\
-0.20 & 0.39 & 0.22 & 0.39 & -0.25 & -0.17 & -0.48 & 0.43 & -0.48 & 0.07 & 1.00
\end{bmatrix}
$$

Investigate the structure of the correlations using both principal components analysis and factor analysis.

18.2 Fit a one-factor model to the following correlation matrix, and comment on the results.

$$\mathbf{R} = \begin{bmatrix} 1.00 & & \\ 0.83 & 1.00 & \\ 0.78 & 0.67 & 1.00 \end{bmatrix}$$

18.3 Repeat 18.2 with the following correlation matrix and again comment on the results:

$$\mathbf{R} = \begin{bmatrix} 1.00 & & \\ 0.84 & 1.00 & \\ 0.60 & 0.35 & 1.00 \end{bmatrix}$$

18.4 The correlations below are for the calculus measurements for the six anterior mandibuler teeth. Find all six principal components of the data, and use a screeplot to suggest how many components are needed to describe the correlations adequately. Can you interpret these components?

$$\mathbf{R} = \begin{bmatrix} 1.00 & & & & & \\ 0.54 & 1.00 & & & & \\ 0.34 & 0.65 & 1.00 & & & \\ 0.37 & 0.65 & 0.84 & 1.00 & & \\ 0.36 & 0.59 & 0.67 & 0.80 & 1.00 & \\ 0.62 & 0.49 & 0.43 & 0.42 & 0.55 & 1.00 \end{bmatrix}$$

Variables are calculus measure on

1. Right canine,
2. Right lateral, incisor,
3. Right central, incisor,
4. Left central, incisor,
5. Left lateral, incisor,
6. Left canine.

18.5 Apply principal factor analysis rather than using the maximum-likelihood approach to the survey of AIDS patients data. Compare the results with those given in the text.

18.6 Investigate alternative rotation methods to varimax for the AIDS data.

19
Cluster Analysis

19.1 Introduction

Cluster analysis is a generic term for a large collection of techniques designed to investigate multivariate data to determine whether the data consist of relatively distinct groups of similar 'individuals' (using individuals as a general term for the variety of entities that may be the subject of the analysis). In medicine, for example, discovering that a large set of patients can be partitioned into a small number of groups or clusters, within which the patients have very similar characteristics may have important implications both for treatment of the disease and for understanding its etiology.

Detailed accounts of clustering techniques are available in Everitt *et al.* (2001) and Gordon (1999). Here, we limit ourselves to consideration of three classes of methods.

- agglomerative hierarchical methods

- *k*-means type methods

- classification maximum likelihood methods

19.2 Agglomerative hierarchical clustering

In a hierarchic classification, the data are not partitioned into a particular number of classes or clusters at a single step. Instead, the classification consists of a series of partitions that may run from n 'clusters,' each containing an individual, to a single 'cluster' containing all individuals. See Display 19.1 for more details. Such methods usually take as their starting point an $n \times n$ matrix of interindividual similarities or distances (see Everitt *et al.*, 2001), and end with a diagram known as a *dendrogram*, which illustrates the fusions made at each successive stage of the analysis. Because all such clustering methods ultimately reduce the data to a single cluster containing all individuals, the question arises as to the 'optimal' number of clusters in the data (see next sub-section).

A variety of agglomerative hierarchical clustering methods arise because of the different ways in which intergroup distance can be defined in terms of the original interindividual distances. Display 19.2 describes three possibilities giving rise to three popular clustering methods of this class.

Display 19.1 Agglomerative hierarchical clustering

- This type of clustering produces a series of partitions of the data, $P_n, P_{n-1}, \cdots, P_1$.

- The first P_n consists of n single-member 'clusters'; the last P_1 consists of a single group containing all n individuals.

- The basic operation of all such methods is similar and is as follows:
  START: Clusters $C_1, C_2, \cdots, C_n$, each containing an individual.

  (1) Find nearest pair of distinct clusters, say c_i and c_j, merge c_i and c_j, delete c_j and decrease number of cluster by one.

  (2) If number of clusters equals one then stop, else return to (1).

- At each particular stage, the methods fuse individuals or groups of individuals that are closest (or most similar).

- Differences between methods arise because of the different ways of defining distances (or similarity) between an individual and a group containing several individuals, or between two groups of individuals— see Display 19.2.

19.2.1   Clustering foodstuffs

We shall illustrate the application of single linkage, complete linkage and group average clustering on the nutrients in foodstuffs data introduced in Chapter 18 (see Table 18.3). To begin, we need to calculate a between foodstuffs distance matrix, but because the variables are on very different scales, we need to first standardize the data in some way. Here, we shall use the sample range and then calculate Euclidean distances. Applying each of the three clustering techniques to the resulting distance matrix leads to the three dendrograms shown in Figure 19.1. Often, 'large' changes in fusion level in the dendrograms are taken as an informal indicator of the optimal number of clusters in the data. Leaving aside the dendrogram for single linkage, which shows the 'chaining' structure characteristic of this method (see Everitt *et al.*, 2001), the other two dendrograms suggest a similar two-

---

Display 19.2 Intergroup distances

- Intergroup distances can be defined in various ways, the most common definitions being *single linkage*, *complete linkage* and *average linkage*.

- **Single linkage**: The distance between two clusters A and B is

$$d_{AB} = \min_{i \in A, j \in B} (d_{ij}) \qquad (1)$$

- **Complete linkage**: The distance between two clusters A and B is

$$d_{AB} = \max_{i \in A, j \in B} (d_{ij}) \qquad (2)$$

- **Average linkage**: The distance between two clusters A and B is

$$d_{AB} = \frac{1}{n_A n_B} \sum_{i \in A} \sum_{j \in B} d_{ij} \qquad (3)$$

where in each case d_{ij} is the distance between individuals i and j and n_A and n_B are the number of individuals in each of the clusters.

TABLE 19.1. Mean nutrients in two clusters of foods

Group 1	HR, BC, CB, CC, BH, LL, BT, VC, FB, AR				
	AC, TC, HF, MB, MC, PF, SC, DC, UC, RC				
Group 2	BB, BR, BS, LS, HS, PR, PS				
	Energy	Protein	Fat	Calcium	Iron
Group 1	156	19	7.6	56	2.4
Group 2	353	19	30	0.7	2.4

group solution to each other. For complete linkage, the foods in the two groups and their mean nutrient profiles are shown in Table 19.1.

The groups are separated primarily on energy, fat and calcium. The second, smaller group consists of high-energy, high fat foods, such as beef, lamb and pork.

19.3 k-means clustering

The k-means clustering technique seeks to partition a set of data into a specified number of groups k by minimising some numerical criterion, low values of which are considered indicative of a 'good' solution. The most commonly used approach, for example, is to try to find the partition of the n individuals into k groups, which minimizes the within-group sum-of-squares over all variables. The problem then appears relatively simple; namely, consider every possible partition of the n individuals into k groups, and select the one with the lowest within-group sum of squares. Unfortunately, the problem in practice is not so straightforward. The numbers involved are so vast that complete enumeration of *every* possible partition remains

Single linkage

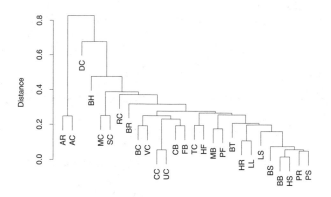

Compact linkage

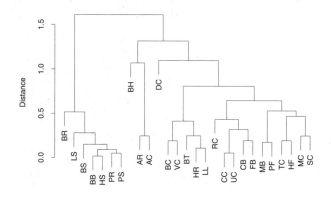

Average linkage

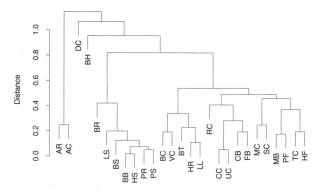

FIGURE 19.1. Agglomerative hierarchical clustering of food data based on single, complete and average linkage.

impossible even with the fastest computer. To illustrate the scale of the problem:

n	k	Number of possible partitions
15	3	2, 375, 101
20	4	45, 232, 115, 901
25	8	690, 223, 721, 118, 368, 580
100	5	10^{68}

The impracticability of examining every possible partition has led to the development of algorithms designed to search for the minimum values of the clustering criterion by rearranging existing partitions and keeping the new one only if it provides an improvement. Such algorithms do not, of course, guarantee finding the global minimum of the criterion. The essential steps in these algorithms are as follows:

1. Find some initial partition of the individuals into the required number of groups. (Such an initial partition could be provided by a solution from one of the hierarchical clustering techniques described in the previous section).

2. Calculate the change in the clustering criterion produced by 'moving' each individual from its own to another cluster.

3. Make the change that leads to the greatest improvement in the value of the clustering criterion.

4. Repeat steps (2) and (3) until no move of an individual causes the clustering criterion to improve.

To illustrate the *k*-means approach with minimization of the within-clusters sum of squares criterion, we shall apply it to the data shown in Table 19.2, which is concerned with the variation of mortality rates among geographical areas. The data correspond to 48 states in alphabetical order; Alaska and Hawaii are not included.

Current residence is widely used for the comparison of incidence or mortality rates among geographical areas. When studying diseases with long latency periods, migration between geographical areas reduces the sensitivity of this method. Beginning in 1979, mortality statistics by state or country of birth were published by the U.S. Federal Government and made available in computerised files. An analysis of residence histories provided in the U.S. 1958 current population survey found that 77.4% of people had not moved from their birthplace by the age of 19. Consequently, birthplace, which is listed on death certificates, provides a reasonably stable measure for geographical comparisons of potential early exposures for cohorts born before 1940, and Betemps and Buncher (1993) investigated state of birth as a possible risk factor for motor neuron disease (MND), Parkinson's disease (PD), multiple sclerosis (MS) and cerebrovascular disease (CVA). Using proportional mortality rates for each of the states in the USA, except

406   19. Cluster Analysis

TABLE 19.2. Mortality rates from motor neuron disease (MND), Parkinson's disease (PD), multiple sclerosis (MS) and cerebovascular disease (CVA) in American states

MND	PD	MS	CVA
12.15	20.29	5.41	942.5
10.62	15.94	7.97	650.7
18.09	25.41	4.62	928.2
28.37	25.85	18.29	797.0
10.98	31.11	20.13	755.9
19.55	24.88	11.26	753.6
18.33	7.33	3.67	645.2
12.83	14.81	7.90	830.5
12.95	18.01	4.42	1004.8
26.80	37.11	16.49	828.9
16.31	24.19	8.76	865.7
12.35	29.05	9.61	974.1
16.32	28.37	9.29	994.8
19.32	32.32	9.48	955.6
17.14	18.72	3.83	915.3
15.95	18.76	1.41	910.3
16.46	22.86	8.23	787.4
12.92	22.46	11.23	712.1
19.33	22.31	10.20	721.9
17.02	20.06	12.77	849.6
21.90	30.55	10.37	1011.3
13.20	23.10	3.85	964.5
14.93	26.45	6.30	942.9
28.21	24.69	12.34	717.7
17.92	32.63	7.81	947.3
12.09	12.09	12.09	677.2
5.25	19.24	8.74	781.7
18.16	19.76	11.75	731.5
21.67	32.51	14.45	680.9
15.95	19.84	10.46	726.2
12.40	21.50	5.79	960.3
22.71	22.71	15.14	848.0
19.24	21.48	11.60	868.3
20.10	23.39	8.77	792.2
23.67	29.89	11.21	833.3
14.44	21.65	8.39	780.2
12.11	24.22	9.42	709.2
9.01	25.10	5.15	914.1
11.24	31.68	19.42	866.6
13.01	16.70	5.04	1007.9
16.31	23.63	5.20	933.6
16.70	44.95	12.84	909.3
11.93	25.84	9.94	783.3
17.35	23.13	3.40	925.5
24.34	21.09	12.97	800.7
12.56	16.37	6.85	781.6
20.46	25.14	8.63	915.1
18.46	18.46	23.07	706.0

Hawaii and Alaska, Betemps and Buncher (1993) found positive correlations between each disease rate and the latitudes and longitudes of the states, apart from CVA. Here, the *k*-means clustering procedure will be used to 'explore' the structure of the mortality rates of the 48 states by forming clusters of states with similar mortality profiles.

The *k*-means approach can be used to partition the states into a pre-specified number of clusters, but the question remains as to the 'optimal' number of clusters for the data. A number of suggestions have been made as to how to tackle this question (see Everitt *et al.*, 2001), but none is completely satisfactory. Here, we shall examine the value of the within-group sum of squares associated with solutions for a range of values of *k*, the number of groups, in the hope of finding some 'sharp' change indicative of the best solution (cf. the screeplots used in Chapter 18). A plot of the within-group sum of squares for the one to six group solutions is shown in Figure 19.2. The plot suggests looking at the two- or three- cluster solution. We shall examine the latter in more detail.

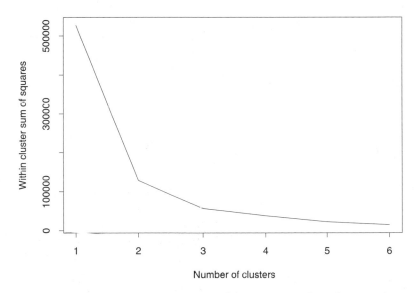

FIGURE 19.2. Within-group sums of squares v number of groups *k*.

The means of each variable in each cluster are given in Table 19.3. Cluster three is characterised by relatively low mortality rates for each of the four diseases. Cluster two has high rates for PD and CVA, but a very low rate for MS. Cluster one has the highest MND rate.

Here, there is a natural way to display the results graphically by placing the cluster label of each state in the relevant position on a map of the USA. This diagram is given in Figure 19.3. (We leave interpretation of this diagram to our readers in the USA!)

TABLE 19.3. Mean profiles of the three-cluster solution

```
Centers:
          MND    PD     MS    CVA
[1,]  17.70  23.64  11.592  818.4
[2,]  15.66  25.46   6.445  950.4
[3,]  16.80  21.20  12.157  706.8
```

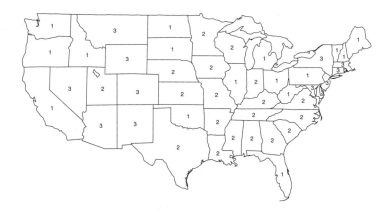

FIGURE 19.3. Map of USA with cluster membership.

19.4 Classification maximum likelihood

Scott and Symons (1971) and Banfield and Raftery (1992) approach the clustering problem by assuming that the population from which the observations arise consists of c subpopulations each corresponding to a cluster, and that the density of a p-dimensional observation from the jth subpopulation is $f_j(\mathbf{x}, \boldsymbol{\theta}_j)$ for some unknown vector of parameters, $\boldsymbol{\theta}_j$. They also introduce a vector $\boldsymbol{\gamma}\prime = [\gamma_1, \cdots, \gamma_n]$, where $\gamma_i = k$ if x_i is from the kth subpopulation; the γ_i label the subpopulation of each observation. The clustering problem now becomes that of choosing $\boldsymbol{\theta} = (\boldsymbol{\theta}_1, \boldsymbol{\theta}_1, \cdots \boldsymbol{\theta}_c)$ and $\boldsymbol{\gamma}$ to maximize the likelihood function associated with such assumptions. This classification maximum likelihood procedure is described briefly in Display 19.3.

To illustrate this approach to clustering, we shall apply it to the data on birthrates and death rates in 69 countries introduced in Chapter 4 (see Table 4.5). We shall assume that clusters have the same covariance matrix and therefore employ the equivalent of minimising $|\mathbf{W}|$ (see Display 19.3). The resulting dendrogram is shown in Figure 19.4. A relatively clear division into two groups is suggested, and the countries contained in each group and the group mean birthrates and death rates are shown in Table 19.4. A graphical display of the results is shown in Figure 19.5; here, two scatterplots of the birthrates and death rates are shown, the first giving the country labels, the second the cluster labels of the two-group solution. The results confirm the division into 'Western' and 'Third World' suggested by the bivariate density function of the data described in Chapter 4.

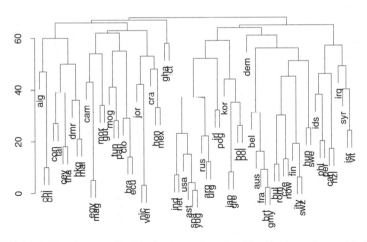

FIGURE 19.4. Dendogram for birthrates using classification maximum likelihood.

Display 19.3 Classification maximum likelihood

- Assume the population consists of c subpopulations, each corresponding to a cluster of observations, and that the density function of a p-dimensional observation from the jth subpopulation is $f_i(\mathbf{x}; \boldsymbol{\theta}_j)$ for some unknown vector of parameters, $\boldsymbol{\theta}_j$.

- Also, assume that $\boldsymbol{\gamma}' = [\gamma_1, \cdots, \gamma_n]$ gives the labels of the subpopulation to which each observation belongs. So $\gamma_i = j$ if $\mathbf{x}_i$ is from the jth population.

- The clustering problem becomes that of choosing $\boldsymbol{\theta}' = [\boldsymbol{\theta}_1, \boldsymbol{\theta}_2, \cdots \boldsymbol{\theta}_c]$ and $\boldsymbol{\gamma}$ to maximize the likelihood

$$L(\boldsymbol{\theta}, \boldsymbol{\gamma}) = \Pi_{i=1}^n f_{\gamma_i}(\mathbf{x}_i; \boldsymbol{\theta}_{\gamma_i}) \qquad (1)$$

- If $f_j(\mathbf{x}; \boldsymbol{\theta}_j)$ is taken as a multivariate normal density with mean vector $\boldsymbol{\mu}_j$ and covariance matrix $\boldsymbol{\Sigma}_j$, this likelihood has the form

$$L(\boldsymbol{\theta}; \boldsymbol{\gamma}) = \text{const} \prod_{k=1}^c \prod_{i \in E_k} |\boldsymbol{\Sigma}_k|^{\frac{1}{2}} \exp\left\{-\frac{1}{2}(\mathbf{x}_i - \boldsymbol{\mu}_k)'\boldsymbol{\Sigma}_k^{-1}(\mathbf{x}_i - \boldsymbol{\mu}_k)\right\} \qquad (2)$$

where $E_j = \{i : \gamma_i = j\}$

- The maximum likelihood estimator of $\boldsymbol{\mu}_j$ is $\hat{\mathbf{x}}_j = n_j^{-1} \sum_{i \in E_j} \mathbf{x}_i$, where n_j is the number of elements in E_j. Replacing $\boldsymbol{\mu}_j$ in (2) with this maximum likelihood estimator yields the following log-likelihood:

$$l(\boldsymbol{\theta}, \boldsymbol{\gamma}) = \text{const} - \frac{1}{2} \sum_{j=1}^c \text{trace}(\mathbf{W}_j \boldsymbol{\Sigma}_j^{-1} + n \ \log |\boldsymbol{\Sigma}_j|) \qquad (3)$$

where $\mathbf{W}_j$ is the $p \times p$ matrix of sums of squares and cross products of the variables for subpopulation j.

- Banfield and Raftery (1992) demonstrate the following:

  - If $\boldsymbol{\Sigma}_k = \sigma^2 \mathbf{I}$ ($k = 1 \cdots c$), then the likelihood is maximised by choosing $\boldsymbol{\gamma}$ to minimize trace($\mathbf{W}$), where $\mathbf{W} = \sum_{k=1}^c \mathbf{W}_k$, i.e., minimisation of the within-group sum of squares.

  - If $\boldsymbol{\Sigma}_k = \boldsymbol{\Sigma}$ ($k = 1 \cdots c$), then the likelihood is maximised by choosing $\boldsymbol{\gamma}$ to minimize $|\mathbf{W}|$, a clustering criterion discussed by Friedman and Rubin (1967) and Mariott (1982).

  - If $\boldsymbol{\Sigma}_k$ is not constrained, the likelihood is maximised by choosing $\boldsymbol{\gamma}$ to minimize $\sum_{k=1}^c n_k \log |\mathbf{W}_k|/n_k$.

  - Banfield and Raftery (1992) derive a number of other criteria that are more general than minimising $|\mathbf{W}|$ but more parsimonious than the completely unconstrained model. For full details, see the original paper.

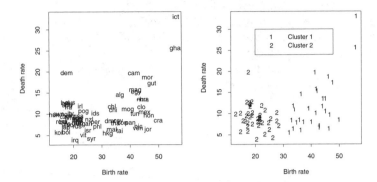

FIGURE 19.5. Scatterplots illustrating two-cluster solution for birthrate data.

TABLE 19.4. Cluster solution for birthrate and death rate data

Group 1:		mean birthrate: 41.57, mean death rate: 12.09						
alg	con	egy	gha	ict	mag	mor	tun	cam
cey	chi	tai	hkg	jor	mal	mog	tha	cra
dmr	gut	hon	mex	nic	pan	bra	chl	clo
ecu	ven							

Group 2:		mean birthrate: 20.32, mean death rate: 9.03						
ind	ids	irq	isr	jap	kor	phl	syr	vit
can	usa	arg	bol	per	urg	aus	bel	brt
bul	cze	dem	fin	fra	gmy	gre	hun	irl
ity	net	now	pol	pog	rom	spa	swe	swz
rus	yug	ast	nzl					

19.5 Summary

Cluster analysis techniques provide a rich source of possible strategies for exploring complex multivariate data. They have been used widely in medical investigations; examples include Everitt *et al.* (1971), Duflou *et al.* (1990) and Wastell and Gray (1987). Increasingly, model-based techniques such as finite mixture densities (see Everitt *et al*, 2001) and classification maximum likelihood, as described in this chapter, are superceeding older methods, such as the single linkage, complete linkage and average linkage methods described in Section 19.2. Two recent references are Fraley and Raftery (1998, 1999).

19.6   Using S-PLUS

19.6.1   Using the S language

Section 19.2

This section uses the `dist()` function to compute Euclidean distances; `hclust()` to apply single, complete and average linkage; and `plclust()` to plot resulting dendograms.

Script for Section 19.2

```
# Read in food data

food<-read.table("food.dat",header=T)

# Now standardize by the range
rge<-apply(food,2,max)-apply(food,2,min)
food.std<-sweep(food,2,rge,FUN="/")

# Get dendrograms for single linkage (Euclidean),
win.graph()
plclust(hclust(dist(food.std),method="connected"),
labels=row.names(food),ylab="Distance")
title("Single linkage")

# Complete linkage (Euclidean)
plclust(hclust(dist(food.std),method="compact"),
labels=row.names(food),ylab="Distance")
title("Complete linkage")

# Average linkage (Euclidean)
plclust(hclust(dist(food.std),method="average"),
labels=row.names(food),ylab="Distance")
title("Average linkage")                          ⟹ ┌──────────────┐
                                                    │ Figure 19.1  │
                                                    └──────────────┘

# Get two-cluster solution from complete linkage
two<-cutree(hclust(dist(food.std),method="compact"),k=2)

# Print out foodstuffs in each cluster
row.names(food)[two==1]
row.names(food)[two==2]

# Find cluster means of this two-group solution

clus1.mean<-apply(food[two==1,],2,mean)
clus2.mean<-apply(food[two==2,],2,mean)
rbind(clus1.mean,clus2.mean)                       ⟹ ┌──────────────┐
                                                     │ Table 19.1   │
                                                     └──────────────┘
```

Section 19.3

Here, `kmeans()` is used to apply cluster analysis by minimising within-group sums of squares. The `usa()` function is used to produce a map of the USA.

Script for Section 19.3

```
# Read mortality data, and name the variables
mortality<-matrix(scan("mort.txt"),ncol=4,byrow=T)
dimnames(mortality)<-list(NULL,c("MND","PD","MS","CVA"))

# Find within-group ss for the data before clustering
n<-length(mortality[,1])
wss1<-(n-1)*(var(mortality[,1])+var(mortality[,2])
   +var(mortality[,3])+var(mortality[,4]))

# Find the within-group ss for two to six groups
# as determined by the k-means method
wss<-numeric(0)
for(i in 2:6) {
   W<-sum(kmeans(mortality,i)$withinss)
   wss<-c(wss,W)
}

# Plot within-group ss against number of groups
wss<-c(wss1,wss)
win.graph()
plot(1:6,wss,xlab="Number of clusters",
   ylab="Within cluster sum of squares",type="l")
```
$\implies$ Figure 19.2

```
# Get three-group solution from kmeans
mortality.kmean<-kmeans(mortality,3)
mortality.kmean
```
$\implies$ Table 19.3

```
# Plot cluster labels on map of USA leaving out Hawaii
# and Alaska
win.graph()
usa(fifty=F)
text(state.center$x[-c(2,11)],state.center$y[-c(2,11)],
   mortality.kmean$cluster, cex=.5)
```
$\implies$ Figure 19.3

Section 19.4

This section uses `mclass()` to apply classification likelihood clustering.

Script for Section 19.4

```
# Read in birthrate-death rate data
birdea<-read.table("birdea.dat",header=T)
attach(birdea)

# Cluster data using determinant criterion
birdea.clus<-mclust(as.matrix(birdea),method="determinant")

# Plot dendrogram of clustering
win.graph()
plclust(birdea.clus$tree,labels=row.names(birdea))
```
$\Longrightarrow$ Figure 19.4

```
# Find countries corresponding to two-group classification
# and get group means
birdea.class<-mclass(birdea.clus,n.clus=2)
class<-birdea.class$classification
row.names(birdea)[class==1]
row.names(birdea)[class!=1]

apply(birdea[class==1,],2,mean)
apply(birdea[class!=1,],2,mean)
```
$\Longrightarrow$ Table 19.4

```
# Produce scatterplots of country labels and cluster labels
class[class==14]<-2
win.graph()
par(pty="s")
# Produces equal scales on both axes
par(mfrow=c(1,2))
plot(as.matrix(birdea),xlab="Birthrate",
    ylab="Death rate",type="n")
text(as.matrix(birdea),labels=row.names(birdea))

plot(as.matrix(birdea),xlab="Birthrate",
    ylab="Death rate",type="n")
text(as.matrix(birdea),labels=class)
legend(locator(1),c("Cluster 1","Cluster 2"),pch="12")
```
$\Longrightarrow$ Figure 19.5

19.7   Exercises

19.1 One of the problems when clustering the nutrients in foodstuffs data is how to standardize. Here, there is actually a 'natural' scaling of each food that might be considered preferable, which arises by expressing the five variables in terms of a percentage of recommended daily allowances, namely, food energy (3200 cal), protein (70 g), calcium (0.8 g), fat (100 g), and iron (10 g). Calculate the relevant percentages, and cluster the new data using complete linkage. Compare your results with those given in the chapter.

19.2 Write a general S-PLUS function that will display a particular partition chosen from a dendrogram on both a scatterplot matrix of the original data and a scatterplot or scatterplot matrix of a selected number of prinicpal components of the data.

19.3 Investigate the use of a criterion other than minimizing $|\mathbf{W}|$ for clustering the birthrate/death rate data with the classification likelihood approach.

19.4 Apply the classification likelihood clustering procedure to the mortality of states in the U.S. data, and produce a series of maps of the USA that show the optimal number of group solutions obtained with different clustering criteria.

20
Discriminant Function Analysis

20.1 Introduction

The aim of cluster analysis, the subject of the previous chapter, is to discover whether multivariate data contains relatively distinct groups of observations. A further aspect of the classification of multivariate data concerns the derivation of rules and procedures for allocating individuals to one of a set of *a priori* defined groups in some optimal fashion. This is the province of *assignment* or *discrimination* techniques. In medicine, for example, patients' conditions may only be able to be diagnosed without error at a postmortem. On the basis of a large number of postmortems, the characteristics of, say, disease and nondisease classes are established. From these *training set* observations, an investigator may wish to establish an allocation rule to be used on patients still alive, in the hope that their conditions can be diagnosed accurately and so treated appropriately. The information used in deriving a suitable allocation rule is the observations made on the training sample. One approach to discrimination or classification is to view the grouping variable as a univariate dependent variable and, in the case of two groups, use logistic regression (Chapter 9) or classifiaction and regression trees (Chapter 15) to predict group membership from a number of explanatory variables. In discriminant analysis, these 'explanatory' variables are viewed as the multivariate dependent variable and the grouping variable as the predictor.

20.2   The linear discriminant function

Fisher (1936) approached the discrimination problem for two groups by seeking a linear function of the variables observed on the members of the training set, which maximised the ratio of the between-group variance of the linear function to its within-group variance. Details are given in Display 20.1. Fisher's method is optimal for discrimination (in the sense of minimizing the number of misclassifications) when the observations in each group each have multivariate normal distributions with the same covariance matrix.

To illustrate the use of Fisher's linear discriminant function, the data shown in Table 20.1 will be used. These data were collected by Spicer *et al.* (1987) in an investigation of sudden infant death syndrome (SIDS). Data are available on 16 SIDS victims and 49 controls. All children had a gestational age of 37 or more weeks and were regarded as full term. Four variables were recorded for each infant as follows.

Group—victim of SIDS (1) or control (0)

HR—heart rate in beats per minute

BW—birthweight in grams

Factor68—heart and lung function

Gesage—gestational age in weeks

The Factor68 variable arises from spectral analysis of 24-hour recordings of the electrocardiograms and respiratory movements made on each child—see Spicer *et al.* (1987) for more details.

To begin with, only the Factor68 and BW variables will be used. Table 20.2 shows the group mean vectors and covariance matrices for these two variables, along with the estimate of the assumed common covariance matrix. A scatterplot of the two variables with cases (labeled 2) and controls (labeled 1) identified is shown in Figure 20.1.

The resulting discriminant function, derived as shown in Display 20.1, is

$$z = 0.001948 \times \text{BW} - 16.0846 \times \text{Factor68} \qquad (20.1)$$

To derive the classification rule associated with z, the group means on the discriminant variable are needed. These are as follows:

- Controls: $\bar{z}_1 = 1.696$

- Cases: $\bar{z}_2 = -0.689$

The classification rule for an individual with discriminant function score z_i is (assuming prior probabilities are the same) as follows:

- Assign to controls if $z_i > \frac{\bar{z}_1 + \bar{z}_2}{2}$
- Assign to cases if $z_i \leq \frac{\bar{z}_1 + \bar{z}_2}{2}$

Display 20.1 Fisher's discriminant function

- The aim is to find a way of classifying observations into one of two known groups using a set of variables $x_1, x_2, \cdots, x_p$.

- Fisher's idea was to find a linear function z of the variables, $x_1, \cdots, x_p$

$$z = a_1 x_1 + a_2 x_2 + \cdots + a_p x_p \tag{1}$$

such that the ratio of the between-group variance of z to its within-group variance is maximised.

- The coefficients $\mathbf{a}' = [a_1, \cdots, a_p]$ have, therefore, to be chosen so that V, given by

$$V = \frac{\mathbf{a}'\mathbf{B}\mathbf{a}}{\mathbf{a}'\mathbf{S}\mathbf{a}} \tag{2}$$

is maximised, where $\mathbf{S}$ is the pooled within-group covariance matrix and $\mathbf{B}$ the covariance matrix of group means; explicitly,

$$\mathbf{S} = \frac{1}{n-2} \sum_{i=1}^{2} \sum_{j=1}^{n_i} (\mathbf{x}_{ij} - \bar{\mathbf{x}}_j)(\mathbf{x}_{ij} - \bar{\mathbf{x}}_j)' \tag{3}$$

$$\mathbf{B} = \sum_{i=1}^{2} n_i (\bar{\mathbf{x}}_i - \bar{\mathbf{x}})(\bar{\mathbf{x}}_i - \bar{\mathbf{x}})' \tag{4}$$

where $\mathbf{x}'_{ij} = (x_{ij1}, x_{ij2} \cdots, x_{ijp})$ represents the set of p variable values for the jth individual in group i, $\bar{\mathbf{x}}_j$ is the mean vector of the jth group, and $\bar{\mathbf{x}}$ is the mean vector of all observations. The number of observations in each group is n_1 and n_2, with $n = n_1 + n_2$.

- The vector $\mathbf{a}$ that maximizes V is given by the solution of the following equation:

$$(\mathbf{B} - \lambda\mathbf{S})\mathbf{a} = 0 \tag{5}$$

- In the two-group situation, the *single* solution can be shown to be

$$\mathbf{a} = \mathbf{S}^{-1}(\bar{\mathbf{x}_1} - \bar{\mathbf{x}_2}) \tag{6}$$

- The allocation rule is now to allocate an individual with discriminate score z to group 1 if $z > \frac{\bar{z}_1 + \bar{z}_2}{2}$, where $\bar{z}_1$ and $\bar{z}_2$ are the mean discriminant scores in each group.

- Fisher's discriminant function also arises from assuming that the observations in group one have a multivariate normal distribution with mean vector $\boldsymbol{\mu}_1$ and covariance matrix $\boldsymbol{\Sigma}$ and those in group two have a multivariate distribution with mean vector $\boldsymbol{\mu}_2$ and, again, covariance matrix $\boldsymbol{\Sigma}$, and assuming that an individual with vector of scores $\mathbf{x}$ is allocated to group one if

$$\mathrm{MVN}(\mathbf{x}, \mu_1, \boldsymbol{\Sigma}) > \mathrm{MVN}(\mathbf{x}, \mu_2, \boldsymbol{\Sigma}) \tag{7}$$

- Substituting sample values for population rules leads to the same allocation rule as that given above.

- The above is only valid if the prior probabilities of each group are assumed to be the same.

TABLE 20.1. SIDS data

Group	HR	BW	Factor68	Gesage
1	115.6	3060	0.291	39
1	108.2	3570	0.277	40
1	114.2	3950	0.390	41
1	118.8	3480	0.339	40
1	76.9	3370	0.248	39
1	132.6	3260	0.342	40
1	107.7	4420	0.310	42
1	118.2	3560	0.220	40
1	126.6	3290	0.233	38
1	138.0	3010	0.309	40
1	127.0	3180	0.355	40
1	127.7	3950	0.309	40
1	106.8	3400	0.250	40
1	142.1	2410	0.368	38
1	91.5	2890	0.223	42
1	151.1	4030	0.364	40
1	127.1	3770	0.335	42
1	134.3	2680	0.356	40
1	114.9	3370	0.374	41
1	118.1	3370	0.152	40
1	122.0	3270	0.356	40
1	167.0	3520	0.394	41
1	107.9	3340	0.250	41
1	134.6	3940	0.422	41
1	137.7	3350	0.409	40
1	112.8	3350	0.241	39
1	131.3	3000	0.312	40
1	132.7	3960	0.196	40
1	148.1	3490	0.266	40
1	118.9	2640	0.310	39
1	133.7	3630	0.351	40
1	141.0	2680	0.420	38
1	134.1	3580	0.366	40
1	135.5	3800	0.503	39
1	148.6	3350	0.272	40
1	147.9	3030	0.291	40
1	162.0	3940	0.308	42
1	146.8	4080	0.235	40
1	131.7	3520	0.287	40
1	149.0	3630	0.456	40
1	114.1	3290	0.284	40
1	129.2	3180	0.239	40
1	144.2	3580	0.191	40
1	148.1	3060	0.334	40
1	108.2	3000	0.321	37
1	131.1	4310	0.450	40
1	129.7	3975	0.244	40
1	142.0	3000	0.173	40
1	145.5	3940	0.304	41
2	139.7	3740	0.409	40
2	121.3	3005	0.626	38
2	31.4	4790	0.383	40
2	152.8	1890	0.432	38
2	125.6	2920	0.347	40
2	139.5	2810	0.493	39
2	117.2	3490	0.521	38
2	131.5	3030	0.343	37
2	137.3	2000	0.359	41
2	140.9	3770	0.349	40
2	139.5	2350	0.279	40
2	128.4	2780	0.409	39
2	154.2	2980	0.388	40
2	140.7	2120	0.372	38
2	105.5	2700	0.314	39
2	121.7	3060	0.405	41

TABLE 20.2. Group mean vectors, covariance matrices and common covariance matrix for SIDS data

```
mean vector for group 1:
   BW Factor68
 3438   0.3108

mean vector for group 2:
   BW Factor68
 2965   0.4018

covariance matrix for group 1:
              BW Factor68
        BW 195270.833 3.244494
Factor68       3.244 0.005842

covariance matrix for group 2:
              BW Factor68
        BW 545304.90 7.759604
Factor68       7.76 0.007275

common covariance matrix:
              BW Factor68
        BW 278612.28 4.319520
Factor68       4.32 0.006183
```

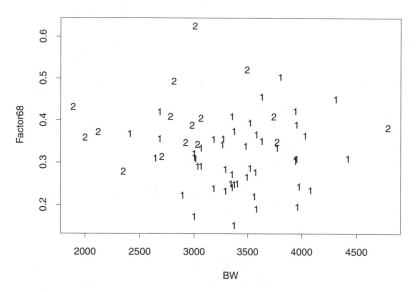

FIGURE 20.1. Scatterplot of BW and Factor68 with group labels.

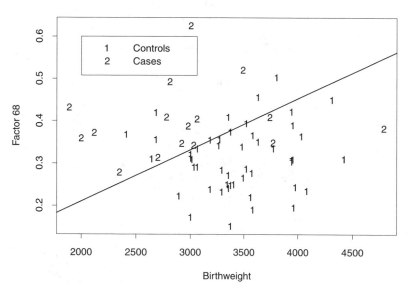

FIGURE 20.2. Scatterplot of BW and Factor68 showing derived linear discriminant function.

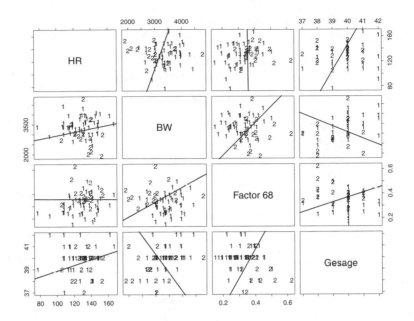

FIGURE 20.3. Scatterplot matrix with linear discriminant functions for all pairs of variables.

The discriminant function can be plotted on the scatterplot of the two variables, the relevant straight line being

$$0.001948 \times \text{BW} - 16.0846 \times \text{Factor68} - \frac{1}{2}(1.696 - 0.689) = 0 \qquad (20.2)$$

The resulting diagram is shown in Figure 20.2. A new infant with BW and Factor68 values that placed them above the line would be considered a possible SIDS case; below the line allocation would be in the non-SIDS group.

For comparison, we might be interested in deriving and displaying the discriminant functions for each pair of variables in the data. This can be done conveniently using the scatterplot matrix of the four variables—see Figure 20.3.

The linear discriminant function for all four variables is given by

$$
\begin{aligned}
z = \quad & 0.000179 \times \text{BW} - 15.533 \times \text{Factor68} \\
& -0.00178 \times \text{HR} + 0.215 \times \text{Gesage}
\end{aligned} \qquad (20.3)
$$

The performance of a discriminant function is evaluated by its misclassification rate. But how should this be estimated? The most obvious method, applying the derived discriminant function to the training set data, is known to be biased, hopelessly in many situations (see Hand, 1998, for details). A more suitable approach to estimating the misclassification rate is to use the so-called 'leaving one out method'. Here, a discriminant function is derived on the basis of $n-1$ of the subjects and then used to classify

TABLE 20.3. Misclassification rate estimates for Fisher's linear discriminant function derived from SIDS data

```
Plug-in classification table:
        1   2 Error Posterior.Error
     1 41   8 0.163              -0.070
     2  3  13 0.188               0.508
Overall       0.175               0.219
(from=rows,to=columns)

Optimal Error Rate:
      1     2 overall
   0.13  0.13    0.13

Rule Mean Square Error: 0.294
(conditioned on the training data)

Cross-validation table:
        1   2 Error Posterior.Error
     1 40   9 0.18               -0.064
     2  4  12 0.250               0.516
Overall       0.217               0.226
(from=rows,to=columns)
```

the individual omitted; the process is then repeated for each individual in turn. The result of both procedures are shown in Table 20.3. Here, there is a relatively small increase in the estimated misclassification rate using the more satisfactory estimation procedure.

20.3 Discriminant functions when group covariance matrices cannot be assumed to be equal

The linear discriminant function described and applied in the previous sections is based on the assumption that the covariance matrices of each group are equal. When this is not the case, it may be necessary to consider a more complex assignment procedure. For example, in the two-group situation, assuming again multivariate normality of the observations but allowing different covariance matrices for each groups leads to a *quadratic discriminant function*, as explained in Display 20.2.

Applying quadratic discrimination to the BW and Factor68 variables in the SIDS data gives the comprehensive results shown in Table 20.4. (Here we have assumed that the prior probabilities are proportional to the sample size.) A plot of the derived discriminant function is shown in Figure 20.4. According to the resubstitution estimation procedure, there is one less misclassification than for the linear discriminant function applied to these data. But when estimated by the 'leaving one out' method, there is an extra ob-

---

Display 20.2 Quadratic discriminant function

- Quadratic discriminant function.

- Suppose we have two groups, within group 1, the observations having a multivariate normal distribution with mean vector $\boldsymbol{\mu}_1$ and covariance matrix $\boldsymbol{\Sigma}_1$, and within group 2, mean vector $\boldsymbol{\mu}_2$ and covariance matrix $\boldsymbol{\Sigma}_2$.

- The assignment rule becomes:

  – Allocate an observation with vector of values $\mathbf{x}$, to group 1 if

$$\text{MVN}(\mathbf{x}, \boldsymbol{\mu}_1, \boldsymbol{\Sigma}_1) > \text{MVN}(\mathbf{x}, \boldsymbol{\mu}_2, \boldsymbol{\Sigma}_2) \tag{1}$$

- This leads to the following sample based quadratic discriminant function rule:

  – Allocate to group one if

$$\mathbf{x}'(\mathbf{S}_2^{-1} - \mathbf{S}_1^{-1})\mathbf{x} - 2\mathbf{x}'(\mathbf{S}_2^{-1}\bar{\mathbf{x}}_2 - \mathbf{S}_1^{-1}\bar{\mathbf{x}}_1) + (\bar{\mathbf{x}}_2'\mathbf{S}_2^{-1}\bar{\mathbf{x}}_2 - \bar{\mathbf{x}}_1'\mathbf{S}_1^{-1}\bar{\mathbf{x}}_1)$$
$$\geq \ln(|\mathbf{S}_2|/|\mathbf{S}_1|) + 2\ln\frac{\pi_1}{\pi_2} \tag{2}$$

  where π_1 and π_2 are the prior probabilities of the two groups and where $\mathbf{S}_1$ and $\mathbf{S}_2$ are the sample covariance matrices of each group.

---

servation misclassified. The problem with quadratic discrimination is the large number of parameters involved that may lead to a poorer performance when applied to new data. Here, the test for homogeneity of covariance matrices given in Table 20.4 suggests that a linear discriminant function is adequate.

20.4   Discriminant analysis with more than two groups

When more than two groups are involved, the assumed density functions of each pair of groups can be compared to derive the required allocation rules. Display 20.3 gives details for the three-group situation.

As an illustration of three-group discrimination, we shall use data collected during the magnetic resonance imaging investigation introduced in Chapter 4. One aim of the investigation was to derive a rule for allocating each voxel in an image into one of three known classes: grey matter, white matter or cerebrospinal fluid (CSF), on the basis of two measures of intensity, PD and T_2, which were recorded during the imaging process.

Class mean vectors and covariance matrices are shown in Table 20.6. Also given in this table are the estimate of the assumed common covariance matrix in the three groups, and the three derived classification functions.

A scatterplot of the data is shown in Figure 20.5; points are labelled by class. The lines representing the three derived classification functions are also shown in this diagram.

TABLE 20.4. Quadratic discriminant function results for SIDS data

```
Covariance Structure: heteroscedastic

Group: 1
            BW Factor68
      BW 195271    3.244
Factor68           0.006

Group: 2
            BW Factor68
      BW 545305    7.760
Factor68           0.007

Constants:
    1     2
 -39.62 -22.62

Linear Coefficients:
           1    2
      BW  0.02  0.0
Factor68 43.83 50.2

Quadratic coefficents:

group: 1
              BW Factor68
      BW -0.000003    0.00
Factor68             -86.38

group: 2
              BW Factor68
      BW -0.0000009   0.00
Factor68             -69.79

Tests for Homogeneity of Covariances:
      Statistic df     Pr
Box.M    7.261   3 0.0640
adj.M    6.886   3 0.0756

Hotelling's T Squared for Differences in Means Between Each Group:
       F df1    df2       Pr
1-2 10.88    2 20.99 0.000572
* df2 is Yao's approximation.

95% Simultaneous Confidence Intervals Using the Sidak Method:
                       Estimate Std.Error Lower Bound Upper Bound
            1.BW-2.BW   473.000   195.000       4.490    942.0000
1.Factor68-2.Factor68    -0.091     0.024      -0.149     -0.0334

                   1.BW-2.BW ****
1.Factor68-2.Factor68 ****
(critical point: 2.4022 )
* Intervals excluding 0 are flagged by '****'

Pairwise Generalized Squared Distances:
    1     2
1 0.000 1.744
2 2.835 0.000

Kolmogorov-Smirnov Test for Normality:
         Statistic Probability
      BW    0.0861      0.7209
Factor68    0.0718      0.8912
```

TABLE 20.4. Quadratic discriminant function results for SIDS data (continued)

```
Plug-in classification table:
          1 2  Error Posterior.Error
      1 46 3 0.0612          0.0547
      2  8 8 0.5000          0.4617
Overall       0.1692          0.1549
(from=rows,to=columns)

Rule Mean Square Error: 0.2261
(conditioned on the training data)

Cross-validation table:
          1 2  Error Posterior.Error
      1 45 4 0.0816          0.0491
      2  9 7 0.5625          0.4667
Overall       0.2000          0.1519
(from=rows,to=columns)
```

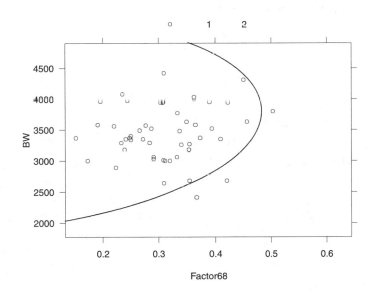

FIGURE 20.4. Quadratic discriminant function based on BW and Factor68.

428   20. Discriminant Function Analysis

Display 20.3 Discriminant analysis for three groups

- Assuming that the observations in the three groups have multivariate normal distributions with different means $\mu_1, \mu_2,$ and μ_3 but a common covariance matrix Σ, the allocation rule becomes:

    - Allocate to group one if an observation with vector of scores $\mathbf{x}$ is such that

    $$\text{MVN}(\mathbf{x}, \mu_1, \Sigma) > \text{MVN}(\mathbf{x}, \mu_2, \Sigma) \tag{1}$$

    and

    $$\text{MVN}(\mathbf{x}, \mu_1, \Sigma) > \text{MVN}(\mathbf{x}, \mu_3, \Sigma) \tag{2}$$

    - Allocate to group two if

    $$\text{MVN}(\mathbf{x}, \mu_2, \Sigma) > \text{MVN}(\mathbf{x}, \mu_1, \Sigma) \tag{3}$$

    and

    $$\text{MVN}(\mathbf{x}, \mu_2, \Sigma) > \text{MVN}(\mathbf{x}, \mu_3, \Sigma) \tag{4}$$

    - Allocate to group three if

    $$\text{MVN}(\mathbf{x}, \mu_3, \Sigma) > \text{MVN}(\mathbf{x}, \mu_1, \Sigma) \tag{5}$$

    and

    $$\text{MVN}(\mathbf{x}, \mu_3, \Sigma) > \text{MVN}(\mathbf{x}, \mu_2, \Sigma) \tag{6}$$

- This leads to sample based allocation rules as follows:

    - Allocate to group one if $h_{12}(\mathbf{x}) > 0$ and $h_{13}(\mathbf{x}) > 0$.
    - Allocate to group two if $h_{12}(\mathbf{x}) < 0$ and $h_{23}(\mathbf{x}) > 0$.
    - Allocate to group three if $h_{13}(\mathbf{x}) > 0$ and $h_{13}(\mathbf{x}) < 0$, where

    $$h_{ij}(\mathbf{x}) = (\bar{\mathbf{x}}_i - \bar{\mathbf{x}}_j)'\mathbf{S}^{-1}[\mathbf{x} - \frac{1}{2}(\bar{\mathbf{x}}_i + \bar{\mathbf{x}}_j)] \tag{7}$$

    where $\mathbf{S}$ is the sample estimate of the assumed common covariance matrix of the three groups and $\bar{\mathbf{x}}_i$ and $\bar{\mathbf{x}}_j$ represent group mean vectors.

TABLE 20.5. Part of the imaging data

PD	T2	Class
124	58	1
107	44	1
98	45	3
87	34	3
129	61	1
99	42	3
142	122	2
96	37	3
99	44	3
144	148	2
133	66	1
122	53	1
98	40	3
99	46	3
97	43	3
99	42	3
103	47	3
120	62	1
97	40	3
117	46	1
96	46	3
119	53	1
133	54	1
120	52	1
100	44	3
100	43	3
94	41	3
116	51	1
120	51	1
98	43	3
113	56	1
123	60	1
98	42	3
99	39	3
101	40	3
146	143	2
95	38	3
146	128	2
99	43	3
147	142	2
128	61	1
120	52	1
131	108	2
126	57	1
103	43	3
114	48	1
98	39	3
118	49	1
122	51	1
101	39	3

TABLE 20.6. Group mean vectors and covariance matrices for imaging data

```
mean vector for group 1:
     PD      T2
   121.6 53.56

mean vector for group 2:
     PD      T2
   134.3 112.2

mean vector for group 3:
     PD      T2
   97.43 40.92

covariance matrix for group 1:
        PD      T2
PD 54.35 37.98
T2 37.98 53.88

covariance matrix for group 2:
        PD      T2
PD 169.5 286.8
T2 286.8 670.2

covariance matrix for group 3:
        PD      T2
PD 16.486 7.927
T2  7.927 9.402

common covariance matrix
        PD      T2
PD 63.14  77.46
T2 77.46 163.54
```

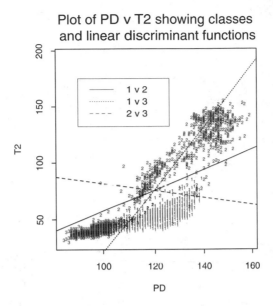

FIGURE 20.5. Linear discriminant functions for imaging data.

Misclassification rates estimated by applying the three classification functions to the training set data and by using the 'leaving out one' method are shown in Table 20.7. Again, the estimated misclassification rate given by each approach is almost identical.

20.5 Summary

Discriminant function analysis is used to derive rules for classifying individuals into one of a number of *a priori* defined groups. The rules result from observations made on a training set whose group membership is known. Fisher's method is most often used, but the discrimination approach can also be applied when there are more than two groups and when the covariance matrices of groups differ. More details of this methodology are given in Hand (1998).

TABLE 20.7. Misclassification rate estimates for imaging data

```
Plug-in classification table:
          1   2    3  Error Posterior.Error
  1 1057   1   69 0.0621          0.0574
  2   32 504   50 0.1399          0.1554
  3    3   0 1120 0.0027         -0.0734
Overall             0.0547          0.0258
(from=rows,to=columns)


Rule Mean Square Error: 0.08721
(conditioned on the training data)

Cross-validation table:
          1   2    3  Error Posterior.Error
  1 1057   1   69 0.0621          0.0574
  2   32 504   50 0.1399          0.1555
  3    3   0 1120 0.0027         -0.0735
Overall             0.0547          0.0258
(from=rows,to=columns)
```

20.6   Using S-PLUS

20.6.1   Using the S language

Section 20.2

The linear discriminant function is derived from first principles using the
var() and apply() functions. Function discrim() is used to get misclassification rates.

Script for Section 20.2

```
# Read in SIDS data
sids<-read.table("sids.dat",header=T)

# Store the group value in group for convenience
# select birthweight and Factor68 for first analysis
group<-sids[,1]
sids2<-sids[,c(3,4)]

# Plot the data
win.graph()
plot(as.matrix(sids2),type="n")
text(as.matrix(sids2),labels=group)                    ⟹  Figure 20.1

# Calculate the discriminant function coefficients
# from first principles

# First calculate the covariance matrices in each group
v1<-var(sids2[group==1,])
v2<-var(sids2[group==2,])

# Calculate group mean vectors
m1<-apply(sids2[group==1,],2,mean)
m2<-apply(sids2[group==2,],2,mean)

# Find number of observations in each group
n1<-length(group[group==1])
n2<-length(group[group==2])

# Estimate common covariance matrix
v<-((n1-1)*v1+(n2-1)*v2)/(n1+n2-2)

# Print results so far
m1
m2
v1
```

```
v2
v
```
$\Longrightarrow$ Table 20.2

```
# Invert common covariance matrix
v<-solve(v)

# Calculate discriminant function coefficients
a<-v%*%(m1-m2)

# Calculate threshold value for disciminant rule
z12<-(m1%*%a+m2%*%a)/2

# Plot the data labelling the members of the two groups,and add
# the discriminant function line and an appropriate legend
win.graph()
plot(sids2[,1],sids2[,2],xlab="Birthweight",
    ylab="Factor68",type="n")
text(sids2[,1],sids2[,2],labels=group)
legend(locator(1),c("Cases","Controls"),pch="12")
abline(z12/a[2],-a[1]/a[2],lwd=2,lty=1)
```
$\Longrightarrow$ Figure 20.2

```
# Produce scatterplot of all variables, and add discriminant
# function to each panel
win.graph()
pairs(sids[,-1],labels=c("HR","BW","Factor68","Gesage"),
    panel=function(x,y) {
        text(x,y,labels=group)
        X<-cbind(x,y,group)
        m1<-apply(X[group==1,-3],2,mean)
        m2<-apply(X[group==2,-3],2,mean)
        x1<-X[group==1,-3]
        x2<-X[group==2,-3]
        S<-((n1-1)*var(x1)+(n2-1)*var(x2))/(n1+n2-2)
        a<-solve(S)%*%(m1-m2)
        z12<-(m1%*%a+m2%*%a)/2
        abline(z12/a[2],-a[1]/a[2],lwd=2,lty=1)
    }
)
```
$\Longrightarrow$ Figure 20.3

```
# Now use S-PLUS discriminant functions to get the coefficients
group<-as.factor(group)
sids2.disc<-discrim(group~.,data=sids2)
plot(sids2.disc)
coefs<-coef(sids2.disc)$linear.coefficients
# a as derived above is now coefs[,1]-coefs[,2]
```

```
# Now repeat analysis for all variables, and get tables of
# misclassification rates and other details from using summary()
sids.disc<-discrim(group~.,data=sids[,-1],prior="uniform")
summary(sids.disc)                              ⟹  Table 20.3


# Discriminant function coefficients obtained as
coefs<-coef(sids.disc)$linear.coefficients
coefs[,1]-coefs[,2]
```

Section 20.3

The discrim() function is used to apply quadratic discrimination.

Script for Section 20.3

```
# Quadratic discriminant for birthweight and Factor68
sids.disc1<-discrim(group~.,data=sids2,
   Classical(cov.structure="heteroscedastic"))
summary(sids.disc1)                             ⟹  Table 20.4

win.graph()
plot(sids.disc1)                                ⟹  Figure 20.4
```

Section 20.4

Discriminant functions for the three-group situation are derived from first principles.

Script for Section 20.4

```
image<-read.table("image.dat", header=T)
attach(image)

# Discriminant function analysis from first principles
m1<-apply(image[Class==1,-3],2,mean)
m2<-apply(image[Class==2,-3],2,mean)
m3<-apply(image[Class==3,-3],2,mean)
# calculates the class mean vectors

l1<-length(Class[Class==1])
l2<-length(Class[Class==2])
l3<-length(Class[Class==3])
print(c(l1,l2,l3))

# Find the number of observations in each class
x1<-image[Class==1,-3]
```

```
x2<-image[Class==2,-3]
x3<-image[Class==3,-3]
# saves the bivariate observations for each class in
# separate matrices for convenience

S123<-((l1-1)*var(x1)+(l2-1)*var(x2)+(l3-1)
    *var(x3))/(l1+l2+l3-3)
# finds the pooled covariance matrix over all three groups


# Print information
m1
m2
m3
var(x1)
var(x2)
var(x3)
S123
```

$\Longrightarrow$ | Table 20.6 |

```
# Find coefficients defining each classification function
a1<-solve(S123)%*%(m1-m2)
a2<-solve(S123)%*%(m1-m3)
a3<-solve(S123)%*%(m2-m3)
# solve(S123) is the inverse of the pooled covariance matrix

z12<-(m1%*%a1+m2%*%a1)/2
z13<-(m1%*%a2+m3%*%a2)/2
z23<-(m2%*%a3+m3%*%a3)/2
# finds the constants in the three classification functions
# halfway between the class means on the discriminant score.

# Scatterplot showing classes-change limit of y-axis to
# allow room for legend
win.graph()
par(pty="s")
ylim<-range(T2)
ylim[2]<-ylim[2]+40
plot(PD,T2,xlab="PD",ylab="T2",type="n",lwd=2,ylim=ylim)
text(PD,T2,labels=as.character(Class),cex=0.5,lwd=2)
title("Plot of PD v T2 showing classes\ n
    and linear discriminant functions",lwd=2)

# Superimpose lines for classification
abline(z12/a1[2],-a1[1]/a1[2],lwd=2,lty=1)
abline(z13/a2[2],-a2[1]/a2[2],lwd=2,lty=2)
abline(z23/a3[2],-a3[1]/a3[2],lwd=2,lty=3)
# adds the required lines corresponding to each of the
# classification functions
```

```
legend(locator(1),c("1 v 2","1 v 3","2 v 3"),lty=1:3)
# adds an appropriate legend
```
$\Longrightarrow$ [Figure 20.5]

```
# now use S-PLUS function to apply same analysis and to
# get misclassification rates
image.disc<-discrim(as.factor(Class)~.,data=image)
summary(image.disc)
```
$\Longrightarrow$ [Table 20.7]

20.7 Exercises

20.1 Investigate the use of the `discrim()` function in S-PLUS on both the SIDS data and the imaging data, with alternative assumptions about the covariance matrices than equality and complete inequality.

20.2 Derive the quadratic discriminant function for the SIDS data from first principles.

20.3 Construct box plots of the discriminant function scores for the cases and controls in the SIDS data.

20.4 By scoring controls 1 and cases -1 in the SIDS data, show the equivalence of a multiple regression model for the response variable 'group', with the discriminant function derived in the text.

Appendix A
The S-PLUS GUI

A.1 Introduction

In this text, we have concentrated on describing how to use the S-PLUS command line language via script files to undertake a wide variety of statistical analyses and to construct many types of graphical display. On the whole, such an approach is essential for more ambitious analyses, but for the relatively routine (and, perhaps, for the slightly less than routine) analyses that may be required, initially, at least, by many researchers, there is an alternative route that can be followed that involves use of the S-PLUS GUI. Use of the GUI involves menus, dialogue boxes and point-and-click graphics, and in this chapter, we will briefly illustrate the approach using a number of examples met earlier in the book.

A.2 Statistical analysis using dialogue boxes

Many statistical techniques can be applied in S-PLUS by using the Statistics Menu and the relevant dialogue box. All such boxes are used in a similar way; so here we will simply illustrate the use of the linear regression dialogue box to analyse the cystic fibrosis data encountered in Chapter 8. (see Table 8.3).

We assume that the cystic fibrosis data are available as a data frame cystic, e.g., by reading it in using

```
cystic<-read.table("cystic.dat",header=T)
```

and that we first wish to regress the response variable PEmax on the nine explanatory variables in the data: Age, Sex, Height, Weight, BMP, FEV, RV, FRC and TLC. To get to the relevant dialogue box, click on Statistics in the tool bar and then on Regression and Linear. A linear regression dialogue box then appears. To proceed, select the cystic data frame in the data set window. Then, in the dependent variables window, select PEmax, and in the independent variables window, highlight the nine explanatory variables for this example (use the Ctrl key to select several variables). This automatically generates the required model formula, which can also be edited directly. Finally, clicking on OK produces the required parameter estimates, standard errors, and so on.

The steps are summarized below and the completed dialogue box is given in Figure A.1.

Statistics
    Linear...
        Data Set: *Cystic*
        Dependent: *PEmax*
        Independent: *Age Sex Height Weight BMP FEV RV FRC TLC*
        OK

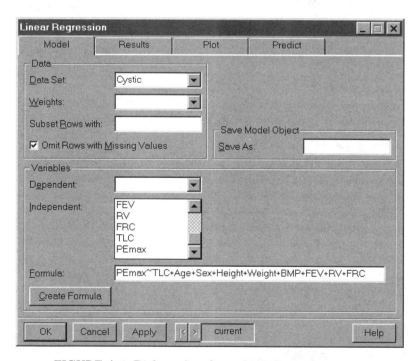

FIGURE A.1. Dialogue box for multiple linear regression.

More detailed results, residual plots, predicted values, and so on, can be found by using options available by clicking on the Results, Plot and Predict tabs of the dialogue box. For example, we might want the correlation matrix of the parameter estimates (check Results tab, and select relevant option) and some diagnostic plots (check Plot tab, and select chosen options). Clicking the OK button will again run the analysis with the selected options.

Several other possibilities are available using the dialogue, such as performing the analysis only on a subset of the data; readers are encouraged to explore these possibilities.

A stepwise regression can be applied to the cystic fibrosis data via the Stepwise Linear Regression dialogue. Click on Statistics, and select Regression and Stepwise. The dialogue in Figure A.2 then appears.

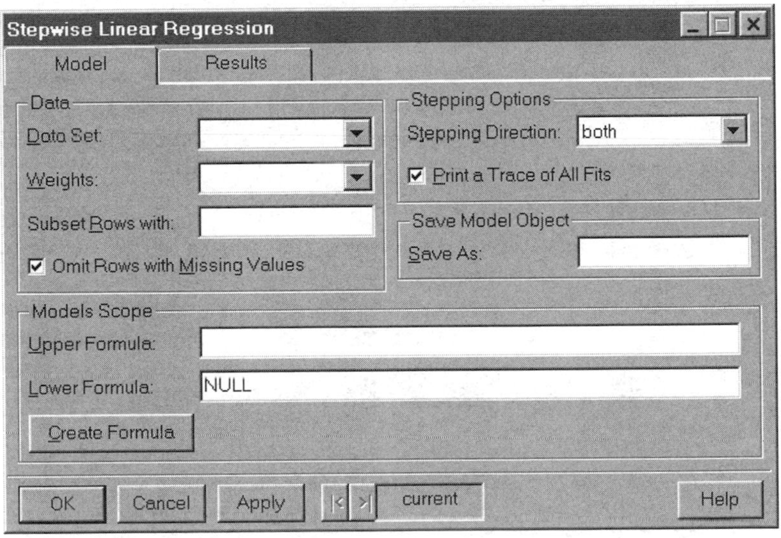

FIGURE A.2. Dialogue box for stepwise linear regression.

Again, select cystic in the data window, and then specify the required upper and lower models for the stepping procedure. This can be done conveniently using the Create Formula option, which when clicked produces the new dialogue shown in Figure A.3.

Highlight PEmax in the Choose Variables window, and click on the Response button. This generates the formula PEmax∼ 1. Now, highlight the explanatory variables in the Choose Variables Window, and click on the Main Effect (+) button. The dialogue will now look like that in Figure A.4.

Click on OK, and the original Stepwise dialogue reappears. Click the OK button, and the required stepwise analysis will be run. The steps are summarized below:

Statistics
    Stepwise...
        Data Set: *Cystic*
        Upper Formula:

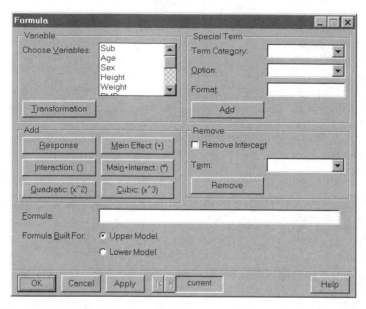

FIGURE A.3. Dialogue box for defining a model formula for stepwise linear regression.

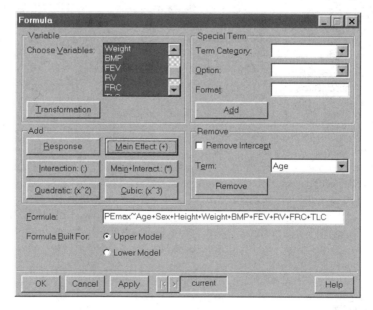

FIGURE A.4. Completed Dialogue box for defining a model formula for stepwise linear regression.

<u>C</u>reate Model Formula
    <u>C</u>hoose Variables: *PEmax*
    <u>R</u>esponse
    <u>C</u>hoose Variables:*Age Sex Height Weight BMP FEV RV FRC TLC*
    <u>M</u>ain Effect: (+)
    | OK |
| OK |

A.3   Graphics using the GUI

The GUI approach to producing S-PLUS graphics is extensive and flexible. Here, only a few basic operations will be illustrated using the data on paint sprayers introduced in Chapter 7 (see Table 7.1). Read the data using

```
paint<-read.table("paint.dat",header=T)
```

To begin with, let us produce a simple scatterplot of HAEMO against PCV. Click on Graph in the tools bar, select 2D Plot, and Scatter Plot is highlighted by default. Click OK, and the Line/Scatter Plot [1] dialogue in Figure A.5 appears.

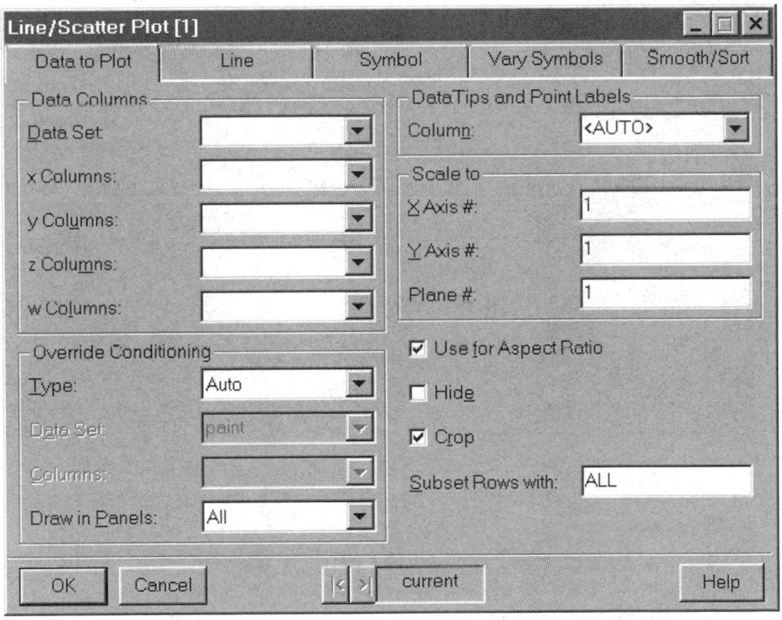

FIGURE A.5. Dialogue box for scatterplot.

Select the paint data set, and select HAEMO for the x column and PCV for the y column. Click on OK, and the required scatterplot appears. The steps are summarized below.

Graph
    2D plot...
        Plot Type: *Scatter Plot(x,y1,y2,...)*
        | OK |
            Data Set: *paint*
            x Column(s): *HAEMO*
            y column(s): *PCV*
            | OK |

By clicking on File, this can be printed or exported to be saved as a file of a particular type.

Now, let us construct a scatterplot matrix for the data. Click on Graph, 2D Plot. Then, in Axes Type, select Matrix and click OK. The Scatter Plot Matrix [1] dialogue in Figure A.6 appears.

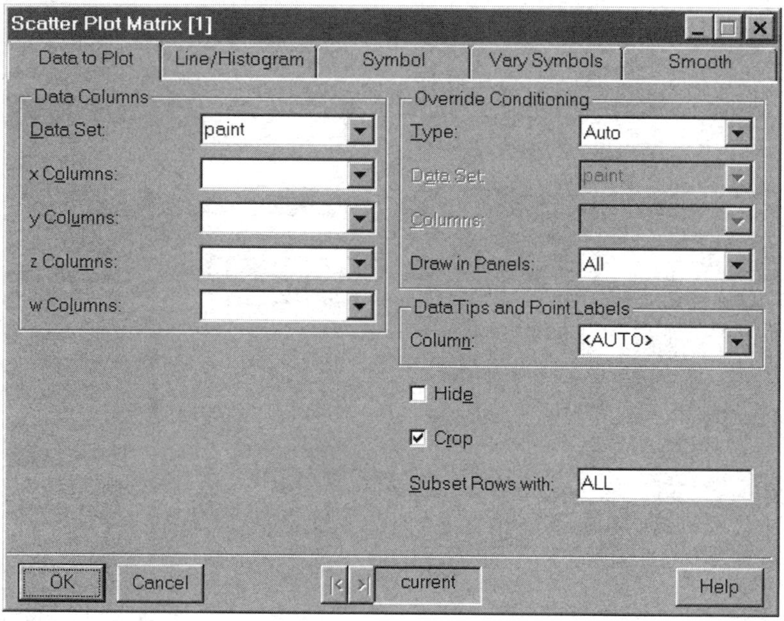

FIGURE A.6. Dialogue box for scatterplot matrix.

Select all variables except row labels in the x columns window. Now, simply click OK to see the resulting scatterplot matrix.

Graphs can also be obtained using the 2D or 3D graphics palettes, which are seen by clicking on (2D) or (3D). For example, first make the 2D palette visible (see Figure A.7).

Open the Object Explorer by clicking into and click into Data . This shows all data frames available in the current session. Click into the

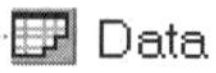

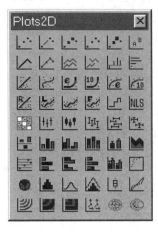

FIGURE A.7. Palette for 2D graphs.

paint data frame to open a spreadsheet window of the data, as shown in Figure A.8

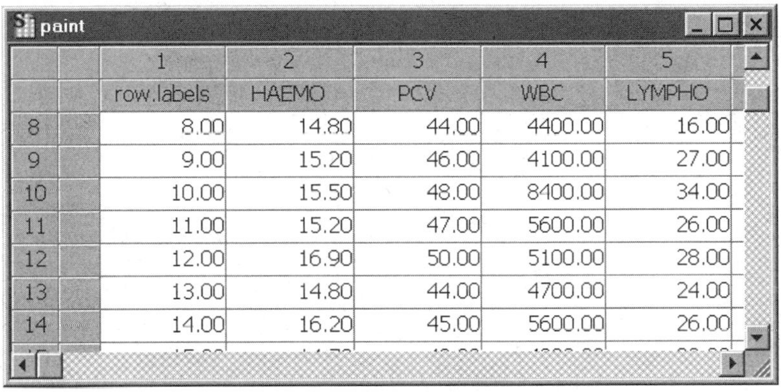

	1	2	3	4	5	
	row.labels	HAEMO	PCV	WBC	LYMPHO	
8	8.00	14.80	44.00	4400.00	16.00	
9	9.00	15.20	46.00	4100.00	27.00	
10	10.00	15.50	48.00	8400.00	34.00	
11	11.00	15.20	47.00	5600.00	26.00	
12	12.00	16.90	50.00	5100.00	28.00	
13	13.00	14.80	44.00	4700.00	24.00	
14	14.00	16.20	45.00	5600.00	26.00	

FIGURE A.8. Paint data frame as a spreadsheet.

Now, click in the top grey cell of the HAEMO column (it will be highlighted), and then hold down the Ctrl key and click on the PCV column. Select the scatterplot option ⬚ from the 2D palette, and the required scatterplot appears.

Now, suppose we would like a coplot of PCV vesus HAEMO conditional on WBC. First, click the conditioning button ⬚. Note that all graphs on the 2D Palette now have a conditioning bar at the top. (Pressing the conditioning button again turns conditioning off.) Now, first click PCV, hold down the control key, and press into HAEMO followed by WBC (the order determines the conditioning variable that is last). Click the scatter option on the 2D palette, and the required coplot is obtained.

Appendix B
Answers to selected exercises

```
# Function to find position of maximum of a matrix
maxpos<-function(X) {
   m<-length(X[,1])
   # store matrix as a vector
   x<-as.vector(X)

   # Find position of maximum in vector
   position<-seq(1,length(x))[x==max(x)]

   # Convert to position in matrix
   col<-position%/%m
   row<-position-col*m
   col<-col+1
   result<-list(row=row,column=col,value=max(x))
}

# Generate matrix,and find position of maximum
X<-matrix(rnorm(500,0,1),ncol=5)
maxpos(X)
```

Script for exercises of Chapter 2

```
## 2.1
stem(heights)
stem(leukaem)

## 2.2
length(heights[heights>=156&heights<=162])

## 2.3
ninrange<-function(data,lower,upper)
    length(data[data>=lower&data<=upper])
ninrange(leukaem,400,500)

## 2.4
hist(heights)
rug(jitter(heights))
```

Script for exercises of Chapter 3

```
## 3.1
cdf.compare(sirdsa,sirdsd)
ks.gof(sirdsa,sirdsd)

## 3.2
# need to scale data to zero mean and unit variance to
# compare with standard normal

cdf.compare(scale(as.matrix(sirdsa)),dist="normal")
cdf.compare(scale(as.matrix(sirdsd)),dist="normal")

## 3.3
# form subjective rating of health table
Table<-c(954,444,78,985,504,87,459,175,43,377,176,
    35,926,503,109)
Table<-matrix(Table,ncol=3,byrow=T)
# contingency table frequencies stored in r x c matrix

# Find row, column and grand total of frequencies.
nrow<-apply(Table,1,sum)
ncol<-apply(Table,2,sum)
N<-sum(nrow)
r<-length(Table[,1])
c<-length(Table[1,])

# Find expected values under independence, and use these to
# find standardized and adjusted residuals
expected<-matrix(rep(nrow,c),ncol=c)*
    matrix(rep(ncol,r),ncol=c,byrow=T)/N
```

```
stand<-(Table-expected)/sqrt(expected)

adjust<-stand/sqrt(matrix(rep(1-nrow/N,c),ncol=c)*
    matrix(rep(1-ncol/N,r),ncol=c,byrow=T))
```

Script for exercises of Chapter 4

```
## 4.1
den<-tdden1(Height,Pulse)
plot(Height,Pulse)
contour(den$seqx,den$seqy,den$den,add=T)

## 4.2
plot(birth,death,type="n")
text(birth,death,labels=row.names(birdea))
abline(lm(death~birth))
lines(lowess(birth,death),lty=2)
legend(locator(1),c("Linear","Lowess"),lty=1:2)
```

Script for exercises of Chapter 6

```
##6.1
# because the na.rm=T is removed, any woman with one or more missing
# values will  have the mean summary measure missing
oestrogen.rmp<-apply(oestrogen.p[,3:8],1,mean)
oestrogen.rma<-apply(oestrogen.a[,3:8],1,mean)
t.test(oestrogen.rmp,oestrogen.rma)

## 6.2
# function for filling in missing values in rows of a matrix
# by LOCF assumes that subject drops out so that a missing
# value is not followed by any genuine observations

locf<-function(X) {
    n<-length(X[,1])
    p<-length(X[1,])
    for(i in 1:n) {
        x<-X[i,]
        y<-x[!is.na(x)]
        N<-length(y)
        if(N!=p) y<-c(y,rep(y[N],p-N))
        X[i,]<-y
    }
    X
}

oestrogen.rmp<-apply(locf(oestrogen.p[,3:8]),1,mean)
oestrogen.rma<-apply(locf(oestrogen.a[,3:8]),1,mean)
t.test(oestrogen.rmp,oestrogen.rma)
```

Script for exercises of Chapter 7

```
## 7.1

# before using stars option in symbol, scale
# matrix so that column values are in 0,1. Here, we
# subtract minimum value and then divide by the range.
symbols(HAEMO,PCV,stars=scale(paint[,4:7],
    center=apply(paint[,4:7],2,min),
scale=(apply(paint[,4:7],2,max)-apply(paint[,4:7],2,min))),
    inches=0.5,xlab="HAEMO",ylab="PCV")

## 7.2

pairs(paint[,-1],panel=function(x,y) {
    jitter(rug(x))
    jitter(rug(y,side=2))
    points(x,y)
})

## 7.5

# function for chisquare plot

chiplot<-function(x) {
    n<-length(x[,1])
    p<-length(x[1,])
    xbar<-apply(x,2,mean)
    S<-var(x)
    S<-solve(S)
    index<-vector(length=n)
    di<-vector(length=n)
    for (i in 1:n) {
        di[i]<-t(x[i,]-xbar)%*%S%*%(x[i,]-xbar)
        index[i]<-i/(n+1)
    }
    win.graph()
    quant<-qchisq(index,p)
    plot(quant,sort(di),ylab="Ordered distances",
        xlab="Chi-square quantile",lwd=2,pch=1)
    abline(1,lwd=2)
}

chiplot(as.matrix(paint[,-1]))
```

Script for exercises of Chapter 9

```
## 9.1

# Read and prepare the data as in Chapter 2
# except that dust and emp are not factors
lung<-matrix(scan("lung.dat"),ncol=7,byrow=T)
dimnames(lung)<-list(NULL,
    c("yes","no","dust","race","sex","smoking","emp"))
lung<-as.data.frame(lung)
lung$race<-factor(lung$race,levels=1:2,
    labels=c("White","Other"))
lung$sex<-factor(lung$sex,levels=1:2,
    labels=c("Male","Female"))
lung$smoking<-factor(lung$smoking,levels=c(2,1),
    labels=c("non-smoker","smoker"))
# reverse levels so that treatment contrast is 1 for smokers
contrasts(lung$smoking) <-contr.treatment(2)

lung.glm<-glm(cbind(yes,no)~I(-dust)+smoking+emp,
    family=binomial(link=logit),data=lung)
# the sign of dust is reversed inside the formula
summary(lung.glm)
# coefficients represent log odds ratio for increasing dustiness,
# smoking (v not) and increasing length of employment.

## 9.2

# polynomial constrasts are the default for ordered factors
lung$dust<-ordered(lung$dust,levels=c(3,2,1),
    labels=c("Low","Medium","High"))
# again reverse order of levels
lung$emp<-ordered(lung$emp,levels=1:3,
    labels=c("<10 years","10-20 years","> 20 years"))

lung.glm<-glm(cbind(yes,no)~dust+smoking+emp,
    family=binomial(link=logit),data=lung)
summary(lung.glm)


## 9.3

# consider adding sex and/or race
lung.glm2<-step(lung.glm,
    scope=list(lower=~.,upper=~.+sex+race),data=lung)
summary(lung.glm2)
# no variables added
```

452   Appendix B. Answers to selected exercises

```
## 9.4

# consider adding all pairwise interactions
lung.glm2<-step(lung.glm,scope=list(lower=~.,upper=~.^2),data=lung)
summary(lung.glm2)
summary.aov(lung.glm2)
# this gives p-values for factors (not split into contrasts)
```

Script for exercises of Chapter 10

```
## 10.1

# Prepare data as before:

lung<-read.table("lungcanc.dat", header=T)
lung1<-lung
death1<-lung$death
death1[death1==1&lung$follow>1]<-0
lung1$death<-death1

attach(lung)

lung2<-lung[follow>=2,]
death1<-death[follow>=2]
death1[death1==1&lung2$follow>2]<-0
lung2$death<-death1
lung2$age<-lung2$age+1

lung3<-lung[follow>=3,]
death1<-death[follow>=3]
death1[death1==1&lung3$follow>3]<-0
lung3$death<-death1
lung3$age<-lung3$age+2

lung4<-lung[follow>=4,]
death1<-death[follow>=4]
death1[death1==1&lung4$follow>4]<-0
lung4$death<-death1
lung4$age<-lung4$age+3

lung5<-lung[follow>=5,]
death1<-death[follow>=5]
death1[death1==1&lung5$follow>5]<-0
lung5$death<-death1
lung5$age<-lung5$age+4

lung6<-lung[follow>=6,]
death1<-death[follow>=6]
death1[death1==1&lung6$follow>6]<-0
```

```
lung6$death<-death1
lung6$age<-lung6$age+5

Lung<-rbind(lung1,lung2,lung3,lung4,lung5,lung6)

# Exclude over 80s
Lung<-Lung[Lung$age<=80,]

attach(Lung)

# Collapse data.
age1<-as.vector(tapply(age,
   list(age=age,cigscat=cigscat),FUN=mean))
smoker1<-as.vector(tapply(smoker,
   list(age=age,cigscat=cigscat),FUN=mean))
cigscat1<-as.vector(tapply(cigscat,
   list(age=age,cigscat=cigscat),FUN=mean))
death1<-as.vector(tapply(death,
   list(age=age,cigscat=cigscat),FUN=sum))
freq1<-as.vector(tapply(freq,
   list(age=age,cigscat=cigscat),FUN=sum))

# define cigscat1 as a factor
cigscat1<-factor(cigscat1,levels=0:2,
   labels=c("none","moderate","strong"))

# set constrasts to treatments
contrasts(cigscat1)<-contr.treatment(3)

# fit model
lung.glm4<-glm(death1~cigscat1+age1+I(age1^2)
   +offset(log(freq1)),family=poisson)
summary(lung.glm4)
# strong smokers seem to be at less risk than moderate ones!

## 10.2
# set up Helmert contrast with levels ordered
# from strong to none
cigscat1<-factor(cigscat1,levels=c(2,1,0),
   labels=c("strong","moderate","none"))
contrasts(cigscat1)<-contr.helmert(3)
contrasts(cigscat1)
lung.glm5<-glm(death1~cigscat1+age1+I(age1^2)
   +offset(log(freq1)),family=poisson)
summary(lung.glm5)
# significant difference between moderate and strong smokers

## 10.3
inc<-death1/freq1
```

```
win.graph()
plot(age1, inc, type="n",ylab="Incidence rate",xlab="Age")
points(age1[cigscat1=="none"],inc[cigscat1=="none"],pch=1)
points(age1[cigscat1=="moderate"],inc[cigscat1=="moderate"],
    pch=2)
points(age1[cigscat1=="strong"],inc[cigscat1=="strong"],
    pch=3)

# define data frame for predictions
new<-data.frame(age1=rep(35:80,3),cigscat1=rep(0:2,each=46),
    freq1=rep(20,138))

# defince cigscat as factor as for lung.glm4
new$cigscat1<-factor(new$cigscat1,levels=0:2,
    labels=c("none","moderate","strong"))
contrasts(new$cigscat1)<-contr.treatment(3)

# compute predictions
pred<-predict(lung.glm4,newdata=new,type="response")/20

lines(35:80,pred[1:46])
lines(35:80,pred[47:92])
lines(35:80,pred[93:138])
legend(40,.035,legend=c("non-smoker","moderate smoker",
    "strong smoker"),marks=c(1,2,3))

## 10.4
# compute residuals
resids<-residuals(lung.glm4,type="deviance")

# plot residuals
plot(age1,resids,type="n",ylab="Deviance residuals",xlab="age")
points(age1[cigscat1=="none"],resids[cigscat1=="none"],pch=1)
points(age1[cigscat1=="moderate"],resids[cigscat1=="moderate"],
    pch=2)
points(age1[cigscat1=="strong"],resids[cigscat1=="strong"],
    pch=3)

## 10.5

# revert to treatment contrasts

cigscat1<-as.vector(tapply(cigscat,
    list(age=age,cigscat=cigscat),FUN=mean))
cigscat1<-factor(cigscat1,levels=0:2,
    labels=c("none","moderate","strong"))
contrasts(cigscat1)<-contr.treatment(3)
contrasts(cigscat1)
lung.glm4<-glm(death1~cigscat1+age1+I(age1^2)
```

```
    +offset(log(freq1)),family=poisson)
summary(lung.glm4)


# test for higher order terms of age
# use poly() for convenience
lung.glm6<-glm(death1~cigscat1+poly(age1,3)
    +offset(log(freq1)),family=poisson)
anova(lung.glm4,lung.glm6)
# ns.


# test for interaction between smoking intensity and age
lung.glm7<-glm(death1~cigscat1*poly(age1,2)
    +offset(log(freq1)),family=poisson)
anova(lung.glm4,lung.glm7)
1-pchisq(87.56,4)
# highly significant
summary(lung.glm7)


# to interpret interaction, plot raw ans fitted residuals
# by repeating the steps in 10.3 using lung.glm7 in the
# predict() function
pred<-predict(lung.glm7,newdata=new,type="response")/20
```

Script for exercises of Chapter 11

```
## 11.1
pefr<-read.table("pefr.dat",header=T)
y<-as.vector(as.matrix(pefr[,2:5]))
meth<-c(rep(1,34),rep(2,34))
occ<-rep(c(rep(1,17),rep(2,17)),2)
id<-rep(pefr[,1],4)
pefr2<-data.frame(id=id,y=y,meth=meth,odd=occ)


pefr.lme<-lme(fixed=y~1,random=~1|id,subset=meth==1,
    data=pefr2)
intervals(pefr.lme)
# the estimates are not very different from mini Wright
# meter considering the widths of the confidence intervals


# reliability coefficient
r<-117^2/(117^2+15.31^2)
r
# appears to be more a little reliable than mini Wright meter


## 11.2
pefr.lme2<-lme(fixed=y~meth,random=~1|id,data=pefr2)
summary(pefr.lme2)
# ns.
```

```
# likelihood ratio test (must use method=ML)
pefr.lme3<-lme(fixed=y~1,random=~1|id,data=pefr2,
    method="ML")
pefr.lme4<-lme(fixed=y~meth,random=~1|id,data=pefr2,
    method="ML")
anova(pefr.lme3,pefr.lme4)


## 11.3

estrogen<-matrix(scan("estrogen.dat"),ncol=9,byrow=T)
estrogen[estrogen==-9]<-NA

# Reshape data matrix for analysis using lme()
depress<-as.vector(estrogen[,-1])
# stacks eight columns into a single column

subject<-1:nrow(estrogen)
id<-rep(subject,8)
# creates subject ids corresponding to elements in depress

group<-rep(estrogen[,1],8)
time<-rep((1:8)-4.5,times=1,each=nrow(estrogen))
estlong<-data.frame(id,group,time,depress)

# remove missing observations
estlong<-estlong[!is.na(depress),]

# Simple random effects model
est.lme1<-lme(fixed=depress~group*time,random=~1|id,
    data=estlong,method="ML")
summary(est.lme1)
est.lme2<-lme(fixed=depress~group*poly(time,2),
    random=~1|id,data=estlong,method="ML")
anova(est.lme1,est.lme2)


## 11.4
est.lme3<-lme(fixed=depress~group*poly(time,2),
    random=~time|id,data=estlong,method="ML")
anova(est.lme2,est.lme3)
# sig.


## 11.5
# Reshape data matrix for analysis using lme()
depress<-as.vector(estrogen[,-(1:3)])
# exclude first three columns
# (columns 2 and 3 are baseline measures)

# create baseline vector
base<-apply(estrogen[,2:3],1,mean)
```

```
base<-rep(base,6)

subject<-1:nrow(estrogen)
id<-rep(subject,6)

group<-rep(estrogen[,1],6)
time<-rep((1:6)-3,times=1,each=nrow(estrogen))
estlong2<-data.frame(id,group,time,depress,base=base)

# remove missing observations of dependent variable
estlong2<-estlong2[!is.na(depress),]
# remove missing observations of baseline variable
estlong2<-estlong2[!is.na(estlong2$base),]

# Simple random effects model
est.lme1<-lme(fixed=depress~base+group*time,random=~1|id,
    data=estlong2,method="ML")
summary(est.lme1)
est.lme2<-lme(fixed=depress~base+group*poly(time,2),
    random=~1|id,data=estlong2,method="ML")
anova(est.lme1,est.lme2)
est.lme3<-lme(fixed=depress~base+group+time,
    random=~1|id,data=estlong2,method="ML")
anova(est.lme1,est.lme3)
# group by time not significant, but main effect of group
#   can be interpreted as treatment effect

est.lme4<-lme(fixed=depress~base+group+time,
    random=~time|id,data=estlong2,method="ML")
anova(est.lme3,est.lme4)
# significant variations in slope
```

Script for exercises of Chapter 12

```
## 12.1

estrogen<-matrix(scan("estrogen.dat"),ncol=9,byrow=T)
estrogen[estrogen==-9]<-NA

# Reshape data matrix for analysis using lme()
depress<-as.vector(estrogen[,-(1:3)])

# create baseline vector
base<-apply(estrogen[,2:3],1,mean)
base<-rep(base,6)

subject<-1:nrow(estrogen)
id<-rep(subject,6)
```

```
group<-rep(estrogen[,1],6)
time<-rep((1:6)-3,times=1,each=nrow(estrogen))
estlong2<-data.frame(id,group,time,depress,base=base)

# remove missing observations of dependent variable
estlong2<-estlong2[!is.na(depress),]
# remove missing observations of baseline variable
estlong2<-estlong2[!is.na(estlong2$base),]

# Simple random effects model
est.lme3<-lme(fixed=depress~base+group+time,
    random=~1|id,data=estlong2,method="ML")

# without random slope
est.lme1<-lme(fixed=depress~base+group+time,
    random=~1|id,data=estlong2,method="ML")
oest.lme2<-lme(fixed=depress~base+group+time,random=~1|id,
  correlation=corAR1(form=~time|id),data=estlong2)
anova(est.lme1,est.lme2)

# with a random slope
est.lme3<-lme(fixed=depress~base+group+time,
    random=~time|id,data=estlong2,method="ML")
oest.lme4<-lme(fixed=depress~base+group+time,random=~time|id,
    correlation=corAR1(form=~time|id),data=estlong2)
anova(est.lme3,est.lme4)

## 12.3

# Read hearing loss data
hear<-matrix(scan("hear.dat"),ncol=9,byrow=T)

# Stack responses into a vector
loss<-as.vector(hear[,2:9])

# Create identifiers for id and ear
id<-rep(hear[,1],8)
ear<-c(rep(1,400),rep(2,400))

# Create frequency variable
freq<-rep(rep(1:4,each =100),2)

# Put data into data frame
hear2<-data.frame(id=id,ear=ear,freq=freq,loss=loss,
    lloss=log(loss+11))

# look at relationship between hearing loss and frequency
tapply(hear2$lloss,hear2[,2:3],FUN=mean)
win.graph()
```

```
plot(freq,loss,data=hear2)

# fit three-level models
hear.lme1<-lme(lloss~freq, random = list(id =~1,ear=~1),
   data=hear2,method="ML")

# treat frequency as a factor
hear.lme2<-lme(lloss~as.factor(freq),
    random = list(id =~1,ear=~1),data=hear2,method="ML")
hear.lme3<-lme(lloss~as.factor(freq)+ear,
    random = list(id =~1,ear=~1),data=hear2,method="ML")

# include random slope for frequency
hear.lme4<-lme(lloss~as.factor(freq),
    random = list(id =~freq,ear=~1),data=hear2,method="ML")
anova(hear.lme2,hear.lme4)
summary(hear.lme3)
```

Script for exercises of Chapter 13

```
## 13.2

# Get predicted values from required models
y1<-predict(lm(Ventilation~Oxygen))
y2<-predict(lm(Ventilation~Oxygen+I(Oxygen*Oxygen)))
y3<-predict(gam(Ventilation~s(Oxygen)))
y4<-predict(gam(Ventilation~lo(Oxygen)))

# set range of y

ylim<-range(y1,y2,y3,y4)
plot(Oxygen,Ventilation,ylim=ylim,type="p")
lines(Oxygen,y1,lty=1)
lines(Oxygen,y2,lty=2)
lines(Oxygen,y3,lty=3)
lines(Oxygen,y4,lty=4)

# add suitable legend

legend(locator(1),c("Linear","Quadatic","Lowess","Spline"),
    lty=1:4)
```

Script for exercises of Chapter 14

```
## 14.2

# Calculate likelihood ratio test using the
# function L given below
```

```
L1<-LL(c(p,mu1,sigma1,mu2,sigma2),onsetw)
# likelihood for 2 component mixture

# Get mean and sd for age of onset data; ml estimator
# of variance used
mu<-mean(onsetw)
sig<-var(onsetw,unbiased=F)

L2<-LL(c(1,mu,sig,1,1),onsetw)
# likelihood for single component

chi<-2*(L2-L1)
print(1-pchisq(chi,3))

# Function LL computes log-likelihood
LL<-function(x, data)
{
    # x contains the five parameter values
    # data contains the observations
    p <- x[1]
    mu1 <- x[2]
    sig1 <- x[3]
    mu2 <- x[4]
    sig2 <- x[5]
    t1 <- dnorm(data, mu1, sig1)
    t2 <- dnorm(data, mu2, sig2)
    f <- p * t1 + (1 - p) * t2
    llike <- sum(log(f))
    -llike
}
```

Script for exercises of Chapter 15

```
## 15.2

attach(birthwt)
birthwt.fit<-lm(bwt~age+lwt+race+smoke+ptl+ui+ftv)
summary(birthwt.fit)

## 15.3

birthwt.fit<-aov(bwt~smoke+race)
summary(birthwt.fit)

birthwt.fit<-aov(bwt~smoke*race)
summary(birthwt.fit)
```

Script for exercises of Chapter 16

```
## 16.1
leuk<-matrix(scan("leuk.dat"),ncol=3,byrow=T)
leuk<-data.frame(wbc=leuk[,1],ag=leuk[,2],surv=leuk[,3],
   status=rep(1,nrow(leuk)))
# status = 1 for all observations because there is no censoring

# Log-rank test
survdiff(Surv(surv,status)~ag,data=leuk)
# significant difference

## 16.3
breast<-read.table("breast.dat",header=T)

# Breslow estimates
bresurv<-survfit(Surv(time,status)~stain,type="fl",data=breast)

# Kaplan-Meier estimates
kapsurv<-survfit(Surv(time,status)~stain,data=breast)
# default is Kaplan-Meier

# Plot curves
win.graph()
par(mfrow=c(2,1))
plot(bresurv)
plot(kapsurv)

# log-rank test
survdiff(Surv(time,status)~stain,data=breast)
```

Script for exercises of Chapter 17

```
## 17.3
breast<-read.table("breast.dat",header=T)
breast.cox<-coxph(Surv(time,status)~stain,data=breast)
summary(breast.cox)

## 17.4

# assess the proportional hazards assumption graphically
win.graph()
plot(cox.zph(breast.cox))

# test of proportional hazards
cox.zph(breast.cox)
# ns.

## 17.5
```

```
# compute scaled changes in beta
bresid<-resid(breast.cox,type="dfbeta")

# plot values
plot(1:length(bresid),bresid,type="h",xlab="observation",
   ylab="change in coeff")
# observation 1 is most influential, but not too influential
```

Script for exercises of Chapter 18

```
## 18.5

patient.fa1<-factanal(patient,factor=3)
summary(patient.fa1)


## 18.6

patient.fa1<-factanal(patient,factor=3,rotation="promax")
summary(patient.fa1)
```

Script for exercises of Chapter 19

```
# 19.1

food<-read.table("food1.dat",header=T)

# Now find percentage of recommended daily allowances
allow<-c(3200,70,0.8,100,10)
food.std<-100*sweep(food,2,allow,FUN="/")

# Get Euclidean distance  matrix

# now get dendrograms for each of single linkage,
# complete linkage and average linkage based on data
# standardized by daily allowance

win.graph()
par(mfrow=c(1,3))
plclust(hclust(dist(food.std),method="connected"),
   labels=row.names(food),ylab="Distance")
title("Single linkage")
plclust(hclust(dist(food.std),method="compact"),
   labels=row.names(food),ylab="Distance")
title("Complete linkage")
plclust(hclust(dist(food.std),method="average"),
   labels=row.names(food),ylab="Distance")
title("Average linkage")
```

```
# Get two-cluster solution from complete linkage
two<-cutree(hclust(dist(food.std),method="compact"),k=2)

# Print out foodstuffs in each cluster
row.names(food)[two==1]
row.names(food)[two==2]

# Find cluster means of this two group solution
clus1.mean<-apply(food[two==1,],2,mean)
clus2.mean<-apply(food[two==2,],2,mean)
```

Script for exercises of Chapter 20

```
## 20.3

attach(sids)

# Calculate discriminant score for whole sample
z<-0.000179*BW-15.533*Factor68-0.00178*HR+0.215*Gesage
boxplot(z[Group==1],z[Group==2],xlab="Group",
    ylab="Discriminant score",
names=c("Controls","Cases"))
```

References

A. Agresti. *Categorical Data Analysis*. Wiley, New York, 1990.

A. Agresti. *Introduction to Categorical Data Analysis*. Wiley, New York, 1996.

M. Aitkin. The analysis of unbalanced cross-classifications (with discussion). *Journal of the Royal Statistical Society, A*, 41:195–223, 1978.

D. G. Altman. *Practical Statistics for Medical Research*. CRC/Chapman and Hall, London, 1991.

D. F. Andrews and A. M. Herzberg. *Data*. Springer-Verlag, New York, 1985.

J. D. Banfield and R. E. Raftery. Model-based Gaussian and non-Gaussian clustering. *Biometrics*, 49:803–822, 1992.

R. A. Becker, J. M. Chambers, and A. R. Wilks. *New S Language*. Wadsworth & Brooks/Cole, California, 1988.

R. A. Becker and W. S. Cleveland. *S-PLUS Trellis Graphics User's Manual, Version 3.3*. Mathsoft Inc., Seattle, 1994.

E. J. Betemps and C. R. Buncher. Birthplaces as a risk factor in motor neurone disease and Parkinson's disease. *International Journal of Epidemiology*, 22:898–904, 1993.

466   References

J. M. Bland and D. G. Altman. Statistical methods for assessing agreement between two methods of clinical measurement. *Lancet*, Feb 8; 1 (8476):307–310, 1986.

A. Bradford and I. D. Hill. *Principles of Medical Statistics*. Arnold, London, 1991.

A. S. Bryk and S. W. Raudenbush. *Hierarchical Linear Models*. Sage Publications, Newbury Park, CA, 1992.

P. Burman. Model fitting via testing. *Statistica Sinica*, 6:589–601, 1996.

J. M. Chambers and T. J. Hastie. *Statistical Models in S*. Chapman & Hall, New York, 1993.

S. C. Choi, J. P. Muizelaar, and T. Y. Barnes. Prediction tree for severely head-injured patients. *Journal of Neurosurgery*, 75:251–255, 1991.

D. Clayton and M. Hills. *Statistical Models in Epidemiology*. Oxford University Press, Oxford, 1993.

D. Clayton and J. Kaldor. Empirical Bayes estimates of age-standardized relative risks for use in mapping. *Biometrics*, 43:671–681, 1987.

W. S. Cleveland. Robust locally weighted regression and smoothing scatterplots. *Journal of the American Statistical Association*, 74:829–836, 1979.

W. S. Cleveland. *The Elements of Graphing Data*. Hobart Press, Summit, N.J., 1985.

W. S. Cleveland. *Visualizing Data*. Hobart Press, Summit, N.J., 1993.

D. Collett. *Modelling Binary Data*. Chapman & Hall, London, 1991.

D. Collett. *Modelling Survival Data in Medical Research*. Chapman & Hall, London, 1994.

D. Collett and A. A. Jemain. Residuals, outliers and influential observations in regression analysis. *Sains Malaysiana*, 4:493–511, 1985.

R. D. Cook and S. Weisberg. *Residuals and Influence in Regression*. Chapman & Hall, London, 1982.

R. D. Cook and S. Weisberg. *Residuals and Influence in Regression*. Chapman & Hall, London, 1994.

N. A. C. Cressie and D. D. Keightly. Analysing data from hormone-receptor assays. *Biometrics*, 37:235–249, 1981.

B. F. Cullen and G. van Belle. Lymphocyte transformation and changes in leukocyte count; effects of anesthesia and operation. *Anesthesiology*, 43:577–583, 1975.

P. J. Diggle, K-Y Liang, and S. L. Zeger. *Analysis of Longitudinal Data*. Oxford University Press, Oxford, 1994.

N. R. Draper and H. Smith. *Applied Regression Analysis (3rd Edition)*. Wiley, New York, 1998.

G. Dunn. Design and analysis of reliability studies. *Statistical Methods in Medical Research*, 1:123–157, 1992.

G. Dunn. *Statistics in Psychiatry*. Arnold, London, 2000.

B. Efron. Bootstrap methods; another look at the jackknife. *Annals of Statistics*, 7:1–16, 1979.

B. Efron and G. Gong. A leisurely look at the bootstrap, the jackknife and cross-validation. *American Statistician*, 37:36–48, 1983.

B. Efron and R. Tibshirani. *An Introduction to the Bootstrap*. Chapman & Hall, London, 1993.

B. S. Everitt. *An Introduction to Optimization Methods and their Application in Statistics*. CRC/Chapman & Hall, London, 1987.

B. S. Everitt. *The Analysis of Contingency Tables*. Chapman & Hall/ CRC Press, London, 1993.

B. S. Everitt and G. Dunn. *Applied Multivariate Analysis*. Arnold, London, 2001.

B. S. Everitt, J. Gourlay, and R. E. Kendall. An attempt at validation of traditional psychiatric syndromes by cluster analysis. *British Journal of Psychiatry*, 119:299–412, 1971.

B. S. Everitt and D. J. Hand. *Finite Mixture Distributions*. CRC/Chapman & Hall, London, 1981.

B. S. Everitt, S. Landau, and M. Leese. *Cluster Analysis (4th Edition)*. Arnold, London, 2001.

B. S. Everitt and A. Pickles. *Statistical Aspects of the Design and Analysis of Clinical Trials*. Imperial College Press, London, 2000.

R. A. Fisher. The use of multiple measurements in taxonomic problems. *Annals of Eugenics*, 7:179–188, 1936.

G. Fraley and A. E. Raftery. How many clusters? Which clustering method? Answers via model-based cluster analysis. *Computer Journal*, 41:578–588, 1998.

G. Fraley and A. E. Raftery. MCLUST Software for model-based cluster analysis. *Journal of Classification*, 16:297–306, 1999.

H. P. Friedman and J. Rubin. On some invariant criteria for grouping data. *Journal of the American Statistical Association*, 62:1159–1178, 1967.

L. Frison and S. J. Pocock. Repeated measures in clinical trials. Analysis using mean summary statistics and its implications for design. *Statistics in Medicine*, 11:1685–1704, 1992.

A. E. Gelfand, S. E. Hills, A. Racine-Poon, and A. F. M. Smith. Illustration of Bayesian inference in normal data models using Gibbs sampling. *Journal of the American Statistical Association*, 85:972–985, 1990.

L. Goldman, F. Cook, P. Johnson, D. Brand, G. Rosian, and T. Lee. Prediction of the need for intensive care in patients who come to emergency departments with acute chest paint. *The New England Journal of Medicine*, 334:1498–1504, 1996.

L. Goldman, M. Wenberg, R. A. Olshen, F. Cook, and R. Sargent. A computer protocol to predict myocardial infarction in emergency department patients with chest pain. *The New England Journal of Medicine*, 307:588–597, 1982.

H. Goldstein. *Multilevel Statistical Models*. Arnold, London, 1995.

A. D. Gordon. *Classification (2nd Edition)*. CRC/Chapman & Hall, London, 1999.

P. Grambsch and T. Therneau. Proportional hazards tests and diagnostics based on weighted residuals. *Biometrika*, 8:515–526, 1994.

A. J. P. Gregoire, R. Kumar, B. S. Everitt, A. F. Henderson, and J. W. W. Studd. Transdermal oestrogen for the treatment of severe post-natal depression. *The Lancet*, 347:930–934, 1996.

D. J. Hand. Discriminant analysis. In P. Armitage and T. Colton, editors, *Encyclopedia of Biostatistics*, volume 2. Wiley, Chichester, 1998.

S. Hannam, D. M. Ingram, S. Rabe-Hesketh, and A. D. Milner. Characterising the Hering-Breuer deflation reflex in the human neonate. *Respiration Physiology*, 124:51–64, 2001.

T. J. Hastie and R. J. Tibshirani. *Generalized Additive Models*. CRC/Chapman & Hall, London, 1990.

M. Hollander and D. A. Wolfe. *Nonparametric Statistical Methods*. Wiley, New York, 1999.

D. W. Hosmer and S. Lemeshow. *Applied Logistic Regression*. Wiley, New York, 1989.

H. Hotelling. Analysis of complex statistical variables into principal components. *Journal of Education Psychology*, 24:417–441, 1933.

J. E. Jackson. *A User's Guide to Principal Components*. Wiley, New York, 1991.

J.P. Klein and M.L. Moeschberger. *Survival Analysis*. Springer, New York, 1997.

E. Kraepelin. *Dementia Pralcox and Paraphrenia*. Livingstone, Edinburgh, 1919.

A. Krause and M Olsen. *The Basics of S and S-PLUS (2nd Edition)*. Springer, New York, 2000.

I. Kreft and J. De Leeuw. *Introducing Multilevel Modeling*. Sage Publications, London, 1998.

W. Krzanowski. *An Introduction to Statistical Modelling*. Arnold, London, 1998.

N. Lange, L. Ryan, L. Biffard, D. Brillinger, L. Conquest, and J. Greenhouse (eds). *Case Notes in Biometry*. Wiley, New York, 1994.

D. E. Levy, J. J. Caronna, and B. H. Singer. Predicting outcome from hypoxic-schemic coma. *Journal of the American Medical Association*, 253:1420–1426, 1985.

R. R. J. Lewine. Sex differences in schizophrenia: timing or subtypes? *Psychological Bulletin*, 90:432–444, 1981.

N. T. Longford. *Random Coefficient Models*. Oxford University Press, Oxford, 1993.

C. L. Mallows. Some comments on C_p. *Technometrics*, 15:661–675, 1973.

C. L. Mallows. More comments on C_p. *Technometrics*, 37:362–372, 1995.

B. Maqs, W. R. Garnett, J. M. Pellock, and T. J. Comstock. A comparative bioavailability study of carbamazepine tablets and a chewable tablet formulation. *Therapeutic Drug Monitoring*, 9:28–33, 1987.

K. V. Mardia, J. T. Kent, and J. M. Bibby. *Multivariate Analysis*. Academic Press, London, 1979.

F. H. C. Mariott. Optimization methods of cluster analysis. *Biometrika*, 69:417–421, 1982.

J. N. S. Mathews, D. G. Altman, M. J. Campbell, and P. Royston. Analysis of serial measurements in medical research. *British Medical Journal*, 300:230–235, 1990.

S. E. Maxwell and H. D. Delaney. *Designing Experiments and Analysing Data*. Wadsworth, California, 1990.

K. M. McConnochie, K. J. Roghmann, and H. Pasternack. Developing prediction rules and evaluating observing patterns using categorical clinical markers: Two complimentary procedures. *Medical Decision Making*, 13:130–142, 1993.

P. McCullagh and J. A. Nelder. *Generalized Linear Models*. Chapman & Hall, London, 1989.

C. R. Mehta and N. R. Patel. A hybrid algorithm for Fisher's exact test on unordered $r \times c$ contingency tables. *Communications in Statistics*, 15:387–403, 1986.

J. A. Nelder. A reformulation of linear models. *Journal of the Royal Statistical Society, A*, 140:48–63, 1977.

K. Pearson. On lines and planes of closest fit to points in space. *Philosophical Magazine*, 2:559–572, 1901.

J. C. Pinheiro and D. M. Bates. *Mixed-Effects Models in S and S-PLUS*. Springer, New York, 2000.

R. Rickman, N. Mitchell, J. Dingman, and J. E. Dalen. Changes in serum cholesterol during the Stillman diet. *Journal of the American Medical Association*, 228:54–58, 1974.

A. B. Rifland, V. Canale, and M. I. New. Antipyrine clearance in homozygous beta-thalassemia. *Clinical Pharmaceuticals and Therapeutics*, 20:476–483, 1976.

P. J. Rousseeuw. Multivariate estimation with high breakdown point. In W. Grossmann, G. Pflug, I. Vincze, and W. Wertz, editors, *Mathematical Statistics and Applications*. Reidel, Dordrecht, 1985.

S. O'Neill and F. Leahy and H. Pasterkamp and A. Tal. The effects of chronic hyperfunction, nutritional status and posture on respiratory muscle strength in cystic fibrosis. *American Review of Respiratory Disorders*, 128:1051–1054, 1983.

D. L. Sackett, R. B. Haynes, G. H. Guyatt, and P. Tugwell. *Clinical Epidemiology*. Little Brown & Company, Massachusetts, 1991.

D. S. Salsburg. Personal communication in Hollander and Wolfe, 1999.

H. A. Scheffé. A method for judging all possible contrasts in the analysis of variance. *Biomctrika*, 40:87–104, 1953.

A.J. Scott and M. J. Symons. Clustering methods based on likelihood ratio criteria. *Biometrics*, 27:387–398, 1971.

S. Senn. *Statistical Issues in Drug Development*. Wiley, Chichester, 1997.

B. Silverman. *Density Estimation*. CRC/ Chapman & Hall, London, 1986.

T. A. B. Snijders and R. J. Bosker. *Multilevel Analysis*. Sage Publications, London, 1999.

G. W. Somes and K. F. O'Brien. Mantel-Haenzel Statistics. In S. Kotz, N.L. Johnson, and C.B. Read, editors, *Encyclopediu of Statistical Sciences*, volume 5. Wiley, New York, 1985.

C. C. Spicer, G. J. Lawrence, and D. P. Southall. Statistical analysis of heart rates and subsequent victoms of sudden infant death syndrome. *Statistics in Medicine*, 6:159–166, 1987.

S. D. Steffman, P. Boffetta, and L. Garfinkel. Smoking habits of 800,000 American men and women in relation to their occupation. *American Journal of Industrial Medicine*, 13:43–58, 1988.

D. L. Streiner and G. R. Norman. *Health Measurement Scales*. Oxford University Press, Oxford, 1989.

N. R. Temkin, R. Holubkov, J. E. Machamer, H. R. Winn, and S. S. Dickme. Classification and Regression Trees (CART) for prediction of function at 1 year following head trauma. *Journal of Neurosurgery*, 82:764–771, 1995.

T. M. Therneau and P. M. Grambsch. *Modeling Survival Data*. Springer, New York, 2000.

E. R. Tufte. *The Visual Display of Quantitative Information*. Graphics Press, Cheshire, CT, 1983.

B. Üstün and N. Sartorius. *Mental illness in General Helath Care: An International Study*. Wiley, Chichester, 1995.

W. N. Venables and B. D. Ripley. *Modern Applied Statistics with S-Plus*. Springer, New York, 1997.

A. P. Verbyla, B. R. Cullis, M. G. Kenward, and S. J. Welham. The analysis of designed experiments and longitudinal data using smoothing splines (with discussion). *Applied Statistics*, 48:269–312, 1999.

D. G. Wastell and R. Gray. The numerical approach to classification: a medical application to develop a typology of facial pain. *Statistics in Medicine*, 6:137–164, 1987.

H. Zhang and B. Singer. *Recursive Partitioning in the Health Sciences*. Springer, New York, 1999.

Index

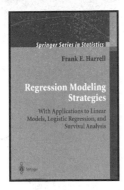
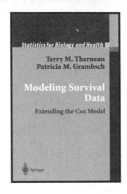
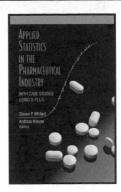
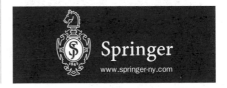